Good Clinical Practice in Assisted Reproduction

This practical, user-friendly book comprehensively covers all aspects of the investigation and treatment of infertility, from clinical assessment of the male and female to the latest assisted technology. Chapters deal with IVF, intracytoplasmic sperm injection (ICSI), techniques of sperm retrieval and clinical aspects of pre-implantation genetic diagnosis (PGD). Guidance is given on how to set up and run a successful IVF programme. With its clinical focus, this book will be invaluable to doctors, embryologists and nurses working in the field of reproductive medicine, whether they are established specialists or in training.

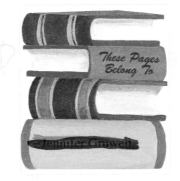

These Pages Belong To

Jennifer Criwell

Good Clinical Practice in Assisted Reproduction

Edited by

Paul Serhal

University College London Hospitals

and

Caroline Overton

St. Michael's Hospital and the
Bristol Royal Infirmary

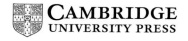

PUBLISHED BY THE PRESS SYNDICATE OF THE UNIVERSITY OF CAMBRIDGE
The Pitt Building, Trumpington Street, Cambridge, United Kingdom

CAMBRIDGE UNIVERSITY PRESS
The Edinburgh Building, Cambridge CB2 2RU, UK
40 West 20th Street, New York, NY 10011–4211, USA
477 Williamstown Road, Port Melbourne, VIC 3207, Australia
Ruiz de Alarcón 13, 28014 Madrid, Spain
Dock House, The Waterfront, Cape Town 8001, South Africa

http://www.cambridge.org

First published 2004

Printed in the United Kingdom at the University Press, Cambridge

Typefaces Minion 10.5/14 pt., Formata and Formata BQ   *System* LATEX 2$_\varepsilon$ [TB]

A catalogue record for this book is available from the British Library

Library of Congress Cataloguing in Publication data

Good clinical practice in assisted reproduction/edited by Paul Serhal, Caroline Overton.
     p.   cm.
Includes bibliographical references and index.
ISBN 0 521 00091 2 (paperback)
1. Human reproductive technology.   2. Infertility – Treatment.   I. Serhal, Paul, 1954–
II. Overton, Caroline.
[DNLM: 1. Reproductive Techniques, Assisted WQ 208 G646 2003]
RC889.G655 2003
616.6′9206 – dc21   2003044039

ISBN 0 521 00091 2 paperback

Contents

List of contributors   *page* vii
Foreword by Bob Edwards   xi
Preface   xv

1   Clinical assessment of the woman for assisted conception   1
Domenico Massimo Ranieri

2   Clinical assessment and management of the infertile man   19
Suks Minhas and David J. Ralph

3   Laboratory assessment of the infertile man   59
R. John Aitken

4   Donor insemination   86
Mathew Tomlinson and Chris Barratt

5   Treatment options prior to IVF   100
Roger Hart and Melanie Davies

6   Strategies for superovulation for IVF   112
Adam Balen

7   Techniques for IVF   129
Tim Child, Imran R. Pirwany and Seang Lin Tan

8   Ovarian hyperstimulation syndrome   146
Botros Rizk and Mary George Nawar

9   Early pregnancy complications after assisted reproductive technology   167
Eric Jauniaux and Natalie Greenwold

10   Oocyte donation   186
Paul Serhal

11   Surrogacy   199
Peter R. Brinsden

12   Clinical aspects of preimplantation genetic diagnosis   209
     Joyce C. Harper and Joy D. A. Delhanty

13   Controversial issues in assisted reproduction   226
     Caroline Overton and Colin Davis

14   Alternatives to in vitro fertilization: gamete intrafallopian
     transfer and zygote intrafallopian transfer   256
     Ehab Kelada and Ian Craft

15   Counselling   266
     Jennifer Clifford

16   Good nursing practice in assisted conception   277
     Kathy Boon, Leigh Oliphant and Elizabeth Fleming

17   Setting up an IVF unit   289
     Alpesh Doshi and Caroline Overton

18   Information technology aspects of assisted conception   310
     René van den Berg

19   Assisted reproductive technology and older women   319
     Paul Serhal

20   Ethical aspects of controversies in assisted reproductive technology 332
     Françoise Shenfield

     Index   342
     Colour plates between pages 130 and 131

Contributors

Professor R. John Aitken
ARC Centre of Excellence in
    Biotechnology and Development
Discipline of Biological Sciences
University of Newcastle
Newcastle Drive
Callaghan
NSW 2308
Australia

Mr Adam Balen
Department of Reproductive Medicine
Leeds General Infirmary
Leeds LS2 9NS
UK

Professor Chris Barratt
Assisted Conception Unit
Birmingham Women's Hospital
Edgbaston
Birmingham B15 2TG
UK

Mrs Kathy Boon
The Assisted Conception Unit
University College London Hospitals
25 Grafton Way
London WC1E 6DB
UK

Mr Peter Brinsden
Bourn Hall Clinic
Bourn
Cambs CB3 7TR
UK

Dr Tim Child
Women's Centre
John Radcliffe Hospital
Headington
Oxford OX3 9DU
UK

Mrs Jennifer Clifford
10 Alwyne Place
London N1 2NL
UK

Professor Ian Craft
London Gynaecology and Fertility Centre
Cozens House
112a Harley Street
London WC1G 7JH
UK

Dr Melanie Davies
Reproductive Medicine Unit
Elizabeth Garrett Anderson and
    Obstetric Hospital
University College Hospital
Huntley Street
London WC1E 6AU
UK

Mr Colin Davis
Department of Gynaecology
St Barts and the London
Hospitals
W Smithfields
London EC1A 7BE
UK

Professor Joy Delhanty
Department of Obstetrics and
  Gynaecology
University College London
86–96 Chenies Mews
London WC1E 6HX
UK

Alpesh Doshi
Assisted Conception Unit
University College London Hospitals
25 Grafton Way
London WC1E 6DB
UK

Ms Elizabeth Fleming
The Assisted Conception Unit
University College London Hospitals
25 Grafton Way
London WC1E 6DB
UK

Dr Natalie Greenwold
Department of Obstetrics and
  Gynaecology
University College London
86–96 Chenies Mews
London WCIE 6HX
UK

Dr Joyce Harper
Department of Obstetrics and
  Gynaecology
University College London
86–96 Chenies Mews
London WC1E 6HX
UK

Dr Roger Hart
UWA School of Women's and
  Infant's Health
University of Western Australia
King Edward Memorial Hospital
374 Bagot Road
Subiaco
WA 6008
Australia

Professor Eric Jauniaux
Department of Obstetrics and
  Gynaecology
University College London
86–96 Chenies Mews
London WC1E 6HX
UK

Ehab Kelada
London Gynaecology and Fertility
  Centre
Cozens House
112a Harley Street
London WC1G 7JH
UK

Mr Suks Minhas
Department of Uro-andrology
Middlesex Hospital
Mortimer Street
London WIT 3AA
UK

Professor Mary George Nawar
Department of Obstetrics and
  Gynecology
University of South Alabama College
  of Medicine
Mobile
Alabama 36688
USA

Miss Leigh Oliphant
The Assisted Conception Unit
University College London Hospitals
25 Grafton Way
London WC1E 6DB
UK

Dr Caroline Overton
St. Michael's Hospital and the Bristol
    Royal Infirmary
Southwell Street
Bristol BS2 8EG
UK

Dr Imran Pirwany
McGill Reproductive Centre
Royal Victoria Hospital
67 Pine Avenue West
Montreal
Quebec H3A 1A1
Canada

Mr David Ralph
Department of Uro-andrology
Middlesex Hospital
Mortimer Street
London W1T 3AA
UK

Dr Domenico Ranieri
The Assisted Conception Unit
University College London Hospitals
25 Grafton Way
London WC1E 6DB
UK

Professor Botros Rizk
Department of Obstetrics and
    Gynecology
University of South Alabama College
    of Medicine
Mobile
Alabama 36688
USA

Dr Paul Serhal
The Assisted Conception Unit
University College London Hospitals
25 Grafton Way
London WC1E 6DB
UK

Dr Françoise Shenfield
Reproductive Medicine Unit
Elizabeth Garrett Anderson and
    Obstetric Hospital
University College Hospital
Huntley Street
London WC1E 6AU
UK

Professor Seang Lin Tan
McGill Reproductive Centre
Royal Victoria Hospital
67 Pine Avenue West
Montreal
Quebec H3A 1A1
Canada

Dr Mathew Tomlinson
Assisted Conception Unit
Birmingham Women's Hospital
Edgbaston
Birmingham B15 2TG
UK

Mr René van den Berg
Infertility Database Systems Ltd
Omnibus Business Centre
39–41 North Road
lslington
London N7 9DP
UK

Foreword

Assisted human reproduction continues its worldwide spread as increasing numbers of patients are treated annually, and more clinicians and scientists enter the field each year. Demand for new knowledge remains insatiable whether on the web, in conferences or textbooks. Demand comes from so many quarters, from medical and scientific professionals, teachers, nurses, counsellors, patients and students, each needing information for their own particular ends. Comprehensive texts covering this wide demand are rare, new books mostly being highly specialised to a particular topic or technique.

Good Clinical Practice in Assisted Reproduction offers this comprehensive approach to the clinical aspects of assisted reproduction. It is unusual among the many books covering this field of biomedicine. Setting out to make data available using a simple form of presentation enabling easy searching, data are presented in 20 straightforward but detailed chapters, each debating topics essential to this form of treatment. Stressing clinical care rather than the scientific aspects of human embryology and their application, successive chapters have a simple and attractive style grouping data under sub-headings at regular intervals. Browsing is made easy without any need for constant recourse to indices or other textbooks. Tables are well laid out and direct, diagrams redrawn to a single style giving a highly attractive layout to the book. References are numerous and complete, present full details to chosen articles and offer advanced knowledge to provide data to more advanced readers in the field. Such simple and direct means of projecting its contents make this book attractive to a wide readership searching for an easy-to-read and easily accessible yet responsible text.

Standards are also high because the editors chose the right authors for each successive chapter: they must have issued clear instructions to authors to present data in a compelling and comprehensive manner. The uncomplicated nature of the texts throughout the book make it even more likely to appeal to wide and diverse readers. Contents of individual chapters begin with the clinical assessment and practice of IVF in women and men, presented by Ranieri, and by Minhas and Ralph.

Its excellent contents reveal the width of current approaches, culminating in the collection of testicular spermatozoa for ICSI. Two further chapters, by Aitken, and by Tomlinson and Barratt, cover laboratory assessments of infertile men and donor insemination. These are more scientific, traversing the field from beginning analyses of sperm quality, through various tests of sperm function and the endocrinology of spermatogenesis to the effects of oxidative stress, including DNA damage to spermatozoa. Donor recruitment, their screening, preparing and cryopreserving spermatozoa are described in turn. Five successive chapters then deal with IVF practice, presenting data essential to the daily routine in IVF clinics. Superovulation, practical techniques, ovarian stimulation and complications of early pregnancy are presented by Hart and Davis, Balen, Child *et al.*, Rizk and Nawar, and Jauniaux and Greenwold. Particular topics are well presented and in sufficient detail, for example options for IVF before it is undertaken – including controlled ovulation and IUI – and regimens involving LHRH agonists and antagonists combined with HMG or recombinant gonadotrophins. Aspects of oocyte retrieval, in vitro insemination, GIFT and embryo transfer are discussed. Risks of hyperstimulation, its prevention and management, and aspects of early pregnancy loss, miscarriage, ultrasound detection of anomalies and fetal reduction complete this section of the book.

More unusual aspects of IVF are then introduced. These open with oocyte donation, its indications, screening participants, their hormonal regulation and embryo replacement in cyclic recipients. The chances of implantation and pregnancy are presented. The complexities of surrogacy require detailed assessment and counselling of hosts and genetic mothers, monitoring pregnancies, and complicated counselling associated with this complex form of treatments, yet it offers reasonable pregnancy rates. Clinical aspects of preimplantation diagnosis include detailed counselling and cover laboratory methods, embryo biopsy and diagnosing single gene disorders or chromosomal anomalies in embryos with modern molecular and cytological techniques. Controversies arise in the application of surgical methods designed to improve assisted conception, identify uterine anomalies, manage the ovary and its precious reserve of oocytes, and ensure a well-developed endometrium. Alternatives to IVF are considered in some detail, including GIFT and ZIFT and their respective values. Again, distinguished authors include Serhal, Brinsden, Harper and Delhanty, Overton and Davis, and Kaleda and Craft.

The final six chapters move beyond operating theatres and laboratories to cover essential related matters. Diverse skills include counselling as a fundamental aspect of treatment, described by Clifford. She deals with its various forms and definitions, and demands on counsellor and those counselled. Nursing receives responsible attention from Boon *et al.*, describing the specialist nurse; coordination and planning; the background of couples attending for treatment; and wider relations with counsellors, physicians and others involved in the treatment. Planning, costing, financing, and the nature of the clinical and laboratory set-ups including layout, equipment and practice including quality control are well discussed by Doshi and Overton. The impact of information technology, assessed by van den Berg, presents details of data processing, statistical methods and necessary software. How to treat older women patients, the problems of declining follicle numbers and oocyte donation in post-menopausal patients is well discussed by Serhal, who covers available treatments, improving embryo quality and pregnancy complications. Last, but far from least, Shenfield deals with the unrelenting ethics of the field, including gamete donation, whether offspring should be told, how preimplantation genetic diagnosis raises the ethics of designer babies, and lastly physicians' rights to decline treatment to patients.

The progress of this textbook should prove highly interesting. Its comprehensive contents, and highly competent and distinguished authors, have presented few errors or mishaps in its 20 chapters. Who will be the primary buyers? Advanced professionals perhaps, yet it should appeal to newcomers to the field, those searching for answers to their own disorders and others with a duty of care in treating them. Such a wide appeal should prove successful and rewarding to editors and authors for their dedication and cooperation.

R. G. Edwards
Chief Editor, Reproductive BioMedicine Online

Preface

The last decade has witnessed striking progress in assisted reproductive technology (ART) and over the past few years the success rate of ART has increased significantly due to the introduction of novel technologies and improved embryo culture systems. Along with this rapid pace of development comes the need for clinicians to keep abreast.

This book brings fresh insights into the pathophysiology of human reproduction, providing up-to-date and practical information on the clinical and laboratory management of subfertility. Particular emphasis is placed on the clinical appraisal of the current and potential strategies to improve the management of the subfertile couple, as well as the various therapeutic options available for the management of subfertility.

The preparation of this book was driven by a desire to provide a hands-on, practical guide to assisted reproduction that would be accessible to those practising in the field of Assisted Reproduction, those working on the establishment and day-to-day running of an IVF clinic, and those with a more general interest in assisted reproduction. The contributing authors include internationally renowned clinicians and scientists actively involved in the field of reproductive medicine and those who are acknowledged in their own fields.

We are most grateful to all who have made the publication of this book possible.

Clinical assessment of the woman for assisted conception

Domenico Massimo Ranieri

Assisted Conception Unit, UCLH, London, UK

In the last four decades significant progress has been made in the diagnosis and treatment of infertile couples. It is currently estimated that about 90% of women will achieve pregnancy in the first year of trying to conceive and 95% within the second year, following which the chances of natural conception are lower. The remaining 5–10% can be defined as infertile and requiring investigation and treatment (WHO, 1992; ESHRE Capri Workshop, 1996). This timeframe can be shorter in women with risk factors such as previous history of pelvic inflammatory disease (PID), pelvic surgery, ectopic pregnancy, family history of premature ovarian failure and in women aged 35 years and over due to the natural age-related decline in fertility (van Noord-Zaadstra et al., 1991). Increasing numbers of women are delaying childbearing to an age when they are more likely to encounter problems with conceiving, and public awareness of the scientific progress made in the field of assisted conception has led to an increased number of people seeking treatment.

The first consultation between an infertile couple and the clinician specializing in infertility is a crucial starting point for collecting the medical history, clinical examination and the evaluation of the appropriateness of a range of investigations to establish the cause of infertility, following which a strategy for treatment can be planned. When infertile couples present at tertiary assisted conception centres often they will have been referred by a general practitioner or gynaecologist and may already have completed basic infertility assessment. In this event it is often possible to discuss treatment strategies during the first consultation.

First consultation:
- Medical history.
- Clinical examination.
- Investigations:
  - cause of infertility;
  - strategy of treatment.

Good Clinical Practice in Assisted Reproduction, ed. P. Serhal & C. Overton.
Published by Cambridge University Press. © Cambridge University Press 2004.

Medical history

It takes about half an hour to glean a complete medical history and this should include the following areas.

Age and duration of infertility

Female fecundity declines with age, therefore reducing the chances of conceiving either naturally or with the help of assisted reproductive technologies (van Noord-Zaadstra *et al.*, 1991; ESHRE Capri Workshop, 1996).

Menstrual history

- Women with regular periods are likely to have ovulatory cycles (van Zonneveld *et al.*, 1999).
- Primary amenorrhoea can be caused by gonadal dysgenesis and/or chromosome abnormalities such as Turner syndrome and mosaicism (see Table 1.2).
- Secondary amenorrhoea can be caused by disturbances in the hypothalamic pituitary ovarian axis, most commonly polycystic ovary syndrome (PCOS), hyperprolactinaemia, premature ovarian failure or drastic weight changes and uterine abnormalities such as Asherman's syndrome.
- Severe dysmenorrhoea is often associated with endometriosis. Particular attention should be given to heavy periods, which can be caused by submucous fibroids.

Contraception

The absence of natural conception in sexually active women who have not used contraception may indicate a severe unidentified cause of infertility. If a woman has used contraception, it is important to focus on the previous form of contraception. The intrauterine contraceptive device (IUCD) can be associated with PID and tubal damage (Beerthuizen, 1996) and women who have had multiple partners without the use of condoms may be at higher risk of tubal damage caused by PID (Miller *et al.*, 1999).

Obstetric history

- Previous pregnancies should be discussed, particularly whether they miscarried, were terminations or ectopic pregnancies.
- Method of delivery and post delivery complications can be important. The necessity of antibiotic treatment for abdominal pain and high temperature after a delivery or termination of pregnancy can be suggestive of pelvic infection with subsequent tubal damage.
- Previous fertility is sometimes a good prognostic factor in women undergoing assisted conception (Stolwijk *et al.*, 2000).

Gynaecological history

A history of PID, endometriosis, fibroids and abdominal or pelvic surgery are of interest. Cervical cytology can be taken if the patient has not been screened in the preceding three years.

Past medical history

Details of the past medical history should be carefully analysed. Sometimes these are directly related to the cause of infertility, and can also reduce the chances of successful treatment, interfere with the pregnancy and worsen the clinical condition of the patient.

General physical condition

- The woman's body mass index (BMI) should be assessed. The normal range is between 20 and 30. Women who are underweight or obese can have either anovulatory cycles or an abnormal response to ovarian stimulation, and therefore lower chances of conceiving (Norman & Clark, 1998; Katz & Voellenhoven, 2000).
- Heavy cigarette smoking and excessive alcohol intake may be relevant. There is evidence that women who are heavy smokers have reduced fertility when compared to women who are non-smokers (Grodstein *et al.*, 1994; Bolumar *et al.*, 1997; Sharara *et al.*, 1998).
- Rubella status and, for women of specific ethnic origin, the possibility of Tay–Sachs (Jewish), sickle cell trait (Afro-Caribbean) and thalassaemia (Mediterranean) should be investigated.
- Couples should be routinely assessed for human immunodeficiency virus (HIV), hepatitis B virus (HBV) and hepatitis C virus (HCV) (Steyaert *et al.*, 2000).

Counselling

The end of the first consultation can be a good opportunity to discuss the advantage of having counselling sessions prior to commencing treatment for assisted conception, particularly for those who will undergo treatment with assisted reproductive technology (ART) (see Chapter 15).

Clinical examination

When the full history has been taken, a clinical examination must be performed. This should include firstly a general examination when any large pelvic masses can be detected at abdominal palpation, and breast examination should be routinely performed.

Vaginal examination is of fundamental importance, as information about the size, shape and position of the uterus can be obtained and sometimes fibroids or adnexal masses (ovarian cysts or hydrosalpinges) can be found. When such abnormalities are detected a sonographic assessment of the pelvis is required to confirm the diagnosis, establish its correlation with the fertility of the patient and to decide on further investigations and treatment.

Investigations

In the last decade, the infertility investigation work-up has expanded (Campana et al., 1995), but when a battery of tests is performed, the chances of false positive results can increase exponentially (Hatasaka et al., 1997; Zayed & Abu-Heija, 1999). It has been suggested that abnormal tests define a cause of infertility only when the treatment of this cause enhances fertility in comparison with no treatment. Therefore, the usefulness of such extensive investigations remains controversial. To avoid unnecessary and expensive tests and treatment, the evaluation of infertile women can be based primarily on the assessment of ovulation and tubal patency (ESHRE Capri Workshop, 1996). As the number of infertile women of advanced reproductive age is increasing, it is also important to include in the preliminary investigations the assessment of the ovarian reserve (Leeton, 1992; Speroff, 1994). (Table 1.1.)

Assessment of ovulation

Subtle ovulation disorders such as anovulation, inadequately timed ovulation or ovulation of a follicle of reduced size are reported in only 4% of the women studied (van Zonneveld et al., 1999). Patients with infertility and regular cycles usually have normal ovulatory cycles. Therefore, intensive hormone monitoring may not be necessary.

Measuring progesterone in the mid-luteal phase appears to be the best test for confirming ovulation (Crosignani & Rubin, 2000), and to predict ovulation, the detection of the LH (luteinizing hormone) surge in the urine can be informative (Martinez et al., 1992). However, ovulation and LH surge may not correspond and false negatives have been noted (Crosignani et al., 1993). Often infertile women will present with basal body temperature (BBT) charts following instruction by their general practitioner. BBT charts are a simple and inexpensive method for determining the production of progesterone and thus confirming ovulation. However, since the role of luteal phase defects as a cause of infertility has been challenged, because they do not necessarily recur in every cycle, the importance of BBT charts has been diminished (Dawood, 1994). Follicular tracking by ultrasound scan may not be cost-effective in women with regular cycles.

Table 1.1. Investigations for infertile women

Ovulation
Basal FSH/LH
Prolactin
Thyroid function tests
Temperature chart
Mid-luteal progesterone
Follicular tracking
Ovarian reserve tests
Static tests:
Basal FSH
Basal oestradiol
Inhibin-B
Dynamic tests:
Clomiphene citrate challenge test
GnRH-agonist stimulation test
FSH GnRH-agonist stimulation test
Ovarian volume
Ultrasound
Tubal and Uterine Factor
Chlamydia
Hysterosalpingography
Hysterosalpingo contrast sonography
Laparoscopy
Hysteroscopy

Note: FSH: follicle stimulating hormone; LH: luteinizing hormone; GnRH: gonadotrophin releasing hormone.

Women with infrequent (oligomenorrhoea) or absent (amenorrhoea) menstruation often have anovulatory cycles and are infertile. Women with primary amenorrhoea in general have usually been evaluated previously, but these investigations are not usually in the context of infertility. Table 1.2 lists the most common causes of primary amenorrhoea:

Patients in this group who can benefit most from ART are those with chromosome abnormalities as, if the uterus is normally formed, egg donation is an option. For women with Rokitansky–Kuster–Hauser syndrome, surrogacy is an option. Kallmann's syndrome can be successfully treated with the gonadotrophin releasing hormone (GnRH) analogue pump or with gonadotrophin (Imai & Tamaya, 1986; Chryssikopoulos *et al.*, 1998). Women with secondary amenorrhoea and

Table 1.2. Causes of primary amenorrhoea

Hypothalamus
Kallmann's syndrome
Hypothalamic tumour or trauma
Hypothalamic amenorrhoea
Anorexia

Gonads
Streak gonads:
    XO Turner's syndrome
    XX or mosaic
    XY gonadal dysgenesis
Testicular feminization
Polycystic ovary syndrome
Galactosaemia

Uterus
Absent
Rokitansky–Kuster–Hauser syndrome
Testicular feminization

Vagina
Absent
Imperforate hymen

Endocrine disorders
Diabetes, thyroid and adrenal abnormalities

oligomenorrhoea are more likely to require investigations and further management because of anovulatory infertility (Table 1.3).

Clinical history and assessment of basal follicle stimulating hormone (FSH), LH and prolactin can be sufficient for the diagnosis of the majority of causes of anovulation listed.

FSH and LH

Hypothalamic dysfunctions related to weight loss, anorexia nervosa, or excessive physical exercise are caused by reduced secretion of luteinizing hormone releasing hormone (LHRH), with FSH and LH levels below the norm (<5 mIU/ml) and very low oestradiol levels (Lachelin & Yen, 1978; Rowe *et al.*, 1993). This condition can be self-limiting if the initiating factors are removed and weight is regained. When amenorrhoea persists for a prolonged time hormone replacement therapy (HRT)

Table 1.3. Causes of secondary amenorrhoea and oligomenorrhoea

---

Hypothalamus
Weight loss/anorexia
Stress, emotional trauma
Excessive physical exercise
Tumour, trauma, craniopharyngioma

Pituitary
Prolactin secreting
Failure: Sheehan's syndrome

Ovaries
Polycystic ovaries
Ovarian failure
Galactosaemia
Chemo-/radiotherapy

Uterus
Asherman's syndrome

Endocrine disorders
Diabetes, thyroid abnormalities

---

is required to prevent loss of bone density (Drinkwater *et al.*, 1984; Rigotti *et al.*, 1984). If pregnancy is desired, ovulation can be successfully stimulated with a GnRH pump or gonadotrophins. Sometimes FSH, LH and oestradiol levels are within the normal ranges and in this case the woman can benefit from the administration of clomiphene citrate.

Premature ovarian failure is defined as the cessation of ovarian activity in women aged <40 years and is caused by exhaustion of the ovarian reserve, with FSH and LH levels of >20–40 mIU/ml. This can be idiopathic, familial in a few cases (Davis *et al.*, 2000), or caused by autoimmune disorders and chemotherapy. In women aged <30 years it is often associated with chromosome abnormalities. When a Y chromosome is identified, the gonads must be surgically removed as there is a 25% risk of malignant tumour formation (Speroff *et al.*, 1989; Conway *et al.*, 1996). Women with ovarian failure need to start HRT immediately. When pregnancy is desired and the uterus is normally formed, oocyte donation is the only option for assisted conception (Serhal & Craft, 1989).

Polycystic ovary (PCO) is a heterogeneous condition that can be associated with endocrine or metabolic disturbances. About 38% of the women with polycystic ovaries are obese, 66% have menstrual disorders, 48% have signs of hyperandrogenism and 73% are infertile because of anovulatory cycles. However, 20% are completely asymptomatic and may be first diagnosed with PCO during their attendance at a fertility clinic when ultrasonography reveals the typical ultrasound appearance of PCO (Polson *et al.*, 1988). In 40% of women with PCO, LH levels can be elevated and when it is >10 mIU/ml it is more likely to be associated with a history of infertility and a higher miscarriage rate (Regan *et al.*, 1990).

Therefore, in women with PCO, infertility needs to be approached by ovulation induction in the first instance, and the first line of treatment should be with clomiphene citrate. If ovulation is not achieved gonadotrophins can be used (Lachelin, 1991). However, the risk of over-response is higher and often the treatment cycle is abandoned because of the risk of multiple pregnancy and hyperstimulation (Jacobs, 1987). In these women or when the LH levels are very high, laparoscopic ovarian diathermy (LOD) is an alternative method of treatment (Farquar *et al.*, 2000).

In vitro fertilization (IVF) finds its place in the treatment of PCO patients when the above methods fail to achieve pregnancy or there are other associated causes of infertility. Women with PCO who need controlled ovarian stimulation for IVF are an unusual group of patients. They need a profound down-regulation with GnRH-analogue, which may result in lower LH levels with improved oocyte quality, higher fertilization rate and significantly reduced miscarriage rate. They also have a high sensitivity to gonadotrophin, which must be used at a lower dose than for non-PCO patients, to reduce the risk of ovarian hyperstimulation syndrome (Balen *et al.*, 1999).

Prolactin

The normal cut-off level for prolactin is 700–800 mIU/l (Lenton *et al.*, 1982) but levels up to 1000 mIU/l are unlikely to be due to a pathological cause as prolactin levels can vary from one assay to another and can be increased by stress (Jeffcoate *et al.*, 1986). Often a rise in prolactin can be driven by psychotherapeutic drugs and high oestrogen levels such as with PCO, oestrogen therapy (pill), or a peri-menopausal state. When a second blood test confirms abnormal levels of prolactin, thyroid function must be checked by measurement of thyroid stimulating hormone (TSH) and thyroxine levels, as primary hypothyroidism that can cause hyperprolactinaemia is not always an easy condition to diagnose clinically (Heyburn *et al.*, 1986). Pituitary adenoma can be diagnosed by magnetic resonance imaging (MRI) (Stein *et al.*, 1989). Microadenoma (<1 cm) can benefit from medical treatment with bromocriptine or cabergoline. Macroadenoma (>1 cm) can be treated medically and/or surgically.

It is important to remember that non-prolactin-secreting pituitary tumours may also be associated with increased prolactin levels because of obstruction of the portal vessels and interference with the control of prolactin release. Therefore, acromegaly and Cushing syndrome must also be looked for. Galactorrhoea may be present in only one-third of women with hyperprolactinaemia and only one-third of women with galactorrhoea will have hyperprolactinaemia (Sakiyama & Quan, 1983). Women planning a pregnancy can be reassured, as there is no evidence of increased risk of miscarriage or malformations if conception occurs when taking bromocriptine (Turkalj *et al.*, 1982). However, it would be prudent to stop the drug when pregnancy is confirmed and commence close follow-up of the patient. When evidence of regrowth of an adenoma occurs, the treatment should be recommenced (Tan & Jacobs, 1986).

Ovarian reserve tests

Ageing of the ovary is characterized by reduction in the number of primordial follicles and a progressively reduced response to exogenous gonadotrophin. The recruitment of a sufficient number of follicles during ovarian stimulation is a crucial factor in the success of ARTs. A good ovarian response yields a larger number of oocytes and provides a wider choice of embryos for transfer (Loumaye *et al.*, 1990; Roest *et al.*, 1996). Failure of the ovaries to respond to gonadotrophin stimulation is a negative prognostic factor because it indicates reduced ovarian reserve. Although this is usually an age-related problem, its onset is highly variable and difficult to detect (Fahri *et al.*, 1997). Age and regularity of cycles are unreliable ways to predict ovarian reserve. The availability of an accurate screening test to identify patients who will respond poorly to ovarian stimulation has always been an attractive proposition to clinicians as it would provide a valuable means to select appropriate fertility treatment. A variety of screening tests to assess ovarian reserve and predict response to gonadotrophin stimulation have been developed.

Static tests

- Basal FSH
  Diminishing of the number of follicles stored in the ovaries is followed by an increase in the FSH level. The measurement of basal FSH has been widely studied and found to be reliable (Muasher *et al.*, 1988; Toner *et al.*, 1991). It is simple and inexpensive and is the most widely used screening test for infertile women (Scott & Hoffman, 1995). However, women with normal basal levels of FSH do not always respond well to ovarian stimulation (Fahri *et al.*, 1997).
- Basal oestradiol (E_2)
  Women with reduced ovarian reserve may have a shorter follicular phase with more advanced follicular recruitment and a higher basal E_2 level. Therefore,

Licciardi *et al.* propose basal E_2 as an accurate predictor of ovarian reserve and IVF outcome (Licciardi *et al.*, 1995), but the accuracy of this test is controversial (Phopong *et al.*, 2000).

- Inhibin-B

  Inhibin-B is a glycoprotein released by granulosa cells, controlling the pituitary secretion of FSH with negative feedback. Low levels of inhibin have been correlated with a reduced ovarian reserve and poor IVF outcome (Seifer *et al.*, 1997) but this is not confirmed in more recent studies (Corson *et al.*, 1999).

Dynamic tests

Dynamic tests have been proposed to reveal poor ovarian reserves in women with an apparently normal static test such as basal FSH.

- Clomiphene challenge test (CCT)

  This is based on the evaluation of the change of FSH levels from days 3 to 10 after administration of clomiphene citrate 100 mg from cycle days 5 to 9 (Navot *et al.*, 1987). When the ΔFSH is >20 there is an increased chance of low ovarian response to stimulation and poor IVF outcome (Scott *et al.*, 1993; Fahri *et al.*, 1997).

- GnRH agonist stimulation test (GAST)

  The administration of a GnRH-a on cycle days 2 and 3 induces an initial surge of FSH, LH, and E_2 (flare-up), followed by pituitary desensitisation. The E_2 response to stimulation reflects the functional integrity of the ovarian follicles. A low E_2 response can be regarded as a consequence of dwindling cohorts of secretory follicles. Therefore, it is a poor prognostic factor for patients undergoing ovarian stimulation for ART (Padilla *et al.*, 1990; Winslow *et al.*, 1991).

- FSH GnRH agonist stimulation test

  Simultaneous evaluation of basal FSH and E_2 response to GnRH-analogue administration (F–G-test) enhances the possibility of predicting ovarian reserve. This was first proposed in 1998 and compared to other tests it has the highest correlation with the ovarian response to stimulation (Ranieri *et al.*, 1998). The importance of this test with the additional evaluation of inhibin was confirmed by Ravhon *et al.* (2000). Recently it has been shown that the F–G-test can be used to individualize the drug regimen in women undergoing ovarian stimulation for IVF (Ranieri *et al.*, 2001).

Ovarian volume

A reduction of ovarian volume and number of antral follicles measured by transvaginal ultrasound scan have been noticed in older women. These changes may be observed earlier than a rise in FSH levels and are correlated with poor response of the ovaries to stimulation and a high cancellation rate in IVF patients (Syrop *et al.*, 1995, 1999).

Tubal and uterine factor

Evaluation of tubal patency and the uterine cavity is of crucial importance in the preliminary assessment of infertile women.

Tubal factor

Chlamydia testing

Chlamydia infection is recognized worldwide as the most prevalent sexually transmitted infection and previous infection has been documented in 20% of asymptomatic women (Eggert-Kruse *et al.*, 1997). Chlamydia is a common cause of urethritis and cervicitis, and the sequelae include PID and tubal factor infertility. Tubal damage was found in 35% of women with high Chlamydia antibody levels (Thomas *et al.*, 2000) and women with an elevated antibody titre may also have lower implantation and pregnancy rates, and a higher early pregnancy loss after ART (Sharara & Queenan, 1999). Therefore, infertile women should be routinely tested for Chlamydia infections and treated prior to undergoing assisted conception.

Hysterosalpingography (HSG)

This is a relatively easy method and provides information on the calibre of the tube and location of occlusion, but HSG cannot distinguish between genuine occlusion and tubal spasm and it fails to identify peritubal lesions (Mol *et al.*, 1996). Therefore, it is possible to have either false positive or false negative results. The accuracy of HSG has been reported as 86% (Holst *et al.*, 1983). An abnormal HSG affecting fecundity was found in about 3% of the cases and was primarily correlated with the finding of bilateral tubal blockage and hydrosalpinges (Stovall *et al.*, 1992). It has also been reported that a large number of women become pregnant after the HSG. This therapeutic effect may be due to the contrast medium mechanically removing mucus plugs and debris during the procedure (De Cherney *et al.*, 1980; Watson *et al.*, 1994). Therefore, HSG is considered a primary investigation method for the morphology and patency of the fallopian tubes (Crosignani & Rubin, 2000).

Hysterosalpingo contrast sonography (HyCoSy)

This is a new method to assess tubal patency by injecting a special echogenic medium (Echovist) under ultrasound control. The results are comparable to HSG and both procedures can be used in the evaluation of tubal pathology (Strandell *et al.*, 1999; Dijkman *et al.*, 2000).

Laparoscopy

Laparoscopy is considered the gold standard for the evaluation of tubal disease but it is an invasive and costly procedure. It should be considered as the first line diagnostic tool for assessing tubal status in infertile women with a previous history of pelvic surgery, PID, or high serum levels of Chlamydia Ab (Crosignani & Rubin, 2000; Thomas *et al.*, 2000). Laparoscopy is the only accurate means of diagnosis and staging of endometriosis. Women with abnormal findings at HSG can have further assessment of the pelvis by laparoscopy. In conjunction with this procedure, tubal surgery for minimal tubal damage can be performed, peritubal adhesion removed and ovaries mobilized to allow transvaginal ultrasound guided oocyte retrieval. Salpingectomy can be performed in women with hydrosalpinges prior to undergoing assisted conception and this may improve IVF outcome (Zeyneloglu *et al.*, 1998; Camus *et al.*, 1999; Cohen *et al.*, 1999).

Uterine factor

Although still subject to some controversy, uterine anomalies may interfere with implantation and pregnancy, causing infertility and pregnancy loss (Bulletti *et al.*, 1996). Uterine malformations, fibroids, intrauterine synaechie and polyps should be detected in infertile women and treated if directly related to the infertility or when reducing the chances of success with ART. HSG is a useful screening method first to assess the uterine cavity and HyCoSy with saline can be helpful.

Hysteroscopy should be performed when:
- Intrauterine lesion is suspected after the previous investigations.
- High risk of intrauterine adhesions (endometritis, PID, D&C).
- History of recurrent miscarriage.
- Repetitive IVF failure despite good quality of embryos.

During hysteroscopy, intrauterine abnormalities can be removed. Uterine septum can cause miscarriage. Polyps and submucous fibroids are associated with infertility, early pregnancy loss and lower pregnancy rate in IVF patients (Richards *et al.*, 1998; Bajekal & Li, 2000; Healy, 2000). Intramural fibroids may also be associated with infertility and lower success rate after ART and can be removed by the abdominal approach (Eldar-Geva *et al.*, 1998; Bulletti *et al.*, 1999). Subserous fibroids not encroaching on the cavity and measuring <7 cm do not seem to interfere with the outcome of IVF or ICSI (Ramzy *et al.*, 1998). When myomectomy is necessary the laparoscopic approach should be favoured if the fibroid does not have a deep intramural growth and there is no risk of opening the cavity (Vercellini *et al.*, 1998; Dubuisson *et al.*, 2000; Fauconnier *et al.*, 2000).

MRI can be useful for the assessment of uterine malformations such as bicornuate or unicornuate uterus. However, surgical treatment may not be required. When IVF treatment is necessary any effort should be made to reduce multiple pregnancy as this can further increase the risk of miscarriage associated with these abnormalities (De Souza *et al.*, 1995; Turnbull *et al.*, 1995).

REFERENCES

Bajekal, N. & Li, T. C. (2000). Fibroids, infertility and pregnancy wastage. *Hum. Reprod. Update* **6**: 614–20.

Balen, A. H., MacDougall, J. & Jacobs, H. S. (1999). Polycystic ovaries and their relevance to assisted conception. In *A Textbook of In Vitro Fertilization and Assisted Reproduction*, 2nd edn, ed. P. R. Brinsden, pp. 109–29. Carnforth: Parthenon Publishing.

Beerthuizen, R. J. (1996). Pelvic inflammatory disease in intrauterine device users. *Eur. J. Contracept. Reprod. Health Care* **1**: 237–43.

Bolumar, F., Olsen, J., Rebagliato, M. & Bisanti, L. (1997). Caffeine intake and delayed conception: a European multicenter study on infertility and subfecundity. European Study Group on Infertility Subfecundity. *Am. J. Epidemiol.* **145**: 324–34.

Bulletti, C., De Ziegler, D., Polli, V. & Flamigni, C. (1999). The role of leiomyomas in infertility. *J. Am. Assoc. Gynecol. Laparosc.* **6**: 441–5.

Bulletti, C., Flamigni, C. & Giacomucci, E. (1996). Reproductive failure due to spontaneous abortion and recurrent miscarriage. *Hum. Reprod. Update* **2**: 118–36.

Campana, A., de Agostini, A., Bischof, P., Tawfik, E. & Mastroilli, A. (1995). Evaluation of fertility. *Hum. Reprod. Update* **1**: 586–606.

Camus, E., Poncelet, C., Goffinet, F. *et al.* (1999). Pregnancy rates after in vitro fertilization in cases of tubal infertility with and without hydrosalpinx: a meta-analysis of published comparative studies. *Hum. Reprod.* **14**: 1243–9.

Chryssikopoulos, A., Gregoriou, O., Papadias, C. & Loghis, C. (1998). Gonadotropin ovulation induction and pregnancies in women with Kallmann's syndrome. *Gynecol. Endocrinol.* **12**: 103–8.

Cohen, M. A., Lindheim, S. R. & Sauer, M. V. (1999). Hydrosalpinges adversely affect implantation in donor oocyte cycles. *Hum. Reprod.* **14**: 1087–9.

Conway, G. S., Kaltass, G., Patel, A. *et al.* (1996). Characterization of idiopathic premature ovarian failure. *Fertil. Steril.* **65**: 337–41.

Corson, S. L., Gutman, J., Batzer, F. R. *et al.* (1999). Inhibin-B as a test of ovarian reserve for infertile women. *Hum. Reprod.* **14**: 2818–21.

Crosignani, P. G. & Rubin, B. L. (2000). Optimal use of infertility diagnostic test and treatments. The ESHRE Capri Workshop Group. *Hum. Reprod.* **15**: 723–32.

Crosignani, P. G., Collins, J., Cooke, I. D. *et al.* (1999). Unexplained infertility. *Hum. Reprod.* **8**: 977–80.

Davis, C. J., Davison, R. M., Payne, N. N., Rodeck, C. H. & Conway, G. S. (2000). Female sex preponderance for idiopathic familial premature ovarian failure suggests an X chromosome defect: Opinion. *Hum. Reprod.* **15**: 2418–22.

Dawood, M. Y. (1994). Corpus luteal insufficiency. *Curr. Opin. Obstet. Gynecol.* **6**: 121–7.

De Cherney, A. H., Kort, H., Barney, J. B. & De Vore, G. R. (1980). Increased pregnancy rate with oil-soluble hysterosalpingography dye. *Fertil. Steril.* **33**: 407–10.

De Souza, N. M., Brosens, J. J. & Schwieso, J. E. *et al.* (1995). The potential value of magnetic resonance imaging in infertility. *Clin. Radiol.* **50**: 75–9.

Dijkman, A. B., Mol, B. W., van der Veen, F., Bossuyt, P. M. & Hogerzeil, H. V. (2000). Can hysterosalpingocontrast-sonography replace hysterosalpingography in the assessment of tubal subfertility? *Eur. J. Radiol.* **35**: 44–8.

Drinkwater, B. L., Nilson, K., Chesnut, C. H., Bremner, W. J., Shainholtz, S. & Southworth, M. B. (1984). Bone mineral content of amenorrheic and eumenorrheic athletes. *New Engl. J. Med.* **311**: 277–81.

Dubuisson, J. B., Fauconnier, A., Chapron, C., Kreiker, G. & Norgaard, C. (2000). Reproductive outcome after laparoscopic myomectomy in infertile women. *J. Reprod. Med.* **27**: 327–37.

Eggert-Kruse, W., Rohr, G., Demirakca, T., Rusu, R., Naher, H., Petzoldt, D. & Runnebaum, B. (1997). Chlamydial serology in 1303 asymptomatic subfertile couples. *Hum. Reprod.* **12**: 1464–75.

Eldar-Geva, T., Meagher, S., Healy, D. L., MacLachlan, V., Breheney, S. & Wood, C. (1998). Effect of intramural, subserosal, and submucosal uterine fibroids on the outcome of assisted reproductive technology treatment. *Fertil. Steril.* **70**: 687–91.

ESHRE Capri Workshop (1996). Guidelines to the prevalence, diagnosis, treatment and management of infertility. *Hum. Reprod.* **11**: 1775–807.

Fahri, J., Homburg, R., Ferber, A., Orvieto, R. & Ben Rafael, Z. (1997). Non-response to ovarian stimulation in normogonadotrophic, normogonadal women: a clinical sign of impending onset of ovarian failure pre-empting the rise in basal follicle stimulating hormone levels. *Hum. Reprod.* **12**: 241–3.

Farquar, C., Vandekerkhove, P., Arnot, M. & Lilford, R. (2000). Laparoscopic "drilling" by diathermy or laser for ovulation induction in anovulatory polycystic ovary syndrome. *Cochrane Database Syst Rev.* No. 2: CD001122.

Fauconnier, A., Dubuisson, J. B., Ancel, P. Y. & Chapron, C. (2000). Prognostic factors of reproductive outcome after myomectomy in infertile patients. *Hum. Reprod.* **15**: 1751–7.

Grodstein, F., Goldman, M. B. & Cramer, D. W. (1994). Infertility in women and moderate alcohol use. *Am. J. Public Health* **84**: 1429–32.

Hatasaka, H. H., Branch, D. W., Kutteh, W. H. *et al.* (1997). Autoantibody screening for infertility: explaining the unexplained ? *J. Reprod. Immunol.* **34**: 137–53.

Healy, D. L. (2000). Impact of uterine fibroids on ART outcome. *Environ. Health Perspect.* **108** (Suppl. 5): 845–7.

Heyburn, P., Gibby, O., Houriham, M., Hall, R. & Scanlon, M. F. (1986). Primary hypothyroidism presenting as amenorrhoea and galactorrhoea with hyperprolactinemia and pituitary enlargement. *BMJ* **292**: 1660–1.

Holst, N., Abyholm, T. & Borgersen, A. (1983). Hysterosalpingography in the evaluation of infertility. *Acta Radiol. Diagn.* **24**: 253–7.

Imai, A. & Tamaya, T. (1986). Kallmann syndrome in females: gonadotropin versus GnRH to induce fertility. *J. Med.* **27**: 237–40.

Jacobs, H. S. (1987). Polycystic ovaries and polycystic ovary syndrome. *Gynecol. Endocrinol.* **1**: 113–131.

Jeffcoate, S. L., Bacon, R. R. A., Beastall, G. H., Diver, M. J., Franks, S. & Seth, J. (1986). Assays for prolactin: guidelines for the provision of a clinical biochemistry service. *Ann. Clin. Biochem.* **23**: 638–51.

Katz, M. G. & Voellenhoven, B. (2000). The reproductive endocrine consequences of anorexia nervosa. *Br. J. Obstet. Gynaecol.* **107**: 707–13.

Lachelin, G. C. L. (1991). *Introduction to Clinical Reproductive Endocrinology*, pp. 73–88. Cambridge: Cambridge University Press.

Lachelin, G. C. L. & Yen, S. S. C. (1978). Hypothalamic chronic anovulation. *Am. J. Obstet. Gynecol.* **130**: 825–31.

Lenton, E. A., Sulaiman, R., Sobowale, E. & Cooke, I. D. (1982). The human menstrual cycle: plasma concentrations of prolactin, LH, FSH, oestradiol and progesterone in conceiving and non-conceiving women. *J. Reprod. Fertil.* **48**: 605–7.

Leeton, J. (1992). Patient selection for assisted reproduction. *Baillières Clin. Obstet. Gynecol.* **6**: 217–27.

Licciardi, F. L., Liu, H. C. & Rosenwaks, Z. (1995). Day 3 estradiol serum concentration as prognosticators of ovarian stimulation response and pregnancy outcome in patients undergoing in vitro fertilization. *Fertil. Steril.* **64**: 991–4.

Loumaye, E., Billion, J. M., Mine, J. M., Psalti, I., Pensis, M. & Thomas, K. (1990). Prediction of individual response to controlled ovarian hyperstimulation by means of a clomiphene citrate challenge test. *Fertil. Steril.* **53**: 295–301.

Martinez, A. R., Voorhorst, F. J. & Shoemaker, J. (1992). Reliability of urinary LH testing for planning of endometrial biopsies. *Eur. J. Obstet. Gynecol. Reprod. Biol.* **43**: 137–42.

Miller, H. G., Cain, V. S., Rogers, S. M., Gribble, J. N. & Turner, C. F. (1999). Correlates of sexually transmitted bacterial infections among U.S. women in 1995. *Fam. Plann. Perspect.* **31**: 4–9, 23.

Mol, B. W., Swart, P., Bossuyt, P. M. M. *et al.* (1996). Reproducibility of the interpretation of hysterosalpingography in the diagnosis of tubal pathology. *Hum. Reprod.* **11**: 1204–8.

Muasher, S. J., Oehninger, S., Simonetti, S. *et al.* (1988). The value of basal and/or stimulated serum gonadotropin levels in prediction of stimulation response and in vitro fertilization outcome. *Fertil. Steril.* **50**: 298–307.

Navot, D., Rosenwaks, Z. & Magalioth, E. J. (1987). Prognostic assessment of female fecundity. *Lancet* **2**: 64–7.

Norman, R. J. & Clark, A. M. (1998). Obesity and reproductive disorders: a review. *Reprod. Fertil. Dev.* **10**: 55–63.

Padilla, S. L., Bayati, J. & Garcia, J. E. (1990). Prognostic value of the early serum estradiol response to leuploride acetate in in vitro fertilization. *Fertil. Steril.* **53**: 288–94.

Phopong, P., Ranieri, D. M., Khadum, I., Meo, F. & Serhal, P. (2000). Basal 17β-estradiol did not correlate with ovarian response and in vitro fertilization treatment outcome. *Fertil. Steril.* **74**: 1133-6.

Polson, D. W., Wadsworth, J., Adams, J. & Franks, S. (1988). Polycystic ovaries: a common finding in normal women. *Lancet* **2**: 870–2.

Ramzy, A. M., Sattar, M., Amin, Y., Mansour, R. T., Serour, G. L. & Aboulghar, M. A. (1998). Uterine myomata and outcome of assisted reproduction. *Hum. Reprod.* **13**: 198–202.

Ranieri, D. M., Phopong, P., Khadum, I., Meo, F., Davis, C. & Serhal, P. (2001). Simultaneous evaluation of basal FSH and oestradiol response to GnRH analogue (F–G-test) allows effective drug regimen selection for IVF. *Hum. Reprod.* **16**: 101–3.

Ranieri, D. M, Quinn, F., Makhlouf, A., Khadum, I., Ghutmi, W., McGarrigle, H., Davies, M. & Serhal, P. (1998). Simultaneous evaluation of basal follicle-stimulating hormone and 17β-astradiol response to gonadotropin-releasing hormone analogue stimulation: an improved predictor of ovarian reserve. *Fertil. Steril.* **70**: 227–33.

Ravhon, A., Lavery, S., Michael, S., Donaldson, M., Margara, R., Trew, G. & Winston, R. (2000). Dynamic assays of inhibin B and oestradiol following buserelin acetate administration as predictors of ovarian response in IVF. *Hum. Reprod.* **15**: 2297–301.

Regan, L., Owen, E. J. & Jacobs, H. S. (1990). Hypersecretion of luteinising hormone, infertility and miscarriage. *Lancet* **336**: 1141–4.

Richards, P. A., Richards, P. D. & Tiltman, A. J. (1998). The ultrastructure of fibromyomatous myometrium and its relationship to infertility. *Hum. Reprod. Update* **4**: 520–5.

Rigotti, N. A., Nussbaum, S. R., Herzog, D. B. & Neer, R. M. (1984). Osteoporosis in women with anorexia nervosa. *New Engl. J. Med.* **311**: 1601–6.

Roest, J., van Heusden, A. M., Mous, H., Zelimaker, G. H. & Verhoeff, A. (1996). The ovarian response as a predictor for successful in vitro fertilization treatment after the age of 40 years. *Fertil. Steril.* **66**: 969–73.

Rowe, P. J., Camhaire, F. H., Hargrave, T. B. & Mellows, H. J. (1993). *WHO Manual for the standardised investigation of the infertile couple.* Cambridge: Cambridge University Press.

Sakiyama, R. & Quan, M. (1983). Galactorrhea and hyperprolactinemia. *Obst. Gynecl. Surv.* **38**: 689–700.

Scott, R. T., Leonardi, M. R. & Hoffman, G. E. (1993). A prospective evaluation of clomiphene citrate challenge test screening in the general infertility population. *Obstet. Gynecol.* **82**: 539–45.

Scott, R. T. & Hoffman, G. E. (1995). Prognostic assessment of ovarian reserve. *Fertil. Steril.* **63**: 1–11.

Seifer, D. B., Gardiner, A. C. & Lambert-Messerlian, G. (1997). Day 3 serum inhibin-B is predictive of assisted reproductive technologies outcome. *Fertil. Steril.* **67**: 110–14.

Serhal, P. F. & Craft, I. L. (1989). Oocyte donation in 61 patients. *Lancet* **i**: 1185–87.

Sharara, F. I., Seifer, D. B. & Flaws, J. A. (1998). Environmental toxicants and female reproduction. *Fertil. Steril.* **70**: 613–22.

Sharara, F. I. & Queenan, J. T. Jr (1999). Elevated serum Chlamydia trachomatis IgG antibodies. Association with decreased implantation rates in GIFT. *J. Reprod. Med.* **44**: 581–6.

Speroff, L. (1994). The effect of ageing on fertility. *Curr. Opin. Obstet. Gynecol.* **6**: 115–20.

Speroff, L., Glass, R. H. & Kase, G. N. (1989). *Clinical Gynecologic Endocrinology and Infertility,* 4th edn, pp. 173–9. Baltimore: Williams & Wilkins.

Stein, A., Levenick, M. N. & Kletzky, O. A. (1989). Computed tomography versus magnetic resonance imaging for the evaluation of suspected pituitary adenomas. *Obst. Gynecol.* **73**: 996–99.

Steyaert, S. R., Leroux-Roels, G. G. & Dhont, M. (2000). Infections in IVF: review and guidelines. *Hum. Reprod. Update* **6**: 432–41.

Stolwijk, A. M., Wetzels, A. M. & Braat, D. D. (2000). Cumulative probability of achieving an ongoing pregnancy after in-vitro fertilization and intracytoplasmic sperm injection according to a woman's age, subfertility diagnosis and primary or secondary subfertility. *Hum. Reprod.* **15**: 203–9.

Stovall, D. W., Christman, G. M., Hammond, M. G. & Talbert, L. M. (1992). Abnormal findings on hysterosalpingography: effects on fecundity in a donor insemination program using frozen semen. *Obstet. Gynecol.* **80**: 249–52.

Strandell, A., Bourne, T., Bergh, C., Granberg, S., Asztely, M. & Thorburn, J. (1999). The assessment of endometrial pathology and tubal patency: a comparison between the use of ultrasonography and X-ray hysterosalpingography for the investigation of infertility patients. *Ultrasound. Obstet. Gynecol.* **14**: 200–4.

Syrop, C. H., Wilhoite, A. & Van Voorhis, B. J. (1995). Ovarian volume: a novel outcome predictor for assisted reproduction. *Fertil. Steril.* **64**: 1167–71.

Syrop, C. H., Dawson, J. D., Husman, K. J. *et al.* (1999). Ovarian volume may predict assisted reproductive outcomes better than follicle stimulating hormone concentration on day 3. *Hum. Reprod.* **14**: 1752–56.

Tan, S. L. & Jacobs, H. S. (1986). Rapid regression through bromocriptine therapy of a suprasellar extending prolactinoma during pregnancy. *Int. J. Gynaecol. Obst.* **24**: 209–15.

Thomas, K., Coughlin, L., Mannion, P. T. & Haddad, N. G. (2000). The value of Chlamydia trachomatis antibody testing as part of routine infertility investigations. *Hum. Reprod.* **15**: 1079–82.

Toner, J. P., Philput, C. B., Jones, G. S. & Muasher, S. J. (1991). Basal follicle-stimulating hormone level is a better predictor of in vitro fertilization performance than age. *Fertil. Steril.* **55**: 784–91.

Turkalj, I., Braun, P. & Krupp, P. (1982). Surveillance of bromocriptine in pregnancy. *J. Am. Med. Assoc.* **247**: 1589–91.

Turnbull, L. W., Lesny, P. & Killik, S. R. (1995). Assessment of uterine receptivity prior to embryo transfer: a review of currently available imaging modalities. *Hum. Reprod. Update* **1**: 505–14.

van Noord-Zaadstra, B. M., Looman, C. W. N., Alsbach, H., Habbema, J. D. F., te Velde, E. R. & Karbaat, J. (1991). Delaying childbearing: effect of age on fecundity and outcome of pregnancy. *BMJ* **302**: 1361–4.

Van Zonneveld, P., Koppeschaar, H. P., Habbema, J. D., Fauser, B. C. & te Velde, E. R. (1999). Diagnosis of subtle ovulation disorders in subfertile women with regular menstrual cycles: cost-effective clinical practice? *Gynecol. Endocrinol.* **13**: 42–7.

Vercellini, P., Maddalena, S., De Giorgi, O., Aimi, G. & Crosignani, P. G. (1998). Abdominal myomectomy for infertility: a comprehensive review. *Hum. Reprod.* **13**: 873–9.

Watson, A., Vandekerckhove, P., Lilford, R. *et al.* (1994). A meta-analysis of the therapeutic role of oil soluble contrast media at hysterosalpingography: a surprising result? *Fertil. Steril.* **61**: 470–7.

Winslow, K. L., Toner, J. P., Brzyski, R. G., Oehninger, S. C., Acosta, A. & Muasher, S. J. (1991). The gonadotropin-releasing hormone agonist stimulation test-a sensitive predictor of performance in the flare-up in vitro fertilization cycle. *Fertil. Steril.* **56**: 711–17.

World Health Organization (1992). *Recent Advances In Medically Assisted Conception,* WHO Technical Report Series No. 820. Geneva: World Health Organization Publications.

Zayed, F. & Abu-Heija, A. (1999). The management of unexplained infertility. *Obstet. Gynecol. Surv.* **54**: 492–99.

Zeyneloglu, H. B., Arici, A. & Olive, D. L. (1998). Adverse effects of hydrosalpinx on pregnancy rates after in vitro fertilization-embryo transfer. *Fertil. Steril.* **70**: 492–499.

2

Clinical assessment and management of the infertile man

Suks Minhas and David J. Ralph

Department of Uro-andrology, Middlesex Hospital, London, UK

Introduction

Of the 10% of couples who are unable to conceive, approximately 20% are affected entirely by the male alone and a further 30% by a combination of male and female factors. Therefore, 50% of couples seeking treatment have a male factor as the underlying cause for their infertility.

The last two decades have seen great technological advances in the development and success of IVF techniques. As a consequence, there has been a shift in the emphasis on surgery in the treatment of male factor infertility. Many couples with causes for their infertility that are readily treatable by surgery are now referred directly for IVF.

All male patients, therefore, with infertility should be thoroughly evaluated and investigated prior to referral for assisted conception. Furthermore, they require a multidisciplinary approach in their assessment and management, involving close liaison between an andrologist, embryologist and gynaecologist, ideally working in a specialized and dedicated assisted conception unit.

This chapter deals firstly with the anatomy and physiology of male reproduction and then gives an account of the aetiology and management of male factor infertility.

Functional anatomy of the male reproductive system

The male reproductive system (Figure 2.1) consists of the penis, testes, ejaculatory ducts and accessory sex glands. The accessory sex glands comprise the prostate, seminal vesicles, Cowper's glands and glands of Littre. The accessory sex glands produce important secretions, which are required to maintain the viability of sperm in the male and female reproductive tract.

Good Clinical Practice in Assisted Reproduction, ed. P. Serhal & C. Overton.
Published by Cambridge University Press. © Cambridge University Press 2004.

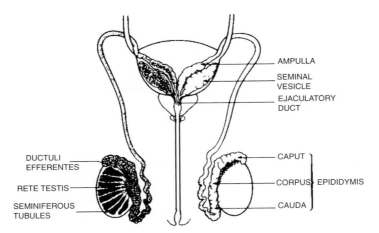

Figure 2.1. Anatomy of the male reproductive system. (Modified from H.N. Whitfield in Hendry, Kirby & Duckett, 1998, p. 1482.)

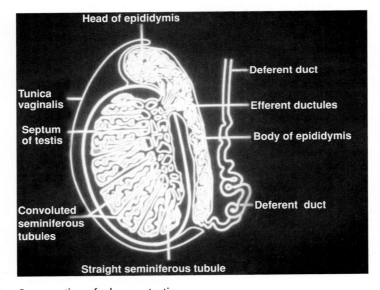

Figure 2.2. Cross-section of a human testis.

Testes

The normal human testis is approximately 15–25 ml in volume and 4.5 cm in length in the adult male. Each testis is oval in shape surrounded by a fibrous layer called the tunica albuginea (Figure 2.2). The epididymis is attached to the posterolateral surface of the testicle in continuity with the vas deferens. The anterior and lateral surfaces of the testicle lie free in a space formed by the overlying tunica vaginalis, a remnant of the fetal processus vaginalis. The blood supply to the testicle is derived from the testicular artery, which is a branch of the aorta, and branches to the epididymis before reaching the posterior surface of the testicle, where it divides into medial and lateral testicular branches. The testis also receives collateral branches from the vasal and cremasteric arteries. Venules from the testicle join to form the pampiniform plexus of veins that surround the testicular artery within the spermatic cord. The intimate relationship of the testicular artery and the pampiniform plexus is thought to create a countercurrent heat exchange that maintains the testicle at 2–4 °C below core body temperature, at which level spermatogenesis can function. The pampiniform plexus forms one to three testicular veins on each side, at the deep internal inguinal ring. The right testicular vein drains directly into the inferior vena cava and the left testicular vein joins the left renal vein.

Ultrastructure of the testis

Each testis is subdivided into discrete lobules by connective tissue septae derived from the tunica albuginea (Figure 2.2). The bulk of each testicle consists of 600–1200 seminiferous tubules and a supportive interstitial connective tissue element. Each seminiferous tubule consists of a loop that ends in a single duct, the tubulus rectus. These ducts anastomose in the rete testis and drain via the ductuli efferentes into the caput of epididymis, where the spermatozoa are stored as they mature.

The interstitial tissue of the testis contains fine connective tissue elements, fibroblasts, mast cells, capillaries and Leydig cells. The Leydig cells produce testosterone and are separated from each seminiferous tubule by a surrounding basement membrane. Directly surrounding the seminiferous tubules are specialized peritubular myoid cells, which secrete paracrine regulatory products and also appear to have contractile effects on the tubules.

Seminiferous tubule

The seminiferous tubules are the primary site for spermatogenesis (Figure 2.3). Each tubule contains germinal cells, which are intimately associated with somatic cells called Sertoli cells. The germinal cells consist of spermatogonia, spermatocytes and spermatids. The spermatogonia divide and mature to form spermatocytes then spermatids, which extend up to reach the tubule lumen where they become spermatozoa.

The Sertoli cells lie on the base of the seminiferous tubules connected by specialized junctional complexes and form the basis of the blood–testis barrier. The blood–testis barrier acts as a barrier to entry of substances into the testis, thus creating optimum conditions for spermatogenesis. The cytoplasm of the Sertoli

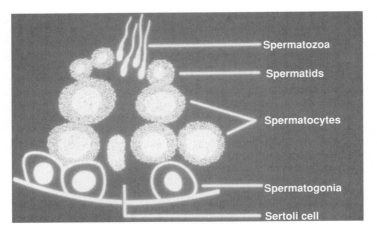

Figure 2.3.   Cross-section of a seminiferous tubule.

cells invests the column of maturing germ cells as it extends towards the tubular lumen. The Sertoli cells not only secrete fluid containing proteins and peptides important in the development and maturation of the spermatozoa, but also nourish the developing sperm. The Sertoli cells are also responsible for the production of inhibin, a glycoprotein involved in the control of follicle stimulating hormone (FSH) secretion.

Spermatogenesis

Throughout the male reproductive life, approximately 100–200 million sperm are produced daily. Each spermatocytic cycle, from the development of the primary spermatogonia to spermatozoa takes approximately 72 days. The origin of these germ cells is still debatable, although they are most likely to arise from specialized stem spermatogonia. These spermatogonia divide mitotically to produce primary spermatocytes, which subsequently undergo a meiotic division to produce secondary spermatocytes, with the result that the secondary spermatocytes contain a haploid number of chromosomes. The secondary spermatocytes undergo further mitosis to produce spermatids, which in turn differentiate to produce spermatozoa. As the germinal cells undergo successive division they move upwards along the adjacent Sertoli cells, which nourish and support them.

During spermiogenesis, the haploid spermatid develops into a mature spermatozoon. Mature spermatozoa are approximately 60 μm in length and are composed of an oval head, middle and tail piece (Figure 2.4). The head contains the nucleus and is covered by a cap, called the acrosome. This vesicular structure contains lytic enzymes required for the absorption and penetration of the outer coat of the female ovum. The middle of the spermatozoa contains mitochondria, which provides the

Table 2.1. The Johnsen mean scoring system

Score	Appearance
10	Many spermatozoa with a central lumen
9	Many spermatozoa but with central sloughing and no lumen
8	Few spermatozoa present
7	No spermatozoa, only spermatids
6	Few spermatids present
5	No spermatids, only spermatocytes present
4	Few spermatocytes
3	Spermatogonia only
2	Sertoli cells only
1	No cells present in the tubules

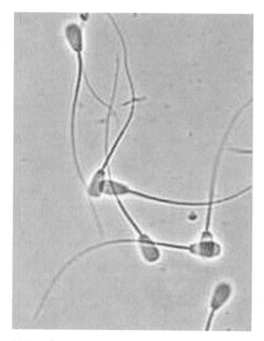

Figure 2.4.   Mature human spermatozoa.

energy source for motility and surrounds a central core of contractile filaments that extend into the tail, allowing propulsion of the spermatozoa. Once released into the seminiferous tubules the spermatozoa remain immotile until they pass into the epididymis, where they are undergo further maturation.

Historically spermatogenesis was quantified histologically on testicular biopsies using mean Johnsen Scores. In this scoring system (Table 2.1) a score between 1 and

10 is designated to each seminiferous tubule on biopsy, depending on the degree of spermatogenesis. This number is divided by the total number of tubules on biopsy to give a mean Johnsen score.

The epididymis

Having been transported from the testis by contractile movements of the ductuli efferentes, the immotile spermatozoa enter the epididymis. The epididymis is divided into the caput (head), corpus (body) and cauda (tail). From animal studies it appears that the epididymis is the final site for maturation and development of the spermatozoa and it is here that they develop the capacity for motility and fertilization. However, the process by which this occurs is not fully understood, although on traversing the epididymis a number of biochemical and molecular changes occur within the spermatozoa. The spermatozoa are transported to the cauda of the epididymis by rhythmic contractions of smooth muscle lining the epididymal tubules. During this stage fluid reabsorption occurs. There is an increase in the concentration of sperm and a number of proteins and chemicals are excreted within the epididymal fluid, including sperm motility and survival factors, glycerophosphocholine, phosphocholine and carnitine. However, the function of these substances still remains obscure.

The sperm are stored in the cauda of the epididymis until ejaculation takes place. Spermatozoa that are not ejaculated deteriorate and are phagocytosed by the lining epididymal cells.

Ejaculation

During ejaculation, sperm are expelled into the urethra by powerful contractions of the smooth muscle lining the epididymis and vas deferens. This results in emission of seminal fluid into the urethra. Once the semen is within the urethra, the preprostatic sphincter closes to prevent retrograde flow of semen into the bladder. Following this, the external sphincter closes and powerful contractions of the bulbo-spongiosus muscle results in forceful ejaculation.

Ejaculatory fluid or semen mainly contains secretions from the seminal vesicles, prostate gland and bulbourethral glands (Table 2.2). The contribution of sperm to the total volume of semen is only 1%. The fluid from the seminal vesicles is rich in fructose and prostaglandins, whereas the prostatic secretion mainly contains proteolytic enzymes, citric acid, zinc and acid phosphatase. The prostate also produces prostatic specific antigen, a serine protease responsible for the liquefaction of semen. Seminal plasma also contains a number of other secretory products and nutrients (Table 2.3). The secretions produced by the accessory sex glands provide an effective transport medium for the spermatozoa.

Table 2.2. Contribution of accessory sex glands to semen volume

Glands	Volume (ml)
Seminal vesicles	2.0
Prostate	0.5
Cowper's glands	0.1

Table 2.3. Main biochemical constituents of seminal plasma

Acid phosphatase
L-carnitine
Citric acid
Fructose
Glucosidase
Glycerophosphocholine
Magnesium
Prostaglandins
Zinc

Hormonal control of male sexual function

Testosterone

Testosterone is the main androgenic hormone produced in the male. The testis produces the majority (6–7 mg/day), although a small amount is also produced by the adrenal glands (20–200 ng/day). Testosterone is a C19 steroid that is synthesized from cholesterol within the interstitial Leydig cells. A description of these metabolic pathways is beyond the scope of this chapter.

Within the circulation, testosterone is mainly bound to sex hormone binding globulin (60%) and the remainder to albumin (38%). A small quantity (2%) of the total circulating testosterone is free. Testosterone is metabolized by conjugation with glucuronic acid in the liver and then excreted by the kidneys.

Free testosterone is converted to dihydrotestosterone intra-cellularly at target tissues, such as the prostate by the enzyme 5-alpha reductase. Dihydrotestosterone acts through nuclear receptors to promote gene activation and specific protein synthesis. Androgen receptors are also found on the Sertoli cells indicating that testosterone has a primary function in spermatogenesis.

At puberty testosterone levels rise in response to luteinizing hormone (LH) and FSH surges leading to development of secondary male characteristics, with the appearance of facial, axillary and pubic hair, enlargement of the genitalia, changes in libido, as well as anabolic effects on skeletal muscle and bone. Levels of testosterone remain constant throughout reproductive years, decreasing later in life as the seminiferous tubules degenerate and the numbers of Leydig cells decrease.

The hypothalamic–pituitary axis

Gonadotrophins

Spermatogenesis and synthesis of testosterone are under control of the anterior pituitary gland, which produces both LH and FSH. Both LH and FSH are produced in a pulsatile fashion in response to stimulation by gonadotrophin releasing hormone (GnRH), which originates from the hypothalamus. GnRH is synthesized in neurosecretory neurons in the median eminence of the hypothalamus and released into the hypophyseal portal system.

FSH promotes spermatogenesis by combining with specific FSH receptors on the Sertoli cells, whilst LH stimulates testosterone production from Leydig cells. Thus both LH and FSH directly and indirectly maintain normal spermatogenesis. Through negative feedback on the hypothalamus and pituitary, testosterone directly inhibits LH and FSH production. FSH production is also inhibited by inhibin, a glycoprotein produced by the Sertoli cells. Studies have demonstrated a good correlation between the plasma levels of FSH and inhibin B and the degree of spermatogenesis on testicular biopsy (see below).

Prolactin is also produced by the pituitary gland and appears to have a direct inhibitory effect on GnRH release.

Definition of infertility

Infertility is defined as *the failure to conceive after one year of unprotected sexual intercourse.*

Epidemiology of male factor infertility

Prior to investigating the infertile male, the clinician must ensure that the female partner has been thoroughly evaluated. On initial consultation with the infertile couple the clinician will be presented with an abnormal semen analysis. Invariably this will show either azoospermia or oligozoospermia. This initial semen analysis will largely dictate subsequent investigations and treatment for the couple.

Table 2.4. World Health Organization (1999) criteria for normal semen quality

Criterion	Value
Volume	>2 ml
pH	>7.2
Sperm concentration	>20×10^6/ml
Total sperm number	>40×10^6
Motility	>50% with space-gaining motility or >25% with rapid progressive motility within 60 minutes of ejaculation
Morphology	>15% normal forms

Table 2.5. Causes of retrograde ejaculation

Neurological
Spinal cord injury
Multiple sclerosis
Diabetes mellitus

Post surgical
Retroperitoneal surgery
Pelvic surgery, e.g. AP resection

Bladder neck dysfunction
Congenital
    Acquired – bladder neck incision
                trans-urethral resection of prostate

Obstruction of urethra
Urethral stricture

Categories of male infertility based on seminal analysis

The World Health Organization has defined the minimal semen parameters for fertility (Table 2.4), which differ from the average seminal analysis quoted in standard texts. These are minimum semen parameters required for fertility.

Terminology of semen analysis

Spermia: volume of semen.
Zoospermia: the spermatozoa in semen.
Asthenozoospermia: reduced sperm motility.

Absent or low volume ejaculate (hypospermia)

This may be due to retrograde ejaculation or anejaculation (Table 2.5). A low volume ejaculant may also be secondary to partial or complete ejaculatory duct

Table 2.6. Causes of ejaculatory duct obstruction

Cause	$n = 87$ (%)
Müllerian duct cyst	20
Wolffian duct malformation	22
Previous surgical trauma	17
Genital infections	22
Tuberculosis	9
Megavesicles	9
Carcinoma of prostate	1

Source: Pryor & Hendry (1991)

obstruction. Ejaculatory duct obstruction is a rare cause of obstructive azoospermia with patients usually presenting with azoospermia or severe oligozoospermia, low volume ejaculate, absent fructose and low pH in their ejaculant. The causes of ejaculatory duct obstruction are listed in Table 2.6.

Azoospermia

This is the absence of spermatozoa in a semen sample. Azoospermia can be divided into obstructive or nonobstructive (secretory) azoospermia.

Obstructive azoospermia

This is the absence of spermatozoa caused by ductal obstruction and accounts for 7% of male factor infertility. The testes are usually of normal size and plasma FSH, LH and testosterone levels are usually normal.

Causes

- Congenital.
- Iatrogenic.
- Infective.

Obstruction may occur anywhere from the efferent ductules to the ejaculatory ducts. The cause may be congenital, for example vasal aplasia, partial or complete absence of ductal structures or acquired, usually post infective or iatrogenic (following surgery).

Congenital bilateral absence of the vas deferens (CBAVD) may occur in approximately 18% of men presenting with azoospermia and can be associated with other genitourinary abnormalities, such as unilateral renal agenesis or pelvic kidneys. Often there is hypoplasia or absence of the seminal vesicles or ampulla. Up to 70% of patients with CBAVD may be carriers of the cystic fibrosis gene and appropriate counselling and screening should be given.

Unilateral vasal aplasia may occur in 5% of men with azoospermia and can be associated with a number of genitourinary abnormalities. Congenital obstruction

Table 2.7. Causes of testicular obstruction

Cause	Incidence %	Aetiology
Caput epididymis	29	Young's syndrome
Cauda epididymis	19	Post infective
Empty epididymis	13	Defective spermatogenesis
Blocked vas	11	Post infective and post surgical
Absent vas		
Bilateral	18	Congenital
Unilateral	5	Mixed
Ejaculatory duct	4	Congenital
obstruction		Traumatic
		Neoplastic

Note: Modified from Hendry *et al.* (1990).

Table 2.8. Causes of epididymitis

Bacteria
  Mycobacterium TB
  Neisseria gonorrhoea
  Chlamydia trachomatis
  Esherichia coli
  Pseudomonas
  Haemophilus
  Streptococcus

of the ejaculatory ducts occurs as a result of Müllerian duct cysts and Wolffian duct anomalies and has already been dealt with above.

Generally, acquired causes of ductal obstruction are the result of surgery or infections and can be unilateral or bilateral (Table 2.7). They can occur anywhere along the seminal ducts, although predominantly in the epididymis. It is important to note that infectious causes of epididymitis (Table 2.8) may not only lead to ductal obstruction but can also result in testicular damage.

Obstructions of the epididymis can be anatomically divided into those affecting the caput or those affecting the cauda, and are either infectious in origin following an episode of epididymitis or post surgical after excision of part or the whole of the epididymis – for example, surgery for epididymal cysts. Less commonly genitourinary infections can cause obstruction at the prostatovesicular junction.

Acquired causes of a blocked vas deferens are either surgical, such as that following herniorrhaphy, or post infective and this can occur with tuberculosis. Of note is the rare chronic respiratory condition known as Young's syndrome, which can lead to obstruction of the caput epididymis due to impaired clearance of viscous epididymal secretions.

Non-obstructive azoospermia (testicular failure)

This is defined as azoospermia caused by failure of spermatogenesis or germ cell failure.

Testicular or germ cell failure is suggested when a patient presents with azoospermia, small volume testes (<15 ml), raised FSH/LH and low serum testosterone. There are a number of pretesticular and testicular causes for this and they are outlined in Table 2.9.

A number of chemicals are known gonadotoxins (Table 2.10). Alcohol may lead to both testicular atrophy and a reduction in germ cells in alcoholics, although studies are not conclusive. Cigarette smoking has been shown to be detrimental to spermatogenesis with a higher number of smokers having abnormal semen parameters compared to non-smokers, although again results are not conclusive.

Chemotherapeutic agents, in particular vinblastine, vincristine and cyclophosphamide, adversely affect spermatogenesis. The germinal cells appear to be particularly prone to damage by alkylating agents, leading to azoo- or oligozoospermia, with an increase in FSH. However, Leydig cell function appears to be spared in these individuals. Therefore, azoospermia can occur in those patients who have undergone previous chemotherapy treatment for Hodgkin's disease or leukaemia.

A number of drugs have also been associated with impaired spermatogenesis and sperm function and these are presented in Table 2.10.

Endocrine causes for testicular failure

These are uncommon and account for only 1–3% of all cases of male factor infertility. Primary hypogonadotrophic hypogonadism occurs in Kallmann's syndrome (hypogonadotrophic hypogonadism associated with anosmia), where there is failure of the hypothalamus to secrete GnRH leading to testicular failure. This syndrome may be autosomal dominantly inherited and is characterized by a delay in the onset of puberty. In the fertile eunuch syndrome there is isolated LH deficiency leading to low levels of plasma LH and testosterone. FSH levels are usually normal and so there some degree of spermatogenesis. Patients present with normal sized testes, hypospermia and severe oligozoospermia/azoospermia. In the rare isolated FSH deficiency, there are normal levels of LH and testosterone, but FSH levels are reduced leading to azoospermia in a normally virilized individual.

Secondary diseases of the pituitary gland can lead to hypogonadotrophic hypogonadism and include infarction, tumours, surgery and irradiation. A number of other rare hormonal diseases have been associated with infertility in the male. Hyperprolactinaemia may be due to a pituitary adenoma, although routine

Table 2.9. Causes of non-obstructive azoospermia (testicular failure)

Germinal aplasia
  Drug induced/ radiotherapy
  Gonadotoxins/chemotherapy
  Klinefelter's syndrome
  XYY syndrome
  Idiopathic
Maturation arrest
  Idiopathic
  XYY syndrome
  Varicocele
Endocrine causes
  Pituitary disease
  Isolated hypogonadotrophic hypogonadism
  Fertile eunuch syndrome
  Isolated follicle stimulating hormone deficiency
  Oestrogens
  Hyperprolactinaemia
Genetic abnormalities
  Kallmann's syndrome
  Klinefelter's syndrome
  XYY syndrome
  XX male
  Androgen insensitivity syndrome
  5-alpha reductase deficiency
Other causes
  Bilateral anorchia
  Bilateral cryptorchidism/torsion
  Sertoli cell only syndrome
  Orchitis
  Immunological

screening is controversial. Other hormonal disorders that may be associated with male infertility include hyperthyroidism and Cushing's disease.

Genetic and chromosomal abnormalities

Overall, approximately 6% of men presenting with infertility will have genetic abnormalities, although this figure increases up to 15% in those who are azoospermic. The majority of these will have Klinefelter's syndrome. This occurs in one in 600 male births and is characterized by an extra X chromosome leading to a 47 XXY

Table 2.10. Drugs associated with infertility

Anabolic steroids
Alcohol
Sulphasalazine
Steroids
Cannabis
Anticonvulsants
Colchicine
Opioids
Antibiotics
    nitrofurantoin, aminoglycosides
Cyproterone acetate
Diethylstilboestrol

karyotype. Typically, individuals present with small firm testes, gynaecomastia with elevated FSH levels and azoospermia. LH levels are usually normal although total plasma testosterone levels may be reduced. Histologically the testis is composed of sclerotic tubules, although the occasional spermatozoa may be found. Other mosaicisms may be present including 46 XY and 47 XXY. Similarly, in the XX male syndrome, patients present with small firm testes, gynaecomastia and azoospermia.

Individuals with XYY syndrome have severe oligo/azoospermia. Histologically there may be maturation arrest to complete germinal aplasia. Serum testosterone and gonadotrophin levels are usually normal, although FSH levels may be elevated.

In Kalmann's syndrome there is failure of gonadotrophin secretion by the hypothalamus leading to testicular failure.

In the partial androgen insensitivity syndrome there is an androgen receptor gene alteration as a result of deletion/mutation of the androgen receptor gene. Clinically, individuals present with a spectrum of phenotypes from females to phenotypic males with azoospermia. In the rare 5-alpha reductase deficiency there is a defect in the peripheral conversion of testosterone into dihydrotestosterone. There is a wide spectrum of phenotypes, but characteristically there is virilization of a phenotypic female at puberty.

The cause of Sertoli cell only syndrome is unknown but is characterized by complete absence of germ cells (Figure 2.5a, b). Clinically this manifests in infertile men with azoospermia, elevated FSH, but normal plasma LH and testosterone as Leydig cell function is preserved.

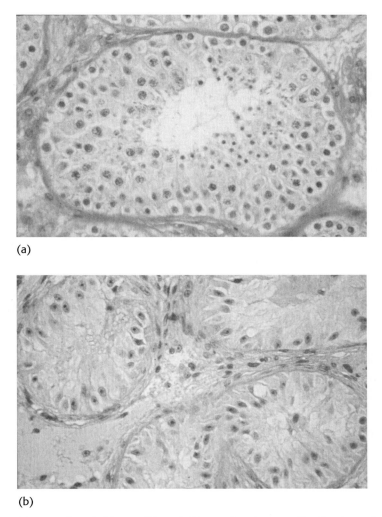

(a)

(b)

Figure 2.5.   (a) Normal testis biopsy; (b) testis biopsy showing Sertoli cell only syndrome.

Asthenospermia

This describes abnormal motility or forward progression of the spermatozoa. Sperm motility is an important factor in male fertility, but often the cause for the impaired motility is not found. Deficiency of sperm motility is not usually isolated but found in combination with necrospermia, congenital defects of the sperm tail or, rarely, abnormalities in seminal biochemistry. Special mention should be made of Kartagener's syndrome, which manifests as situs inversus, dextrocardia and bronchiectasis. Here, the primary motility defect results from an absence of dynein arms in the tail of the sperm.

Causes
- Faulty collection of samples.
- Spermatozoal structural defects, e.g. Kartagener's syndrome, de Kretser's syndrome
- Prolonged abstinence.
- Idiopathic.
- Genital tract infection.
- Antisperm antibodies.
- Testicular hyperthermia, e.g. varicocele.
- Partial ejaculatory duct obstruction.

Oligospermia

This is defined as a sperm concentration of <20 million per ml.
Causes
- Idiopathic.
- Cryptorchidism.
- Varicoceles.
- Drugs and gonadotoxins.
- Chemotherapy.
- Radiotherapy.
- Genitourinary infection.
- Partial ejaculatory duct obstruction.
- Unilateral vasal obstruction.
- Reduced spermatogenesis (hypospermatogenesis).

A reduction in spermatogenesis may be secondary to hypospermatogenesis, where there is a reduction in the number of germinal elements leading to oligozoospermia or maturation arrest. In maturation arrest (Figure 2.6) there is arrest of spermatogenesis at a specific point of maturation. Histologically this can be either complete, often leading to azoospermia, or partial resulting in oligozoospermia. Clinically complete maturation arrest can be difficult to differentiate from testicular obstruction as men with this condition have normal sized testes, normal plasma FSH and azoospermia. It is only when the testes are investigated to exclude an obstruction that empty epididymi are found, associated with the aforementioned testicular biopsy findings.

Teratazoospermia

Teratazoospermia defines a defect in the morphology of the spermatozoa caused by an arrest in the maturation process of spermatogenesis. In these patients it is important to exclude a varicocele.

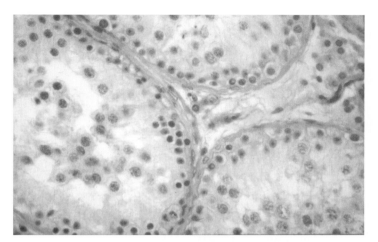

Figure 2.6.   Testis biopsy showing maturation arrest at the spermatocyte level.

Idiopathic

Up to 25% of subfertile men will have no discernible cause for their abnormal semen analysis. There are usually a variety of aetiological factors causing these abnormal semen parameters. Patients may present with a mixture of defects including oligozoospermia, defects of sperm motility and antisperm antibodies.

Other surgical causes of male infertility

Varicocele

A varicocele is the dilatation of the pampiniform plexus of spermatic veins. Approximately 12% of men in the general population will have a varicocele, although this figure increases to 25% of men with infertility. Approximately 90% are left-sided (Figure 2.7) and 10% occur on the right. Various aetiologies have been described to account for varicoceles, including the so-called nutcracker theory due to compression of the left renal vein between the superior mesenteric artery and aorta. The associated testicular dysfunction appears to be the result of raised intrascrotal temperatures leading to defective spermatogenesis.

Invariably serum FSH will be normal but occasionally increased, suggesting a degree of testicular failure. In our experience this is a poor prognostic marker and most of these patients will require assisted conception. Also, there appears to be a direct relationship between the grade of varicocele and sperm count.

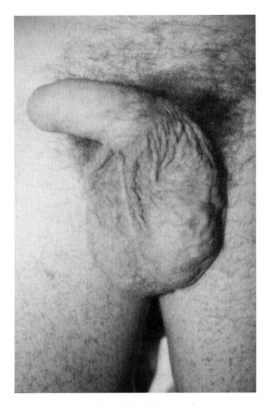

Figure 2.7.   Grade III varicocele of the left testicle.

Grading of varicocele
  I palpable during valsalva
  II palpable on standing
  III visible on standing
In the context of male factor infertility the authors believe there are only two indications for treatment:

- adolescent patients with grade II/III varicoceles associated with a reduction in ipsilateral testicular volume;
- abnormal semen parameters in subfertile men including oligozoospermia $<20 \times 10^6$ per ml, poor motility $<50\%$ progression and abnormal sperm morphology.

The results of varicocele ligation are promising with an overall increase in sperm motility in 70% of cases, sperm concentration in 51% and improved morphology in 44%, whilst conception rates of up to 50% have been reported following varicocele ligation.

Semen characteristics usually improve between three months and one year after surgery. Recurrence rates after surgery have been reported as high as 30%. The authors prefer to use embolization in those cases in which primary surgery has failed. The treatment of a varicocele in men with infertility who are normozoospermic, is of no benefit.

Cryptorchidism

A history of undescended testis, whether unilateral or bilateral, may be the cause of infertility in some men. The incidence of unilateral undescended testis in infants is 4.3% (of which 15% are bilateral). This figure decreases to approximately 1% by one year of age. Most cases of spontaneous descent occur within the first three months of life. If the testis is not in the scrotum by one year of age, irreversible germ cell failure can occur. Oligozoospermia is found in up to 50% of patients with bilateral cryptorchidism and up to 30% of those with unilateral. Very occasionally men with infertility will present at examination with an undescended testis and in this event the testicle may either be removed because of the risk of malignant tranformation or simply observed regularly (if palpable).

Investigation of the male

Medical history (Table 2.11)

Sexual history

This should include a history of the present relationship including length of time of sexual relations with and without contraception, how often coitus is performed and its timing with the female cycle. The age of the couple should also be documented as this may dictate subsequent treatment. A past sexual history, including a history of previous sexually transmitted diseases, pregnancies and miscarriages and any previous history of infertility evaluations or treatments should be sought.

Table 2.11. Pertinent points to ascertain in the medical history

- Age
- Occupation
- Sexual history
- Developmental history
- Surgical history
- Medical history
- Drugs
- Social history
- Family history

Developmental history

Pertinent questions in the developmental history should include the age of puberty, with delayed onset or absent puberty suggesting an endocrine or androgen deficiency cause for infertility. Problems with gynaecomastia may suggest prolactin or oestrogen abnormalities.

A history of congenital anomalies of the genitourinary tract should also be sought. Patients presenting with congenital hypoplasia or total absence of the vas deferens and seminal vesicles will present with absence or low volume ejaculate and should be differentiated from those with retrograde or anejaculation. Congenital syndromes that affect the cilia such as Kartagener's syndrome may present with a history of sinusitis and bronchiectasis or chronic respiratory infections as occurs in cystic fibrosis and Young's syndrome.

Surgical history

A history of cryptorchidism has been shown to reduce fertility significantly and should be assessed in all men presenting with infertility. Previous pelvic or retroperitoneal surgery can lead to damage of both erectile and ejaculatory neurological pathways. At the time of hernia repair, the vas deferens may be damaged or devascularized. Testicular surgery may also lead to damage or testicular trauma and torsion can cause not only testicular atrophy but can lead to the production of antisperm antibodies (see below), which may be implicated in male factor infertility.

Medical history

A history should be sought of previous genitourinary infections and may include a history of recurrent urinary tract infections, orchitis, epididymitis, prostatitis or sexually transmitted diseases. Although a prepubertal episode of mumps does not affect fertility, postpubertal infection by the virus with associated orchitis increases the chance of male infertility. A history of a recent febrile illness may also be associated with an abnormal semen analysis, with impaired spermatogenesis occurring up to three months following a viral infection. Thus patients with such a history should undergo repeated semen analysis after three and six months to allow adequate time for spermatogenesis to recover.

Chronic medical conditions can also be the cause of infertility. Diseases such as diabetes mellitus and multiple sclerosis may cause both erectile and ejaculatory dysfunction. Patients with chronic renal disease may be infertile and have a higher incidence of erectile dysfunction. As previously mentioned, tumours of the pituitary gland can present with infertility and symptoms such as headaches, galactorrhea or impairment of the visual fields may be indicative of this.

Drug history

Many different drugs and chemicals can affect fertility, thus it is important to take a complete drug history including previous treatment with chemotherapeutic agents. A history of recreational drug taking is also important as drugs such as cocaine, marijuana, nicotine and caffeine can all affect spermatogenesis. Fertility can recover once these drugs are stopped.

The overuse of anabolic steroids can lead to hypogonadotrophic hypogonadism, which in most cases reverts once the drug has stopped, although the effects may be permanent.

Both smoking and alcohol has been shown to affect spermatogenesis.

Social history

The patient's occupation may be relevant for the cause of infertility. Pesticides can cause sterility, thus farm workers and workers at the factory of origin may be at particular risk. For normal spermatogenesis and motility the testicular temperature must remain below body temperature. Patients having regular hot baths or wearing tight underpants may present with abnormal semen analysis.

Family history

Patients with a family history of intersex may have androgen receptor abnormalities. Other disorders such as testicular atrophy, hypogonadism, cryptorchidism and midline defects can also be familial.

Examination

All patients should be fully examined and a note made of general body stature and the presence of secondary sexual characteristics, including the distribution of body and pubic hair. Any surgical scars should be also noted. The size of the testis can be measured with a Prader orchidometer although generally a testis that is less than 15 ml in volume is usually indicative of primary testicular failure. The vasa and epididymis are palpated making note of their presence and consistency. The epididymi may be full in cases of unilateral or bilateral ejaculatory duct obstruction or the vasa may be absent in congenital absence of the vas deferens. The presence of a varicocele should also be noted. All patients should undergo a rectal examination for signs of prostatitis.

Investigations

Clinical examination combined with empirical investigations such as semen analysis and hormonal assay will be diagnostic in the vast majority of patients. More complex

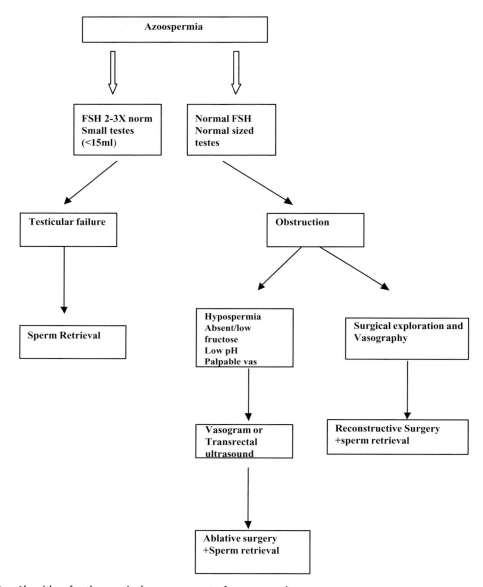

Figure 2.8.   Algorithm for the surgical management of azoospermia.

investigations can be specifically used to discern various aetiologies. Figure 2.8 is a useful algorithm for the investigation of azoospermia.

Laboratory tests

Semen analysis

This has been dealt with earlier in this chapter. The World Health Organization has established standard recommendations for normal values (Table 2.4). When giving semen samples for analysis patients should be provided with strict and comprehensive instructions on how to provide a sample. To maintain accuracy in the analysis of the semen, several samples need to be assessed. Ideally, each should be taken after a constant interval of sexual abstinence, eliminating changes in the quality of the sample. Semen may be collected by either masturbation or from a specifically designed condom. Ideally, analysis should be performed within the first hour of collection, to allow accurate estimation of viable spermatozoa.

More detailed semen analysis such as mixed antiglobulin reaction (MAR test) can be undertaken at the same time as the initial semen analysis. Basic seminal biochemistry such as fructose levels and pH measurement may be indicative of the aetiology of obstructive causes of azoospermia.

Detection of pyospermia

The association of infertility and genital infection has already been discussed. The presence of leukocytes in a concentration $>10^6$ per ml may be indicative of a genitourinary tract infection and the patient should be appropriately screened for a urinary tract infection (including prostatitis) or a sexually transmitted disease.

Hormonal assays

All patients presenting with azoospermia or oligozoospermia should have plasma levels of FSH, LH and serum testosterone determined, as hormonal assays are usually diagnostic in differentiating those with obstructive from non-obstructive causes of infertility. Evidence indicates that those men with an FSH level twice the normal range are more likely to have smaller testes and lower Johnsen mean scores on subsequent histology at testicular biopsy. Thus, in patients with primary testicular failure or hypergonadotrophic hypogonadism, there are usually elevated levels of FSH and LH with low or normal testosterone, associated with azoospermia and small testes. Therefore, these patients are likely to undergo assisted conception with intracytoplasmic sperm injection (ICSI) and an isolated diagnostic testicular biopsy is not indicated.

Likewise men with normal FSH, LH and testosterone and normal sized testes are more likely to have obstructive azoospermia and should undergo further evaluation with testicular exploration and vasography (see below). However, it is important to note that men with complete maturation arrest will also present with normal sized testes and normal LH/FSH levels. It is only at the time of scrotal exploration with a view to tubal reconstruction that a non-obstructed epididymis is found in these cases.

Hypogonadotrophic hypogonadism is characterized by low serum FSH, LH and testosterone levels. These patients should be referred to an endocrinologist for further investigations prior to commencing treatment of their infertility.

In patients with primary testicular failure inadequate Sertoli cell function reduces the production of inhibin. This reduction in inhibin levels alters the negative feedback pathway on the anterior pituitary gland and results in an increase in FSH levels in the presence of low or normal testosterone levels. It has been suggested that inhibin B may be used as a diagnostic marker in the differentiation of those patients with obstructive azoospermia and primary testicular failure. Patients with normal spermatogenesis have higher levels of inhibin compared to those with spermatogenic failure (Lee *et al.*, 2001).

Antisperm antibodies

These are present in the serum of 2% of fertile and 8–13% of infertile men. In the male, the blood–testis barrier normally prevents exposure of the sperm to antibodies in the immune system. A number of conditions can lead to disruption of the blood–testis barrier leading to the appearance of antibodies such as IgG and IgA in the serum, seminal plasma or bound to the spermatozoa.

Causes of antisperm antibodies

- Acquired or congenital ductal obstruction (unilateral or bilateral).
- Vasectomy.
- Testicular/epididymal infections.
- Testicular torsion/trauma.
- Cryptorchidism.
- Varicoceles.

Antisperm antibodies may not only appear in the serum of patients but may also be attached to the individual's spermatozoa. There is still some controversy regarding the importance of antibodies in the serum, with some investigators arguing that antibodies on the sperm themselves are more important as the cause of infertility.

Antisperm antibodies can lead to a number of effects on sperm function including abnormal cervical mucus penetration, premature acrosome reaction, and interference with fertilization. They may also be the cause of oligozoospermia/asthenozoospermia. Antisperm antibodies can be detected by a number of immunological assays and there appears to be a good correlation between individual tests. We routinely perform a MAR test and supplement this with the Kibrick test if positive. Also, it should be noted that antisperm antibodies might occur in the female partner.

Antisperm antibody tests

- Gelatin agglutination test (GAT).
- Tray agglutination test (TAT) – detects antibodies in patients serum or seminal plasma.

- The mixed antiglobulin reaction (MAR test) – detects antibodies on patients' spermatozoa.

Postcoital test (PCT)

For conception to occur, sperm must be able to penetrate the partner's cervical mucus. More than 10 motile sperm per high-power field should be observed in a sample of the partner's postcoital ovulatory mucus. A PCT is usually performed in those males with normal semen parameters who are unable to conceive. A normal semen analysis with a poor PCT is suggestive of the presence of anti-sperm antibodies and both the male and female partner should be evaluated for these. If an abnormal PCT is found, more complex in vitro cervical mucus interaction tests should be performed to further evaluate this. In patients with unexplained infertility, more complex in vitro sperm function tests, such as an acrosome reaction or sperm penetration tests (listed below), can be performed if fertilization is deemed to be the problem. These tests are described in more detail in Chapter 7.

Sperm penetration tests comprise:
- Computer assisted sperm analysis (CASA).
- Zone free hamster penetration test (HEPT).
- Zona binding test.
- Reactive oxygen species.

Chromosomal analysis

Overall, 4.6% of men with oligozoospermia and 13.7% with azoospermia will have an abnormality in karyotype. In men with azoospermia, sex chromosome abnormalities such as 47 XXY or mosaics of 46 XY/47XXX occur in up to 22.1%, whilst autosomal abnormalities are found in up to 3.7%. When performing such tests, patients must be counselled appropriately.

Transrectal ultrasonography (TRUS)

TRUS will allow direct visualization of the ejaculatory ducts and seminal vesicles to exclude ejaculatory duct obstruction and is indicated in those individuals with:
- Low semen volume – <1 ml.
- Acidic seminal plasma – pH <7.0.
- Azoospermia.
- Absent fructose.
- Palpable vas deferens.

Dilated ejaculatory ducts and seminal vesicles indicate obstruction on TRUS (Figure 2.9). In patients with congenital bilateral absence of the vas deferens (CBAVD), hypoplasia or absence of the seminal vesicles, TRUS will confirm the clinical findings of an absent vas deferens.

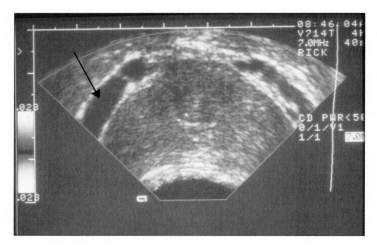

Figure 2.9.   Transrectal ultrasound scan (arrow points to a seminal vesicle).

Ultrasonography

With Doppler flow analysis may be performed to confirm the clinical diagnosis of a varicocele, and spermatic venous reflux may be detected in the absence of a clinical varicocele.

Testicular biopsy

As already discussed, an isolated testicular biopsy is no longer indicated to differentiate between an obstructive or non-obstructive aetiology for male infertility. Therefore, a testicular biopsy should only be performed in the context of a testicular exploration and sperm extraction (TESE) for assisted conception. For this reason biopsies should be performed only in a tertiary referral centre with appropriate facilities for sperm recovery, and cryostorage if the sperm is not being immediately used for ICSI. In non-obstructive azoospermia a testicular biopsy is usually undertaken prior to the woman embarking on IVF to ensure that sperm can be retrieved. The testicular tissue is cryopreserved and used subsequently for ICSI.

Vasography

Vasography is performed to exclude ductal obstruction and for this reason should be performed only in a centre equipped with facilities for microsurgery. Sperm retrieval should be performed at the time of any reconstructive procedure. Vasography is commonly indicated in those men with:
- Azoospermia.
- Normal sized testes.
- Normal FSH.

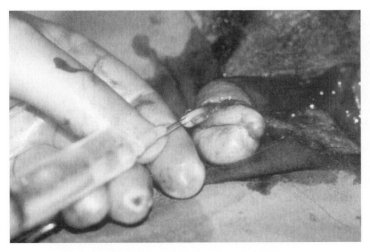

Figure 2.10. Technique of vasography (note the dilated epididymis).

Occasionally vasography is undertaken in those individuals who present with severe oligozoospermia in whom a unilateral obstruction is suspected.

Technique of vasography

Both testes are explored through either infra-pubic incision or bilateral scrotal incisions. The authors prefer to use an infra-pubic incision so both testes can be delivered and inspected at the same time and allow a definitive tension free reconstructive to be performed if required. On delivery of each testis the epididymis is inspected for signs of obstruction as indicated by macroscopic evidence of dilatation of the tubules within the head or tail of the epididymi.

A number of different techniques for vasography have been described, although the authors prefer to use fine needle vasography as, in our experience, it appears to be associated with fewer complications. Using a 25 G needle on a 10 ml syringe containing a 50% diluted solution of radio-contrast medium, such as urograffin, is injected into the lumen of the vas deferens at the junction of its straight and convoluted portion (Figure 2.10). An X-ray film is then performed (Figure 2.11). If an obstruction (Figure 2.12) is demonstrated at the level of the ejaculatory ducts either at the time of vasography or preoperative TRUS, methylene blue can be injected into both vasa facilitating subsequent transurethral resection of the ejaculatory ducts.

Management

The infertile male should be managed in a tertiary centre where appropriate facilities exist for microsurgery, assisted conception techniques and cryostorage of sperm.

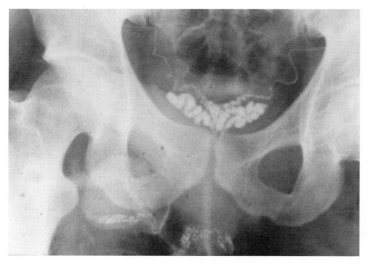

Figure 2.11. Normal vasogram.

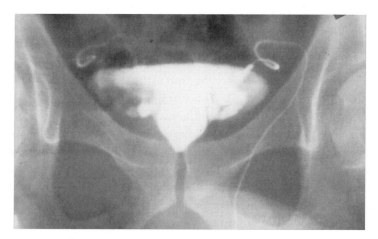

Figure 2.12. Vasogram demonstrating ejaculatory duct obstruction secondary to a Müllerian duct cyst.

In this context the uro-andrologist should work closely with other trained staff including a gynaecologist and embryologist with appropriate expertise.

Medical management

Endocrinopathies

The medical management of the infertile male is controversial, although men who present with hypogonadotrophic hypogonadism appear to respond the best and should be managed in a specialized endocrine unit. Treatment with human chorionic gonadotrophins (HCG) alone or HCG with human menopausal

Table 2.12. Drugs used in the treatment of male factor infertility

Class of drug	Drug
Anti-oestrogens	Tamoxifen/clomiphene
Androgens	Testosterone
Bromocriptine	
Kinin enhancing drugs	Kallikrein
Anti-oxidants	Vitamin E
Mast cell blockers	Tranilast
Alpha blockers	Bunazosin
Steroids	Medroxyprogesterone

gonadotrophins (HMG) is usually given three times per week. In a study of 21 men with hypogonadotrophic hypogonadism, serum testosterone increased in all, whilst sperm counts normalized in 13 (Finkel *et al.*, 1985). In a further study 24 men with isolated hypogonadotrophic hypogonadism, 22% achieved fertility during gonadotrophin treatment leading to a total of 40 pegnancies (Burris *et al.*, 1988).

The role for bromocriptine in the treatment of infertility secondary to hyper-prolactinaemia is unclear, although libido and potency will improve and levels of prolactin fall on treatment.

Infection of the genitourinary tract

Any urinary tract infections including prostatitis and epididymitis should be treated with appropriate antibiotics pending culture and sensitivity. However, there appears to be no evidence that pyospermia resolves with antibiotic treatment or that anti-biotics improve semen parameters in these patients.

Idiopathic infertility

Men with idiopathic oligozoospermia and/or asthenozoospermia have previously been treated with a number of agents, including anti-oestrogens, androgens and bromocriptine (Table 2.12), to improve semen quality. A recent meta-analysis indicates that whilst anti-oestrogens may improve sperm concentration and motility there is no significant increase in pregnancy rate following treatment (Vandekerckhove *et al.*, 1998). Similarly, the role of androgen treatment in the management of men with idiopathic oligozoospermia and/or asthenozoospermia remains controversial. However, a number of studies have suggested improvements in sperm parameters and in pregnancy rates for men with oligozoospermia and/or asthenozoospermia treated with drugs such as anti-oxidants, mast cell blockers and alpha blockers. However, further prospective randomized control trials are needed to evaluate the possible beneficial effects of these drugs. In view of this, the authors do not currently advocate the prescribing of these drugs for the treatment of idiopathic oligozoospermia and/or asthenozoospermia.

The role of steroids in the treatment of infertile men is also controversial. Although, studies have reported improved pregnancy rates for patients with anti-sperm antibodies treated with steroids such as methylprednisolone, trials have been largely uncontrolled and the benefits of treatment appear to be outweighed by the side effects of taking long-term steroids.

Ejaculatory failure

Men with retrograde ejaculation can be treated with ephedrine or imipramine with approximately one-third responding to treatment. Alternatively, sperm may be recovered from the urine and used for either intrauterine insemination (IUI) or IVF. In men with anorgasmia, electro-ejaculation may be combined with IUI or IVF. As a last resort sperm may be collected by microsurgical vasostomy and used for IUI or IVF.

Surgical management

The uro-andrologist will perform surgery on infertile men in situations of:
- Clinical varicocele associated with abnormal semen quality.
- Obstructive azoospermia (including ablative surgery for ejaculatory duct obstruction and reversal of vasectomy).
- Sperm retrieval in men with primary testicular failure or failure of surgical reconstruction.

Varicocele

The effects of varicocele and its surgical treatment on semen quality and a number of surgical approaches for the treatment of varicoceles have been described earlier.

The *scrotal* approach to a varicocele should no longer be practised. Not only are there multiple pampiniform veins at the level of the scrotum but the testicular artery has an intimate relationship with the plexus at this level and is more prone to damage.

Laparoscopic repair has been used in the treatment of varicoceles. Although attractive because it is a minimally invasive technique and allows direct visualization of the testicular artery, it has not gained popularity, probably because it requires specialized training in laparoscopic techniques.

The *Palomo* technique is a retroperitoneal approach to the spermatic vein at the level of the internal inguinal ring. The advantage of this technique is that at this proximal level only one or two spermatic veins are present and fewer veins need to be ligated compared to the inguinal approach.

In the *inguinal* approach for ligation of a varicocele, the inguinal canal is opened and all the external and internal spermatic veins and gubunacular branches are ligated. This means there is less chance of missing collateral vessels. More recently a microsurgical technique has been described in which all the spermatic veins are ligated. This technique is associated with a lower incidence of hydrocoele formation and varicocele recurrence.

Radiographic embolization is a technique requiring considerable expertise and is time consuming. Furthermore there is a potential for serious complications such as femoral vein perforation/thrombosis and pulmonary embolization occurring. Using a cut down technique over the femoral vein the internal spermatic vein is occluded with either a balloon or coil.

Complications of surgical varicocele repair

- Hydrocoele.
- Damage to testicular artery.
- Varicocele recurrence.

Transurethral resection of the ejaculatory ducts

The diagnosis of ejaculatory duct obstruction (partial or complete) is made either preoperatively in men undergoing TRUS with abnormal semen parameters and absent or low fructose in the presence of at least one palpable vas deferens, or perioperatively in men undergoing vasography. TRUS may be used to aspirate sperm from dilated ejaculatory ducts and seminal vesicles for cryopreservation or injection of contrast medium prior to performing ablative surgery. More commonly, the vasa are injected with methylene blue at the time of scrotal exploration and vasography performed prior to undertaking a transurethral resection of the ejaculatory ducts. Resection is carried out at the level of the verumontanum with the appearance of methylene blue confirming successful ablation. A post resection vasogram will confirm patency. In one study, patients with ejaculatory duct obstruction treated by transurethral resection there was an improvement in both semen parameters with good pregnancy rates (Paick *et al.*, 2000).

Complications of transurethral resection of the ejaculatory ducts

- Urinary reflux.
- Epididymitis.
- Retrograde ejaculation.

Surgical reconstruction for testicular obstruction

This procedure is performed under general anaesthesia with antimicrobial pro-phylaxis. The principles of surgical reconstruction for testicular obstruction are to ensure proximal patency and distal patency of the ductal system. At the same time as potential reconstructive surgery, the couple may wish to proceed with a cycle of ICSI with sperm retrieved at the time of surgery.

Proximal patency is indicated by obtaining sperm proximal to the obstruction either from the vas deferens or the epididymis on a wet preparation. Distal patency will have been confirmed by vasography. At the time of attempted reconstruction it may become obvious that the results of surgery will be poor, particularly in cases of caput epididymal blocks or failure to obtain sperm proximally. In these cases sperm retrieval must be performed for cryopreservation. A number of different techniques have been described for tubule reconstruction, although the principles for each remain much the same:

- General
  A dedicated unit with modern facilities – including operating microscope and microsurgical instruments and trained microsurgeon with ancillary staff.
  Facilities available for sperm retrieval, assisted conception techniques and cryo-preservation of sperm.
- Specific
  Ensure distal patency – vasography.
  Ensure proximal patency – sperm on wet preparation.
  Tension free/leak proof anastomosis.
  Good anastomotic technique.

Vaso-vasostomy

Indications

- Reversal of vasectomy.
- Isolated vasal blockages – iatrogenic, e.g. hernia repair; infective, e.g. *Neisseria*, gonorrhoea, tuberculosis.

The commonest indication for a vaso-vasostomy is for reversal of vasectomy and perioperative vasography is not performed in these cases. Vaso-vasostomy can be performed either side to side or end to end (Figure 2.13a, b, c), with either a microsurgical two-layered closure or anastomosing the mucosa and adventitia of the vas deferens, with 10/0 and 8/0 non-absorbable sutures respectively. Alternatively, the anastomosis can be performed macroscopically with a single layered side-to-side anastomosis using 6/0 prolene. If the vasal gap is particularly large the convoluted vas deferens may be mobilized to gain additional length.

Vaso-epididymostomy (VE)

Indications

- Obstruction of the epididymis with distal patency.
- Reversal of vasectomy.

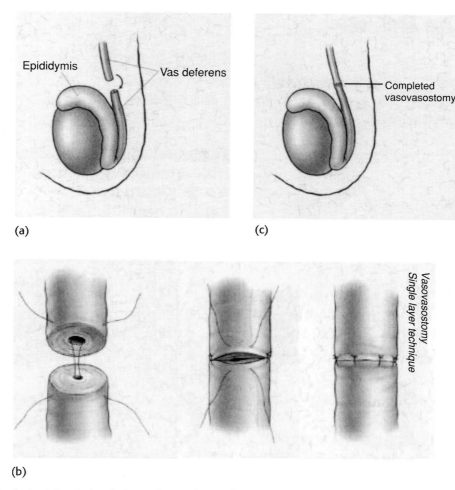

Figure 2.13. (a, b, c) Surgical technique of an end-to-end vaso-vasostomy.

At the time of surgical exploration the epididymis may be seen to consist of dilated tubules. The lowest portion of the dilated tubules is incised and the vas deferens is anastomosed to the epididymis. This can be performed either end to end (Figure 2.14a, b, c) or end to side. An end-to-end VE is preferably performed for caudal blocks or for vasectomy reversal, where vasal length may be short and the epididymis is obstructed distally. The end to side VE is used for proximal obstructions. In both techniques a two-layered anastomosis is performed using a non-absorbable suture. At the same time as performing a VE, a micro-epididymal sperm aspiration (MESA) should be performed to allow sperm to be stored for any future IVF.

Trans-vasovasostomy

This is rarely indicated and only performed in two circumstances:

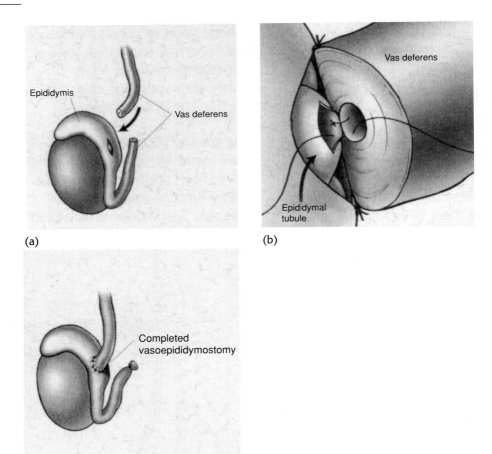

(a)   (b)

(c)

Figure 2.14. (a, b, c) Surgical technique of a vasoepididymo-vasostomy.

- Unilateral inguinal obstruction with an atrophic contralateral testis.
- Unilateral obstruction/aplasia of the vas or ejaculatory duct obstruction with contralateral epididymal obstruction.

Complications of surgery

Early
- Haematoma.
- Wound infection.

Late
- Sperm granuloma.
- Stricture.

Table 2.13. Results of reconstructive surgery for testicular obstruction

Anastomosis	*n*	Patency (%)	Pregnancy (%)
Epididymovasostomy (caput)	90	12	3
Epididymovasostomy (cauda)	60	52	38
Post infective vasal blocks	11	73	27
Trans-vasovasostomy	11	9	0
Vasectomy reversal	130	90	45

Source: Hendry *et al.* (1990).

Results of reconstructive surgery

The results of reconstructive surgery have been reported by Hendry *et al.* (1990) in a large series of patients. In this series the best results were obtained in men undergoing reversal of vasectomy (Table 2.13). Men with caputal blocks did particularly poorly, with three-quarters of this group having Young's syndrome. Of 11 men undergoing trans-vasovasostomy, patency was achieved in nine, but with no resulting pregnancies.

Sperm retrieval techniques (PESA/MESA/TESA/TESE)

Prior to the development of assisted conception techniques, CBAVD was an untreatable condition. However, now pregnancies are possible using epididymal sperm obtained during percutaneous epididymal sperm aspiration (PESA) and ICSI treatment. In fact in one study PESA was successful in 89% and pregnancy rates of 36% were achieved in patients with CBAVD (Meniru *et al.*, 1997).

Even men with severe testicular failure may achieve paternity. In all the methods of sperm extraction described below, sperm retrieval may be performed at the time of an IVF cycle or cryopreserved for future use.

The indications for sperm retrieval in the infertile male include:

- CBAVD.
- Sperm storage – at vasectomy reversal or as a definitive procedure for azoospermia following vasectomy.
- At the time of surgical reconstruction for obstructive azoospermia.
- Definitive treatment for testicular failure.

Percutaneous epididymal aspiration of sperm (PESA)

Indications:

- CBAVD or in men who do not wish to undergo reversal of vasectomy.
- Obstructive azoospermia.
- Reconstruction not possible.

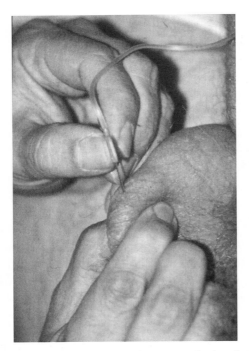

Figure 2.15. Percutaneous epididymal sperm aspiration (PESA).

Technique

With the patient lying supine, a high spermatic cord block is performed by infiltrating the spermatic cord and surrounding skin with local anaesthetic. A 21 G butterfly is then passed into the superior pole of the epididymis, whilst an assistant aspirates a 10 ml syringe containing sperm buffer and connected to the butterfly (Figure 2.15).

PESA is associated with very few complications and appears to be well tolerated.

Micro-epididymal sperm aspiration (MESA)

The main reason for performing MESA is intra-operative sperm retrieval at the time of reconstructive surgery. Using an operating microscope an incision is made over a dilated epididymal tubule and sperm can be aspirated using either a micropipette or a plastic cannula attached to a 2 ml syringe. Gentle squeezing of the testicle and epididymis may enhance sperm retrieval from the incision in the epididymis (Figure 2.16).

Testicular sperm retrieval

Indications:
- Failure to retrieve sperm using epididymal aspiration.
- Men with testicular failure

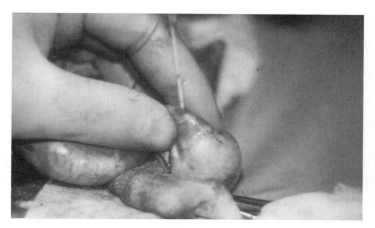

Figure 2.16. Micro-epididymal sperm aspiration (MESA).

Techniques of testicular sperm retrieval

- Percutaneous aspiration.
- Percutaneous biopsy.
- Open testis biopsy.

Testicular sperm can be retrieved using three different techniques. We do not routinely use percutaneous aspiration for harvesting sperm. If used, this technique is best for men who have normal spermatogenesis, such as men with obstructive azoospermia. Furthermore, this method of testicular sperm retrieval has been demonstrated to be inferior compared to more conventional open techniques (Ezeh *et al.*, 1998). A 21G needle is passed percutaneously into the testis and sperm can be retrieved by aspiration, which can be used for ICSI. Alternatively, a percutaneous testicular biopsy may be used to retrieve sperm. This is performed under local anaesthetic using a size 16G trucut biopsy needle. The authors use this technique only in those cases where PESA has been unsuccessful.

Testicular exploration and sperm extraction (TESE) is currently used therapeutically to retrieve sperm from men who have abnormal spermatogenesis and wish to proceed to ICSI. Alternatively, TESE is offered to men who have obstructive azoospermia and in whom sperm retrieval has failed by MESA/PESA or testicular exploration and sperm aspiration (TESA). TESE can be performed under general or local anaesthesia at the same time as an IVF cycle, or sperm may be frozen for future IVF (Figure 2.17).

Overall, sperm retrieval success rates are in the order of 50%, although rates may be improved by testicular mapping where multiple (sextant biopsies) are performed (Altay *et al.*, 2001). Recently, the technique of microdissection, whereby individual tubules are identified microscopically has been shown to improve the results of sperm retrieval in men with non-obstructive azoospermia (Schlegel, 1999). However, TESE is not without complications and it has been shown that biopsy will

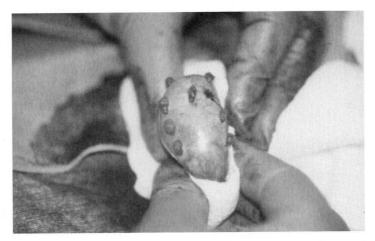

Figure 2.17. Sperm extraction (by testicular exploration and sperm extraction – TESE) for freezing.

reduce the seminiferous tubule volume adjacent to the testicular biopsy site, thus compromising future attempts at sperm extraction (Tash & Schlegel, 2001). Furthermore, TESE results in significant inflammation and haematoma at the biopsy site and repeat TESE is more likely to retrieve sperm if the second attempt is made six months after the first (Schlegel & Su, 1997). Finally serum testosterone levels may fall significantly after TESE.

Results of sperm retrieval rates in the infertile male

The results of sperm retrieval in the male depend upon the technique used and the underlying aetiology. Overall sperm retrieval rates and outcome are higher in cases of obstructive compared to non-obstructive azoospermia. There appears to be no difference in fertilization or pregnancy rates using epididymal or testicular sperm for ICSI, although this remains controversial. The most successful combination for sperm retrieval and assisted conception techniques appears to be the combination of MESA and ICSI, with fertilization and pregnancy rates as high as 45% and 56% respectively. Overall there also appears to be no difference in fertilization rate or pregnancy rates with ICSI between cryopreserved or fresh spermatozoa. Table 2.14 summarizes the most recent results from the University College Hospital Assisted Conception Unit.

Summary

- The introduction and development of assisted conception techniques has revolutionized the management of male factor infertility. For this reason the sub-fertile male should be managed in a tertiary referral unit with close liaison between

Table 2.14. Summary of the combined results of sperm retrieval (MESA/PESA/TESE) with IVF/ICSI. Assisted conception unit, University College Hospital London between 01/01/2000 and 28/02/2001

Number of treatment cycles	76
Number of patients	67
Average age of patient at treatment	33.64
Number of cancelled cycles	1 (1.32%)
Number of oocyte retrievals	75 (98.68%)
Fertilization rate	71.37%
Number of embryo transfers	73 (96.05%)
Average number of oocytes retrieved	10.48
Average number of embryos transferred	2.92
Cycles with one embryo transferred	0
Cycles with two embryos transferred	8
Cycles with three or more embryos transferred	63
Total number of embryos transferred	205
Total number of pregnancies	35
Pregnancy rate per cycle	46.05%
Pregnancy rate per oocyte retrieval	46.67%
Pregnancy rate per embryo transfer	47.95%
Implantation rate	24.39%
Total number of live births	33
Live birth rate per cycle	43.42%
Live birth rate per oocyte retrieval	44.00%
Live birth rate per embryo transfer	45.21%

a multiprofessional team, including a uro-andrologist who has been trained in microsurgery.

- The aetiology of male factor infertility should be readily diagnosed in the majority of men by clinical examination, semen analysis and endocrine tests.
- There is no role for the isolated testicular biopsy for diagnosis of male factor infertility.
- Drug treatment for idiopathic infertility remains controversial. However, in hypogonadotrophic hypogonadism drug treatment can be successful.
- Reconstructive surgery in men with obstructive azoospermia and varicocele ligation in men with astheno/oligozoospermia offer effective treatment with improved postoperative pregnancy rates.
- Even in men with testicular failure, sperm retrieval combined with assisted conception techniques offers a good chance of paternity.

REFERENCES

Altay, B., Hekimgil, M., Cikili, N., Turna, B. & Soydan, S. (2001). Histopathological mapping of open testicular biopsies in patients with unobstructive azoospermia. *Br. J. Urol. Int.* **87**(9): 834–7.

Burris, A. S., Rodbard, H. W., Winters, S. J. & Sherins, R. J. (1988). Gonadotropin therapy in men with isolated hypogonadotropic hypogonadism: the response to human chorionic gonadotropin is predicted by initial testicular size. *J. Clin. Endocrinol. Metab.* **66**: 1144–51.

Ezeh, U. I., Moore, H. D. & Cooke, I. D. (1998). A prospective study of multiple needle biopsies versus a single open biopsy for testicular sperm extraction in men with non-obstructive azoospermia. *Hum. Reprod.* **13**(11): 3075–80.

Finkel, D. M., Phillips, J. L. & Snyder, P. J. (1985). Stimulation of spermatogenesis by gonadotropins in men with hypogonadotropic hypogoadism. *New Engl. J. Med.* **313**: 651–5.

Hendry, W. F., Kirby, R. S. & Duckett, J. W. (Eds) (1998). *Textbook of Genito-Urinary Surgery*, vol. 2, 2nd edn. Oxford: Blackwell Sciences Ltd.

Hendry, W. F., Levison, D. A., Parkinson, M. C., Parslow, J. M. & Royale, M. G. (1990). Testicular obstruction: clinicopathological studies. *Ann. Roy. Coll. Surg. Engl.* **72**: 396–407.

Lee, P. A., Coughlin, M. T. & Bellinger, M. F. (2001). Inhibin B: comparison with indexes of fertility among formerly cryptorchid and control men. *J. Clin. Endocrinol. Metab.* **86**(6): 2546–84.

Meniru, G. I., Gorgy, A., Podsiadly, B. T. & Craft, I. L. (1997). Results of percutaneous epididymal sperm aspiration and intracytoplasmic sperm injection in two major groups of patients with obstructive azoospermia. *Hum. Reprod.* **12**(11): 2443–6.

Paick, J., Kim, S. H. & Kim, S. W. (2000). Ejaculatory duct obstruction in infertile men. *Br. J. Urol.* **85**(6): 720–4.

Pryor, J. P. & Hendry, W. F. (1991). Ejaculatory duct obstruction in subfertile males: analysis of 87 patients. *Fertil. Steril.* **56**: 725–30.

Schlegel, P. N. (1999). Testicular sperm extraction: microdissection improves sperm yield with minimal tissue excision. *Hum. Reprod.* **14**(1): 131–5.

Schlegel, P. N. & Su, L. M. (1997). Physiological consequences of testicular sperm extraction. *Hum. Reprod.* **12**(8): 1688–92.

Tash, J. A. & Schlegel, P. N. (2001). Histologic effects of testicular sperm extraction on the testicle of men with non-obstructive azoospermia. *Urology* **57**(2): 334–7.

Vandekerckhove, P., Lilford, R. & Hughes, E. (1998). The medical treatment of idiopathic oligo/asthenospermia: anti-oestrogens versus placebo or no treatment (Cochrane Review). In *The Cochrane Library*, Issue 2. Oxford: Update Software.

3

Laboratory assessment of the infertile man

R. John Aitken

ARC Centre of Excellence in Biotechnology and Development, University of Newcastle, New South Wales, Australia

Semen analysis

Approximately one in four male patients attending infertility clinics possess an overt defect in their semen profile (Hull *et al.*, 1985).

The paucity of human semen quality sets us apart from most, if not all, other mammalian species. Even in normal fertile men a majority of the spermatozoa may exhibit abnormalities in their morphology and motility.

The first step in the laboratory assessment of male fertility is to create a traditional semen profile according to the criteria set out in the World Health Organization's laboratory manual for the examination of human semen and sperm–cervical interaction (World Health Organization, 1999). This analysis consists of a preliminary macroscopic examination of the semen followed by a detailed microscopic assessment of the cellular components of the ejaculate (Figure 3.1).

Macroscopic inspection

The initial macroscopic investigation of semen should take account of the volume of the ejaculate, the completeness of liquefaction viscosity, odour, colour, and the presence of blood, gelatinous bodies and mucous streaks. Contamination with urine, as may happen with patients exhibiting disturbances of bladder neck function, results in a yellow discoloration of the sample. Yellow discoloration of the semen is also common in jaundiced patients.

The consistency of the semen, also known as viscosity, refers to the fluid nature of the entire sample (Figure 3.2). Highly viscous samples are difficult to analyse and are associated with infertility since the migration of the spermatozoa into cervical mucus is impaired.

Particular attention should also be paid to the liquefaction status of the semen. Under normal circumstances a human semen sample should coagulate on

Good Clinical Practice in Assisted Reproduction, ed. P. Serhal & C. Overton.
Published by Cambridge University Press. © Cambridge University Press 2004.

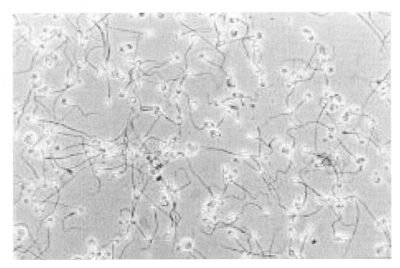

Figure 3.1.   Typical human ejaculate, showing a high incidence of spermatozoa with defective morphology.

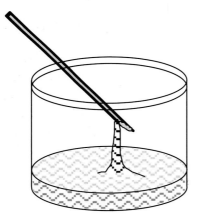

Figure 3.2.   High viscosity samples are examined by immersing the tip of a 1 ml plastic pipette or glass rod in the semen sample and raising it >2 cm from the surface. The formation of a thread indicates the existence of a viscous sample.

ejaculation and then liquefy within 5–15 minutes at room temperature. If liquefaction fails to occur, subsequent microscopic assessment of the spermatozoa will be extremely difficult and the fertility of the sample will be compromised.

Poor liquefaction results in a heterogeneous ejaculate consisting of gelatinous material in a fluid base. Exposure of the sample to bromelain, a mixture of cysteine proteases from pineapple stems, can be used to induce complete liquefaction and facilitate the subsequent microscopic examination of the semen.

Microscopic examination

The microscopic examination of human semen is normally done with the aid of a phase contrast microscope. The purpose of the microscopic semen profile is to give an overall indication of the quality of the ejaculate on the basis of sperm number motility and morphology. As a diagnostic technique it is often poorly understood and badly interpreted.

The semen profile is meant to give an indication of the underlying quality of the spermatogenic process. If low numbers of poorly motile, malformed spermatozoa are present in the ejaculate, it suggests that spermatogenesis is defective and that even the apparently normal cells in the ejaculate are dysfunctional.

Although the semen profile places emphasis on the number of morphologically normal, motile spermatozoa in the ejaculate, this should not be interpreted to mean that fertility is a question of sperm number. Normal men rendered oligo-zoospermic by exogenous steroid treatment may be fertile even though they have sperm counts well within the infertile range, i.e. less than 5×10^6/ml (Wallace *et al.*, 1992). However, such cases differ from the infertile patient population in that while sperm counts are low, the spermatozoa that are present in the ejaculate are normal.

Thus the semen profile is an indirect way of revealing the fundamental normality of spermatogenesis. While thresholds for gauging the normality of a semen profile have been developed and formalized by the World Health Organization (1999), the values given are only an approximate guide. Recent studies have revealed significant regional variation in semen quality. As a consequence, it will be important for individual clinics to establish their own thresholds of normality based upon analyses of the local fertile population. Table 3.1 shows the values suggested by the World Health Organization. According to this Table a man can be considered normal if

Table 3.1. World Health Organization (1999) criteria for normal semen quality

Criterion	Value
Volume	>2 ml
pH	>7.2
Sperm concentration	$>20 \times 10^6$/ml
Total sperm number	$>40 \times 10^6$
Motility	>50% with space-gaining motility or >25% with rapid progressive motility within 60 minutes of ejaculation
Morphology	>15% normal forms

his ejaculate contains more than 40 million spermatozoa, with 50% motility and at least 15% normal morphology.

Leukocytes

Spermatozoa are not the only cellular constituents of human semen. Every human semen sample is contaminated with leukocytes. On average 30 000 leukocytes/ml are found in normal human semen samples, the predominant cell type being the polymorph. The threshold for pathological leukocytic infiltration of the ejaculate (leukocytospermia) has been set at 1×10^6 white cells/ml (World Health Organization, 1999). These cells are powerful generators of toxic oxygen metabolites and may be damaging to the spermatozoa. Post ejaculation, the latter are protected by the powerful antioxidants that are present in seminal plasma. However, as soon as the seminal plasma is removed (e.g. during the preparation of spermatozoa for IVF therapy) then the leukocytes can inflict considerable damage on the spermatozoa affecting both the integrity of sperm DNA and the fertilizing potential of these cells (Twigg *et al.*, 1998b).

Leukocytes can be accurately detected by immunocytochemistry using a monoclonal antibody against CD45 (Figure 3.3), the common leukocyte antigen. This method detects all leukocyte species including lymphocytes, macrophages and polymorphonuclear leukocytes. More specific detection of the latter can be achieved using histochemical methods based on the presence of peroxidase activity in the

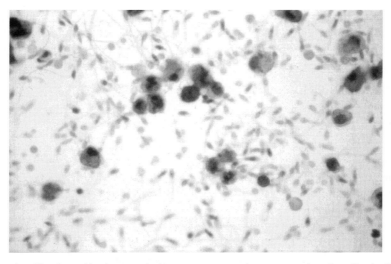

Figure 3.3.   Identification of leukocytes in human semen using a monoclonal antibody directed against CD45 – *the common leukocyte antigen.* Leukocytospermia is considered significant if the white cell count exceeds 1×10^6/ml.

secretory granules. The protocol recommended by the World Health Organization (1999) uses orthotoluidine blue as the peroxidase substrate – with this reagent granulocytes stain brown.

Leukocytes may inflict damage directly on spermatozoa by virtue of their ability to produce cytotoxic cytokines and reactive oxygen species. Alternatively the presence of these cells may disrupt fertility by virtue of the damage they induce in the male secondary sexual glands such as the seminal vesicles (Gonzales *et al.*, 1992). Clearly persistent leukocytospermia should be followed up by attempts to culture the causative organism and initiation of the appropriate antibiotic therapy. It should be noted, however, that the leukocytospermic condition shows a strong tendency for spontaneous resolution, in the absence of therapeutic intervention.

Semen profile

The conventional semen profile consists of an analysis of sperm count, motility and morphology in the unfractionated ejaculate. Sperm count and percentage motility are relatively straightforward criteria to assess using protocols set out in the World Health Organization handbook (1999). The most contentious criterion is morphology because its assessment is largely subjective. The value given for percentage normal morphology will depend heavily upon the definition of normality. Since the morphological attributes of a normal spermatozoon (i.e. a sperm capable of fertilization) are not known, the criteria used to define 'normality' are innately variable and inevitably arbitrary. In this context it may be helpful to generate a population of selected 'normal' spermatozoa by recovering cells bound to the surface of the zona pellucida or following migration through a column of cervical mucus (World Health Organization, 1999; Figure 3.4). The trend in recent years has been to adopt

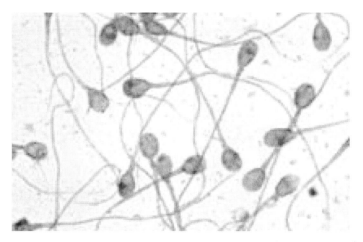

Figure 3.4.   A group of morphologically normal human spermatozoa.

stricter criteria for assessing sperm morphology with the result that the threshold of normality has shifted from 50% in 1987 (World Health Organization 1987) to 15% in 1999 (World Health Organization, 1999).

Computer aided sperm analysis (CASA)

Motility is generally described in terms of the percentage of spermatozoa exhibiting space-gaining motility. The introduction of CASA systems has allowed detailed quantitative analysis of sperm motility to be undertaken that are characterized by high precision (Figure 3.5). The kinematic measurements of greatest significance include the curvilinear and progressive velocity of the cells and the amplitude of lateral sperm head displacement. An adequate progressive velocity and amplitude of lateral sperm head displacement are both essential for the effective penetration of cervical mucus (Feneux *et al.*, 1985; Aitken *et al.*, 1986; Mortimer *et al.*, 1986).

The use of CASA systems also permits the rapid and accurate identification of physiologically important patterns of movement, particularly hyperactivation. The rate at which spermatozoa hyperactivate is highly correlated with fertilization rates in vitro. Sets of validated criteria for the rapid, accurate assessment of forwardly progressive and hyperactivated human spematozoa are given in Table 3.2.

Using the movement characteristics of human spermatozoa, the outcome of in vitro fertilization procedures has been predicted with great accuracy. For example, data describing the incidence of hyperactivated motility after three hours incubation, and the ability of the spermatozoa to exhibit forward progressive motility after 24 hours, could be used to predict whether fertilization rates would be above or below 50%, with 92% accuracy (Sukcharoen *et al.*, 1995).

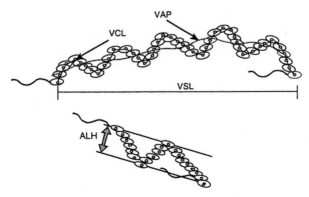

Figure 3.5.   Key attributes of movement defined by computer aided sperm analysis systems. VCL: curvilinear velocity (total distance travelled by the sperm head in Unit time); VAP: average path velocity (5-point average path followed by sperm head in unit time); VSL: straight line velocity (straight line distance travelled by the sperm head in unit time); ALH: Amplitude of lateral sperm head displacement (average lateral movement of sperm head).

Table 3.2. Criteria for automatically categorizing
spermatozoa as forward progressive or hyperactivated

Forward progressive	Hyperactivation
ALH <7 μm	VCL >90 μm/sec
Dancemean <21 μm	LIN <20%
	Dancemean >45.8 μm

Note: ALH: amplitude of lateral sperm head displacement;
VCL: curvilinear velocity;
LIN: linearity;
Dancemean: (ALH/LIN) × 100 μm.
Source: Sukcharoen *et al.*, 1995.

Sperm viability

Assessments of sperm viability are occasionally helpful, particularly where sperm motility is seriously compromised and it is important to determine whether the lack of motion is secondary to cell death or due to a specific flagellar defect. The hypo-osmotic swelling test is a simple means of assessing cell viability. Spermatozoa are exposed to hypo-osmotic conditions and if the plasma membrane is intact and compliant, water will enter the cell and the latter will swell. The increase in intracellular volume allows the sperm tail to curl (white arrows, Figure 3.6)

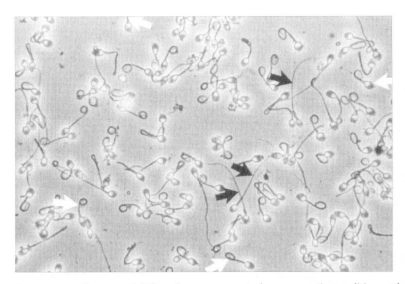

Figure 3.6.   Assessment of sperm viability after exposure to hypo-osmotic conditions. The increase in intracellular volume allows the sperm tail to curl (white arrow), but damaged cells remain with straight tails (black arrows).

whereas cells with damaged plasma membranes possess straight tails (black arrows, Figure 3.6).

Cervical mucus penetration

Cervical mucus is undoubtedly one of the most severe barriers that spermatozoa have to traverse on their route to the site of fertilization in vivo. Moreover, failures of sperm–cervical mucus interaction are clearly responsible for human infertility, largely because of defects on the part of the spermatozoa.

The quality of cervical mucus is assessed according to spinnbarkeit, ferning (crystallization), consistency and pH (Figure 3.7). A scoring protocol has been recommended by the World Health Organization (1999) that gives a maximum cervical mucus quality score of 15. Values above 10 are considered satisfactory for mid-cycle cervical mucus. Conversely, a score below 10 suggests that the quality of the mucus does not favour sperm penetration. A summary of the scoring system proposed by the World Health Organization is presented in Table 3.3. Most of the criteria are self evident and refer to the volume, viscosity, spinnbarkeit formation and cellular contamination. Ferning is described in terms of the level of branching: the primary axis branching once, twice or three times to give secondary, tertiary and quarternary stems. Note that mucus pH is not part of the scoring system, however it should be assessed as an important determinant of sperm–cervical mucus interaction (World Health Organization, 1999).

The quality of the cervical mucus is a critical part of the assessment of the *post coital test* (PCT). This in vivo assay for the effectiveness of sperm–cervical mucus

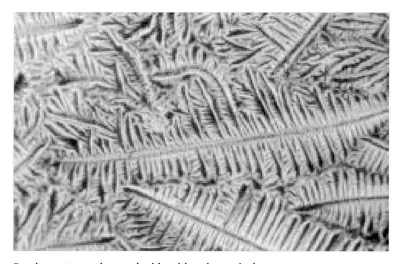

Figure 3.7.   Ferning pattern observed with mid-cycle cervical mucus.

Table 3.3. Cervical mucus scoring system

Criterion	Score
Volume	0 = 0 ml
	1 = 0.1 ml
	2 = 0.2 ml
	3 = 0.3 ml or more
Consistency	0 = thick viscous
(subjective measure of relative	1 = intermediate
viscosity)	2 = mild
	3 = watery
Ferning	0 = no crystallization
(descriptive assessment of	1 = atypical ferning
crystallization on drying)	2 = 1° and 2° ferning
	3 = 3° and 4° ferning
Spinnbarkeit	0 = <1 cm
(length of thread that forms when	1 = 1–4 cm
cervical mucus on a microscope	2 = 5–8 cm
slide is touched by a cover slip	3 = >9 cm
that is then lifted gently)	
Cellularity	0 = >1000 cells/mm^2
	1 = 501–1000 cells/mm^2
	2 = 1–500 cells/mm^2
	3 = 0 cells

interaction that can give valuable prognostic information providing the conditions under which the assay is conducted are carefully controlled. The PCT is a particularly effective predictor of conception where defined female causes of infertility are absent and the duration of infertility is less than three years. Once infertility is prolonged beyond three years, the conception rate is low even with a positive test because a large proportion of couples remaining childless after this period of time have other, unexplained causes for their infertility (Glazener *et al.*, 2000).

The PCT should be conducted as close as possible to the time of ovulation as predicted by cycle length, basal body temperature record, cervical mucus quality and, if available, serum and urinary oestrogen assays and/or ovarian ultrasound scans. The couples should abstain from intercourse for at least two days prior to the test and intercourse should take place the night before the day of analysis. The test involves the aspiration of mucus from the endocervical canal that is then subjected to a microscopic examination for the presence of spermatozoa exhibiting rapid progressive motility. The presence of such cells is indicative of a positive test. Given the many uncontrolled variables associated with the application of this test, it is essential that negative results are repeated. If negative results are consistently found at the optimal stage of the cycle, then cervical hostility or inadequate sperm motility are indicated.

Inadequacies on the part of the spermatozoa can be readily diagnosed using in vitro cervical mucus penetration assays (Figure 3.8). With such methods it is possible to determine with some accuracy the ability of human spermatozoa to penetrate the cervical barrier. Quite specific deficiencies in the movement characteristics of human spermatozoa, such as a low beat amplitude, can lead to a reduction in their ability to penetrate the cervical barrier. Moreover in vitro cervical mucus penetration assays correlate very well with the ultimate ability of human spematozoa to fertilize oocytes in vivo and in vitro. The major problem with in vitro cervical mucus penetration assays is that they depend upon a source of human cervical mucus. This difficulty can be overcome by the use of surrogate media for the penetration assay including bovine cervical mucus and hyaluronate polymers (Aitken et al., 1992).

A method for studying sperm–cervical mucus interaction when the latter is not available in significant quantities is the Sperm–Cervical Mucus Contact test (Figure 3.9). With this assay a drop of cervical mucus is compressed to a depth of 100 μm beneath a cover slide and semen is introduced on either side of the mucus sample. Microscopic examination of this preparation after 30 minutes incubation at 37 °C should reveal the presence of finger-like projections of seminal fluid (phalanges) penetrating into the mucus. Spermatozoa enter the mucus via these phalangeal canals and then fan out and move at random. Penetration of motile spermatozoa deep into the body of the mucus is indicative of a normal sample. Failure of sperm penetration into the mucus or penetration less than 500 μm from the interface is indicative of a poor or negative result. Sperm penetration into the mucus followed by the development of the 'shaking' phenomenon – vigorous agitated movement of spermatozoa trapped in the cervical mucus matrix – is indicative of the presence of antisperm antibodies of the IgA class.

Antisperm antibodies

Up to 10% of cases of male infertility may be associated with the presence of antisperm antibodies. Spermatozoa contain many potential powerful antigens and are generated by the testes long after immunological tolerance has been established. For a variety of reasons including trauma and reproductive tract infections, men may become autoimmunized against their own sperm antigens. These antibodies are predominantly of the IgG or IgA classes. IgG antibodies can fix complement and are responsible for the sperm immobilizing activity found in the sera and cervical

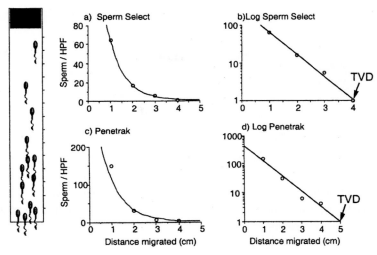

Figure 3.8.   Analysis of sperm–cervical mucus interaction in vitro. Mucus (Penetrak) or hyaluronic acid polymer (Sperm Select) are loaded into capillary tubes and sealed at one end. The open end is then inserted into a reservoir of semen. Following incubation, the number of spermatozoa are counted at regular intervals along the tube. Similar patterns of migration are observed whether hyaluronate (a, b) or bovine cervical mucus (c, d) is used as the penetration medium. Log transformation of the penetration data allows forward extrapolation of the regression line to the point where the number of spermatozoa reaches zero (the Theoretical Vanguard Distance – TVD). This is a robust measure of sperm–cervical mucus interaction that correlates with the functional competence of the spermatozoa.

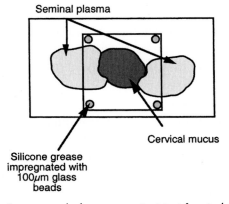

Figure 3.9.   Sperm–cervical mucus contact test for studying the interaction between spermatozoa and cervical mucus.

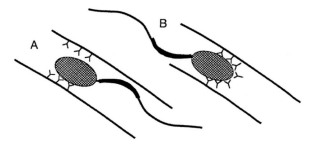

Figure 3.10. Antisperm antibodies and cervical mucus penetration. IgA antisperm antibodies generated by the female (A) or male (B) tracts bind to cervical mucin chains through their Fc region. This interaction impedes the migration of spermatozoa through cervical mucus and is frequently associated with the appearance of the 'shaking' phenomenon as the sperm struggle to disentangle themselves.

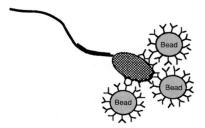

Figure 3.11. Immunobeads (not to scale), coated with antibodies against different human immunoglobulin classes, are incubated with spermatozoa and bind to sites where immunoglobulins are located.

mucus of many isoimmunized women, particularly in Japan (Hjort & Hargreave, 1994). In men, antisperm antibodies of the IgA class seem to be particularly important. The adhesion of such antibodies to the sperm surface impedes the ability of human spermatozoa to penetrate the cervical barrier (Figure 3.10). In addition antisperm antibodies directed against the sperm head can disrupt some of the key cell–cell recognition events involved in fertilization.

Assessment of antisperm antibodies in semen is most conveniently performed with immunobeads – polyacrylamide spheres with covalently bound rabbit antihuman immunoglobulins on their surface (Figure 3.11). With such beads the presence, immunoglobulin class and localization of antisperm antibodies can be determined. The test involves washing spermatozoa free of seminal plasma and then incubating them in a suspension of immunobeads. Spermatozoa with antisperm antibodies on their surface will bind the beads and the percentage of motile, antibody-positive cells can be determined. Since sperm penetration into cervical mucus and in vitro fertilization are not suppressed until more than 50% of the cells are antibody

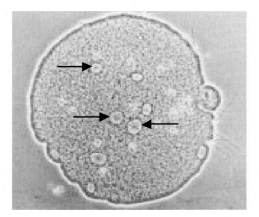

Figure 3.12. Sperm–oocyte fusion as measured by the hamster oocyte assay. Spermatozoa that have fused with the oocyte are characterized by decondensing sperm heads (arrowed).

positive, at least half of the spermatozoa must bind the immunobeads for this test to be considered positive positive (World Health Organization, 1999).

Hamster oocyte pentration assay

The ability of acrosome reacted human spermatozoa to fuse with the vitelline membrane of the oocyte can be assessed by the hamster oocyte penetraton assay (Figure 3.12). The ultrastructural details of sperm–oocyte fusion in this heterologous system are faithful to the homologous situation and the outcome of this is significantly correlated with fertilization in vivo and in vitro (Aitken, 1986, 1994). The assay is complex and difficult to standardize. It probably has more value as a research tool than as a routine method of assessment.

Biochemical assays

The development of simple, biochemical tests of sperm function would obviate the need to use such complex bioassays as the hamster oocyte penetration test. Examples of biochemical parameters that have been used to assess human sperm function include lactic acid dehydrogenase, creatine kinase, superoxide dismutase and glucose-6-phosphate dehydrogenase, all of which are elevated in the ejaculates of infertile men (Huszar *et al.*, 1988; Casano *et al.*, 1991; Aitken *et al.*, 1994; Gomez *et al.*, 1996). It has been proposed that this increase in the cellular content of cytosolic enzymes in the ejaculates of infertile men reflects the retention of excess residual cytoplasm in the midpiece of the spermatozoa (Figure 3.13). Certainly the functional competence of human spermatozoa appears to be negatively impacted by the

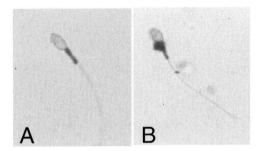

Figure 3.13. Use of diaphorase staining to detect retention of excess residual cytoplasm in the midpiece of human spermatozoa. A, a normal cell showing a cigar shaped area of midpiece cytoplasm in the vicinity of the mitochondria. B, retention of excess residual cytoplasm at the junction between the sperm head and midpiece (Gomez *et al.*, 1996).

presence of excess residual cytoplasm. For example recent studies have demonstrated that the loss of fertility associated with varicocoeles and certain cases of idiopathic male infertility are associated with the retention of excess residual cytoplasm by the spermatozoa, as is the loss of fertility associated with heavy smoking (Mak *et al.*, 2000; Zini *et al.*, 2000). In the case of varicocoele patients, varicocoelectomy has been shown to induce a significant increase in sperm motility in association with a reduction in the percentage of cells carrying cytoplasmic droplets (Zini *et al.*, 1999). Similarly in patients with idiopathic infertility, motility has been shown to be inversely correlated with the presence of cytoplasmic droplets (Zini *et al.*, 1998). Furthermore, independent studies of patients undergoing IVF treatment have revealed a strong negative correlation between the retention of excess residual cytoplasm by the spermatozoa and fertilization rate (Keating *et al.*, 1997).

Oxidative stress

The linkage between cytoplamic droplets and defective sperm function is thought to involve the induction of oxidative stress. Specifically it has been proposed that the cytoplasm contains a family of enzymes responsible for the generation of NADH or NADPH that in turn serve as substrates for NADPH oxidases that drive free radical generation by these cells. There is a set of clear associations between the excessive generation of reactive oxygen species by populations of human spermatozoa and the retention of residual cytoplasm by these cells (Figure 3.14; Gomez *et al.*, 1996). Furthermore the generation of reactive oxygen species is negatively correlated with sperm function (Aitken and Fisher, 1994; Sharma and Agarwal, 1996).

The measurement of reactive oxygen species (ROS) production by spermatozoa can be readily achieved using chemiluminescent techniques based on luminol or

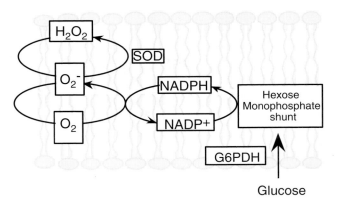

Glucose

Figure 3.14. Proposed scheme for human spermatozoa that provides a link between the presence of excess residual cytoplasm (hence increased amounts of glucose-6-phosphate dehydrogenase: G6PDH) and reactive oxygen species generation. The electrons for superoxide anion generation (O_2^-) could also come from NADPH generated via glycolysis. SOD: superoxide dismutase; H_2O_2: hydrogen peroxide.

lucigenin as probes. The major complication with such analyses is that they can be seriously affected by the presence of leukocytes within the sperm population. The latter must be removed before a meaningful analysis of ROS production by spermatozoa can be undertaken. A convenient method for achieving this is to stimulate the sperm suspensions with FMLP (formyl-methionyl-leucyl-phenylalanine), a leukocyte-specific agonist. If a peak of chemiluminescence is observed then leukocyte contamination is evident and the sample must be processed to remove these cellular contaminants (Figure 3.15). This objective can be readily achieved using paramagnetic beads coated with a monoclonal antibody against the common leukocyte antigen, CD45 (Aitken et al., 1996). Samples that are leukocyte free can be induced to generate a burst of ROS on addition of PMA (12-myristate, 13-acetate phorbol ester), a powerful activator of protein kinase C. The ROS responses elicited by PMA in leukocyte-free sperm suspensions are inversely correlated with semen quality (Figure 3.16). The higher the ROS response, the greater the impairment of sperm quality.

Oxidative stress in human spermatozoa leads to the peroxidation of membrane lipids, a loss of membrane fluidity and a resultant loss of sperm function. The presence of oxidative stress in human sperm populations can be assessed by the measurement of lipid peroxides. The most common method for the measurement of lipid peroxidation involves the spectrofluorometric assessment of malondialdehyde generation following incubation with thiobarbituric acid. This assay involves the incubation of human spermatozoa with a ferrous ion promotor to force the breakdown of pre-existing lipid peroxides and generate malondialdehyde. Recently

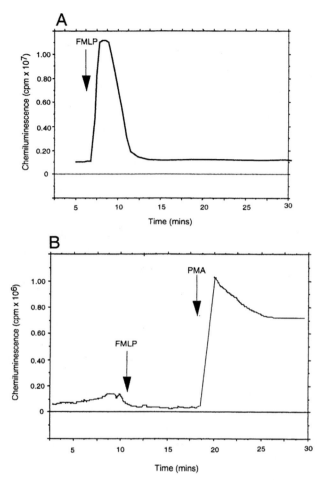

Figure 3.15. Luminol peroxidase enhanced chemiluminescence can be used to monitor leukocyte contamination of human sperm suspensions and the ability of the isolated sperm to generate reactive oxygen species. A, FMLP (formyl-methionyl-leucyl-phenylalanine) – induced chemiluminescence produces an oxidative burst that emanates entirely from the sperm population. B, in leukocyte-free sperm suspensions the spermatozoa can be stimulated to produce an oxidative burst by the addition of 100 nm PMA (12-myristate, 13-acetate phorbol ester).

spectrophotometric assays have been developed for measuring a wider range of lipid peroxidation products including 4-hydroxyalkanals and malondialdehyde. These measures of lipid peroxidation are invariably negatively associated with sperm function (Gomez *et al.*, 1998).

This association is illustrated in Figure 3.17 by reference to the correlation that exists between the degree of motility loss sustained by human spermatozoa following overnight incubation and the accumulation of lipid peroxidation products.

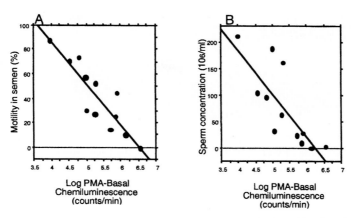

Figure 3.16. PMA (12-myristate, 13-acetate phorbol ester)-induced chemiluminescence responses in leukocyte-free populations of human spermatozoa illustrating the strong negative correlation with semen quality as reflected by (A) motility and (B) sperm count (Gomez *et al.*, 1998).

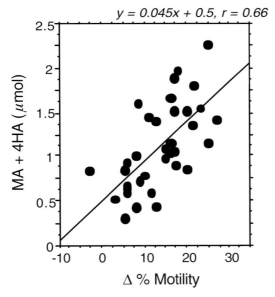

Figure 3.17. Correlation between lipid peroxidation measured by a simple spectrophotometric assay and the loss of motility exhibited by human spermatozoa following their incubation overnight at 37 °C (Gomez *et al.*, 1998). MA + 4HA: malondialdehyde and 4-hydroxy alkenals.

DNA damage

Oxidative stress not only induces peroxidation of unsaturated fatty acids in the sperm plasma membrane, it also induces DNA damage in the sperm nucleus and mitochondria. This damage is inversely correlated with the fertilizing capacity of human spermatozoa in vitro and is a common feature of the semen profile of men

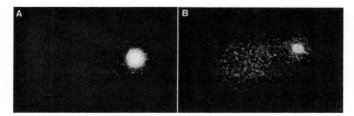

Figure 3.18. COMET assay. A single cell electrophoresis assay that provides information on the stability of sperm DNA in the face of high pH. A, a normal cell, the DNA running as a single cohesive mass. B, a damaged cell, the DNA forming a 'comet' like structure; the relative dimension of the 'tail' indicating the extent to which the DNA is damaged.

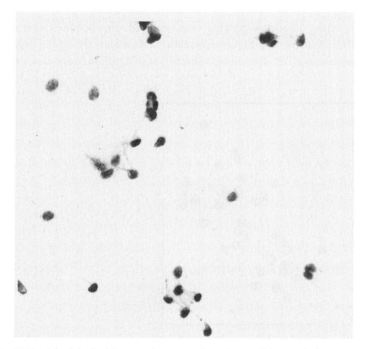

Figure 3.19. DNA nicks labelled in a patient sample using a nick translation assay in which the DNA is partially decondensed prior to the performance of the assay (Twigg *et al.*, 1998b).

attending infertility clinics (Sun *et al.*, 1997; Irvine *et al.*, 2000). The aetiology of such oxidative DNA damage is uncertain although heavy smoking is clearly one lifestyle factor that is capable of precipitating such damage (Aitken & Krausz, 2001). The finding that the offspring of male smokers stand a four- to fivefold increased chance of developing childhood cancer (Ji *et al.*, 1997) emphasizes the importance of monitoring such damage in the spermatozoa of male patients. A variety of techniques have been developed to monitor DNA damage in the germ line including COMET assays (Figure 3.18), nick translation (Figure 3.19) or TUNEL assays and the Sperm Chromatin Stability Assay (SCSA). In addition, biochemical analyses of the degree of oxidative damage to sperm DNA have been used, with 8-hydroxy guanine as an index of oxidative stress (Kodama, 1997).

As yet there is no consensus as to the optimal technique for assessing DNA damage in spermatozoa. COMET and SCSA assays generate results that are highly correlated and appear to provide data on the susceptibility of the chromatin to damage following exposure to extremes of high or low pH, respectively (Aravindan et al., 1997). TUNEL and nick translation assays on the other hand appear to provide information of the presence of double or single DNA strand breaks in the spermatozoa. The advantage of the TUNEL assay is that it can be automated using flow cytometry as an end-point. In this form it appears to be an efficient and effective means of monitoring DNA damage in human spermatozoa. A variation on the nick translation theme has been to relax the DNA structure with reducing agents prior to the performance of the assay. In this way the DNA polymerase or terminal transferase, used for the nick translation and TUNEL assays respectively, are permitted full access to the nick, unhindered by the highly cross linked nature of sperm chromatin (Twigg et al., 1998b).

The highest levels of DNA damage are generally found in the spermatozoa of men with poor semen profiles (Sun et al., 1997; Irvine et al., 2000). Fortunately the collateral oxidative damage inflicted on the plasma membrane of men with poor semen profiles generally means that their spermatozoa, while harbouring a significant level of DNA damage, cannot participate in the normal process of fertilization. This has been demonstrated experimentally in studies in which normal human spermatozoa have been exposed to increasing levels of oxidative stress in the form of hydrogen peroxide (Aitken et al., 1998). At lower levels of oxidative stress the DNA is significant but the fertilizing potential of the spermatozoa is actually enhanced because of the promoting effect of reactive oxygen species on the capacitation of human spermatozoa (Figure 3.20; Aitken et al., 1995).

Intracytoplasmic sperm injection (ICSI)

Although spermatozoa with highly damaged genomes cannot engage in the normal process of fertilization, direct injection of spermatozoa into the ooplasm (ICSI) circumvents this barrier (Figure 3.21). Thus spermatozoa with extremely high levels of oxidative damage to their DNA, induced by high levels of intracellular ROS generation, exposure to hydrogen peroxide or co-incubation with activated leukocytes can fertilize oocytes following ICSI (Twigg et al., 1998a). Since this form of treatment is normally reserved for men with severely abnormal semen profiles whose spermatozoa frequently contain oxidatively induced DNA damage, the risk of transmitting genetic damage to the embryo must be high (Aitken & Krausz, 2001).

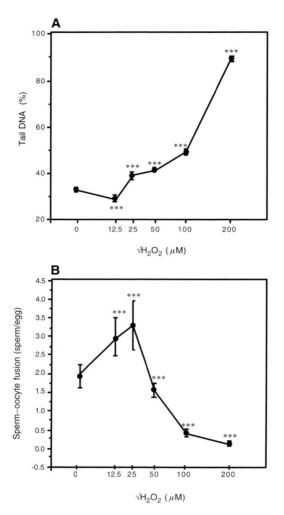

Figure 3.20. Dose response of the impact of hydrogen peroxide H_2O_2 on (A) DNA damage and (B) fertilizing capacity of human spermatozoa. Note that at high levels of oxidative stress the spermatozoa are damaged but the potential for fertilization is suppressed. At lower levels of oxidative stress the DNA is significantly damaged but the fertilizing potential of the spermatozoa is enhanced (Aitken *et al.*, 1998).

The ICSI procedure appears to be extremely forgiving of the quality of the spermatozoa. Higher rates of fertilization are obtained if the spermatozoa selected for ICSI exhibit some residual motility, but otherwise there are no criteria by which to select spermatozoa for this form of treatment. It is not even necessary for the spermatozoa to be recovered from the ejaculate for fertilization to be achieved following intracytoplasmic injection. Spermatozoa recovered surgically from the

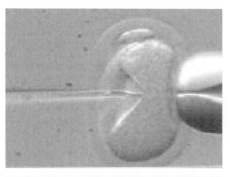

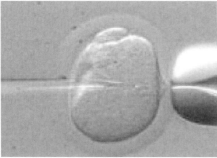

Figure 3.21. Intracytoplasmic sperm injection is commonly used to address the loss of fertility associated with severe male infertility.

epididymis or testes are also suitable for this form of therapy. It is clear from such studies that none of the intricate changes associated with sperm capacitation or the acrosome reaction are necessary for ICSI to be effective. All that is required is that the spermatozoon possesses a haploid genome and a centriole capable of organizing cell division in the embryo. Neither the integrity of the sperm DNA nor the status of the sperm plasma membrane, mitochondria or acrosome have any bearing on the ability of human spermatozoa to fertilize the oocyte.

These findings are of clinical importance because testicular sperm extraction (TESE) in association with ICSI is becoming the standard treatment for non-obstructive azoospermia. The success of ICSI in such cases does not even require that the sperm chromatin is normally protaminated, as conceptions and viable pregnancies have been generated with spermatozoa containing no detectable protamine 2 (Carrell & Liu, 2001). Not only spermatozoa, but also elongated spermatids can apparently support fertilization when ICSI is used, even though such cells, or the nuclei they contain, cannot trigger the normal post-fertilization patterns of calcium oscillation in the oocyte (Yazawa *et al.*, 2001). Round spermatid injection (ROSNI) has also been used clinically with some success although the developmental potential of embryos generated by such means is clearly compromised (Levran *et al.*, 2000; Vicdan *et al.*, 2001).

In cases of obstructive azoospermia, TESE is invariably successful in recovering spermatozoa for injection (Schulze *et al.*, 1999). Even in non-obstructive azoospermia, TESE is successful in recovering spermatozoa in 75% of cases (Schulze *et al.*, 1999). Whether or not a diagnostic testicular biopsy is helpful in determining whether patients with non-obstructive azoospermia are suitable for ICSI treatment is the subject of some debate. Approximately, a 10% false negative rate might be expected on the basis of histological evaluation of semi-thin sections. Elevated FSH levels are also not helpful in predicting those patients with non-obstructive azoospermia for whom TESE is a therapeutic option (Schulze *et al.*, 1999). On the other hand, in all cases of severely impaired spermatogenesis, testicular biopsies are of value in identifying cases of carcinoma in situ.

Y chromosome deletion

One of the major concerns with ICSI as a therapeutic technique is the risk of transmitting genetic mutations to the offspring. Although there is a suspicion that DNA damage in the germ line is associated with childhood cancer in the offspring (Ji *et al.*, 1997), this is a difficult linkage to prove because the aetiology of cancer is so complex. However, one form of mutation that ICSI will definitely propagate is infertility due to DNA damage to the Y chromosome. The Y chromosome is uniquely susceptible to genetic damage because it has no homologue. Whenever double strand breaks occur and genetic information is lost, the Y chromosome cannot retrieve this information via the conventional mechanism of homologous recombination using the information stored on the homologous chromosome. In this sense, the non-recombining region of the Y chromosome is uniquely susceptible to gene deletion. Indeed it is the ultimate evolutionary fate of all genes on this region of the Y chromosome that they will degrade (Figure 3.22).

The ancient homologue of the Y chromosome was the X. However, most of the genes shared with the X chromosome have, by this stage in our evolution, been lost. The Y now contains a cluster of genes involved in male fertility and sex determination. Many of the key fertility regulating genes are located at locus Yq11 and deletions in this region are associated with male infertility (Figure 3.23). The incidence of Y chromosome deletions varies among different studies from 1% to 55% depending on the patient mix. Around 15% of patients with non-obstructive azoospermia are affected in this way, as are 5–10% of cases with severe oligozoospermia.

Because deletions on the Y chromosome lead to infertility, the mutagenic events that are responsible for this condition are largely spontaneous and must have their origins in the germ line of the father. It has been suggested that the primary event

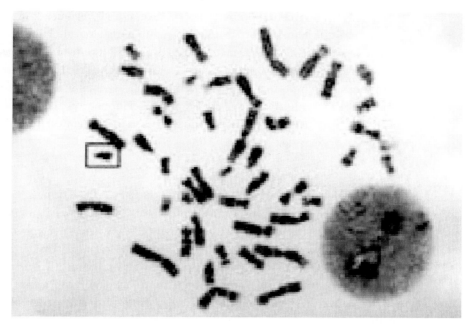

Figure 3.22. Human karyotype. Boxed chromosome is the Y. This chromosome contains many of the key genes involved in sex determination and male fertility. Mutations on the long arm of the Y chromosome may be a key factor in infertility observed in certain patients.

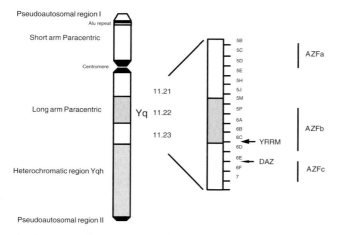

Figure 3.23. The human Y chromosome. A locus on the long arm of the Y chromosome, Yq11, appears to contain genes that are important for spermatogenesis. Gene deletions in this region are associated with infertility.

involves DNA fragmentation in the spermatozoa as a consequence of such factors as aberrant recombination, defective chromatin packaging, abortive apoptosis and oxidative stress (Aitken & Krausz, 2001). This DNA fragmentation constitutes a promutagenic change that may be converted into a gene deletion after fertilization, as the oocyte attempts to repair the genetic damage brought in by the spermatozoon (Aitken & Krausz, 2001). Since Y chromosome deletions are in the germ line, the use of ICSI to treat men with this condition will result in an identical form of infertility in any male offspring.

Cystic fibrosis

Mutations in the cystic fibrosis transmembrane conductance regulator (CFTR) gene are a relatively frequent factor in the aetiology of male infertility. Depending on their molecular consequences, CFTR mutations may result in typical cystic fibrosis (CF) characterized by chronic lung disease, pancreatic exocrine insufficiency, an increase in the concentration of sweat electrolytes and male infertility due to obstructive azoospermia. Alternatively mutations in this gene may result in congenital absence of the vas deferens (bi- or unilateral), bilateral ejaculatory duct obstruction or bilateral obstructions within the epididymides.

Congenital bilateral absence of the vas deferens is found in 1% to 2% of men referred for infertility evaluation, and accounts for 27% of men with primary obstructive azoospermia. Defects in spermatogenesis can also be found among this group of patients. All males with idiopathic obstructive azoospermia bear an increased risk for CF offspring. Couples requesting microsurgical epididymal sperm aspiration and ICSI in the context of obstructive azoospermia should be offered genetic counselling and molecular genetic analysis of the CFTR gene (Stuhrmann & Dork, 2000).

Endocrinology

Male infertility differs from female infertility because it is fundamentally not an endocrine condition. Most infertile men are normogonadotrophic and possess normal androgen levels. Nevertheless, serum FSH levels are often helpful in identifying cases of severe oligozoospermia or azoospermia that are due to defective spermatogenesis. In such cases circulating FSH levels are elevated. If FSH levels are normal, the absence of spermatozoa from the ejaculate is probably indicative of obstruction and CFTR mutations or infection should be considered as causative factors in the patients condition.

Low FSH, usually associated with low LH and testosterone, may be indicative of hypogonadotrophic hypogonadism.

Analysis of testosterone and LH levels is indicated in cases of suspected androgen deficiency, anabolic steroid abuse or steroid secreting lesions such as testicular or adrenal tumours. High LH and testosterone may be indicative of androgen receptor mutations.

Hyperprolactinaemia is not a recognized cause of male infertility but may be a significant factor in the origins of sexual dysfunction (particularly decreased libido). High prolactin levels may also be indicative of pituitary tumours responsible for secondary testicular failure.

Oestrogen determinations are only indicated in cases of gynaecomastia.

REFERENCES

Aitken, R. J. & Fisher, H. (1994). Reactive oxygen species generation and human spermatozoa: the balance of benefit and risk. *Bioessays* **16**: 259–67.

Aitken, R. J. & Krausz, C. (2001). Oxidative stress, DNA damage and the Y chromosome. *Reproduction* **122**: 497–506.

Aitken, R. J., Bowie, H., Buckingham, D. W., Harkiss, D., Richardson, D. W. & West, K. M. (1992). Sperm penetration into a hyaluronic acid polymer as a means of monitoring functional competence. *J. Androl.* **13**: 44–54.

Aitken, R. J., Buckingham, D. W., West, K. & Brindle, J. (1996). On the use of paramagnetic beads and ferrofluids to assess and eliminate the leukocytic contribution to oxygen radical generation by human sperm suspensions. *Am. J. Reprod. Immunol.* **35**: 541–51.

Aitken, R. J., Gordon, E., Harkiss, D., Twigg, J. P., Milne P., Jennings Z. & Irvine, D. S. (1998). Relative impact of oxidative stress on the functional competence and genomic integrity of human spermatozoa. *Biol. Reprod.* **59**: 1037–46.

Aitken, R. J., Krausz, C. & Buckingham, D. W. (1994). Relationships between biochemical markers for residual sperm cytoplasm, reactive oxygen species generation and the presence of leucocytes and precursor germ cells in human sperm suspensions. *Mol. Reprod. Develop.* **39**: 268–79.

Aitken, R. J., Paterson, M., Fisher, H., Buckingham, D. W. & van Duin, M. (1995). Redox regulation of tyrosine phosphorylation in human spermatozoa and its role in the control of human sperm function. *J. Cell Sci.* **108**: 2017–25.

Aitken, R. J., Warner, P. & Reid, C. (1986). Factors influencing the success of sperm-cervical mucus interaction in patients exhibiting unexplained infertility. *J. Androl.* **7**: 3–10.

Aravindan, C. R., Bjordahl, J., Jost, L. K. & Evenson, D. P. (1997). Susceptibility of human sperm to *in situ* DNA denaturation is strongly correlated with DNA strand breaks identified by single-cell electrophoresis. *Exp. Cell Res.* **236**: 231–9.

Carrell, D. T. & Liu, L. (2001). Altered protamine 2 expression is uncommon in donors of known fertility, but common among men with poor fertilizing capacity, and may reflect other abnormalities of spermiogenesis. *J. Androl.* **22**: 604–11.

Casano, R., Orlando, C., Serio, M. & Forti, G. (1991). LDH and LDH-X activity in sperm from normospermic and oligozoospermic men. *Int. J. Androl.* **14**: 257–63.

Feneux, D., Serres, C. & Jouannet, P. (1985). Sliding spermatozoa: a dyskinesia responsible for human infertility? *Fertil. Steril.* **44**: 508–511.

Glazener, C. M., Ford, W. C. & Hull, M. G. (2000). The prognostic power of the post-coital test for natural conception depends on duration of infertility. *Hum. Reprod.* **215**: 1953–7.

Gomez, E., Buckingham, D. W., Brindle, J., Lanzafame, F., Irvine, D. S. & Aitken, R. J. (1996). Development of an image analysis system to monitor the retention of residual cytoplasm by human spermatozoa: correlation with biochemical markers of the cytoplasmic space, oxidative stress and sperm function. *J. Androl.* **17**: 276–87.

Gomez, E., Irvine, D. S. & Aitken, R. J. (1998). Evaluation of a spectrophotometric assay for the measurement of malondialdehyde and 4-hydroxyalkenals in human spermatozoa: relationships with semen quality and sperm function. *Int. J. Androl.* **21**: 81–94.

Gonzales, G. F., Kortebani, G. & Mazzolli, A. B. (1992). Leukocytospermia and function of the seminal vesicles on semen quality. *Fertil. Steril.* **57**: 1058–65.

Hjort T. & Hargreave, T. B. (1994). Immunity to sperm and fertility. In *Male Infertility*, 2nd edn, ed. T. B. Hargreave, pp. 269–90. London: Springer-Verlag.

Hull, M. G. R., Glazener, C. M. A., Kelly, N. J., Conway, D. I., Foster, P. A., Hunton, R. A., Coulson, C., Lambert, P. A., Watt, E. M. & Desai, K. M. (1985). Population study of causes, treatment and outcome of infertility. *BMJ* **291**: 1693–7.

Huszar, G., Vigue, L. & Corrales, M. (1988). Sperm creatine phosphokinase quality in normospermic, variablespermic and oligospermic men. *Biol. Reprod.* **38**: 1061–6.

Irvine, D. S., Twigg, J., Gordon, E., Fulton, N., Milne, P. & Aitken, R. J. (2000). DNA integrity in human spermatozoa: relationship with semen quality. *J. Androl.* **21**: 33–44.

Ji, B. T., Shu, X. O., Linet, M. S., Zheng, W., Wacholder, S., Gao, Y. T., Ying, D. M. & Jin, F. (1997). Paternal cigarette smoking and the risk of childhood cancer among offspring of nonsmoking mothers. *J. Natl. Cancer Inst.* **89**: 238–44.

Keating, J., Grundy, C. E., Fivey, P. S., Elliott, M. & Robinson, J. (1997). Investigation of the association between the presence of cytoplasmic residues on the human sperm midpiece and defective sperm function. *J. Reprod. Fertil.* **110**: 71–7.

Kodama, H., Yamaguchi, R., Fukuda, J., Kasai, H. & Tanaka, T. (1997). Increased oxidative deoxyribonucleic acid damage in the spermatozoa of infertile male patients. *Fertil. Steril.* **68**: 519–24.

Levran, D., Nahum, H., Farhi, J. & Weissman, A. (2000). Poor outcome with round spermatid injection in azoospermic patients with maturation arrest. *Fertil. Steril.* **74**: 443–9.

Mak, V., Jarvi, K., Buckspan, M., Freeman, M. Hechter, S. & Zini, A. (2000). Smoking is associated with the retention of cytoplasm by human spermatozoa *Urology* **56**: 463–6.

Mortimer, D., Pandya, I. J. & Sawers, R. S. (1986). Relationship between human sperm motility characteristics and sperm penetration into human cervical mucus *in-vitro*. *J. Reprod. Fertil.* **78**: 93–102.

Schulze, W., Thoms, F. & Knuth, U. A. (1999). Testicular sperm extraction: comprehensive analysis with simultaneously performed histology in 1418 biopsies from 766 subfertile men. *Hum. Reprod.* **14**: 82–96.

Sharma, R. K. & Agarwal, A. (1996). Role of reactive oxygen species in male infertility. *Urology* **48**: 835–850.

Stuhrmann, M. & Dork, T. (2000). CFTR gene mutations and male infertility. *Andrologia* **32**: 71–83.

Sukcharoen, N., Keith, J. Irvine, D. S. & Aitken, R. J. (1995). Definition of the optimal criteria for identifying hyperactivated spermatozoa at 25Hz using in vitro fertilization as a functional end-point. *Hum. Reprod.* **10**: 2928–37.

Sun, J. G., Jurisicova, A. & Casper, R. F. (1997). Detection of deoxyribonucleic acid fragmentation in human sperm: correlation with fertilization in vitro. *Biol. Reprod.* **56**: 602–7.

Twigg, J. P., Irvine D. S. & Aitken R. J. (1998a). Oxidative damage to DNA in human spermatozoa does not preclude pronucleus formation at ICSI. *Hum. Reprod.* **13**: 1864–71.

Twigg, J., Irvine, D. S., Houston, P., Fulton, N., Michael, L. & Aitken, R. J. (1998b). Iatrogenic DNA damage induced in human spermatozoa during sperm preparation: protective significance of seminal plasma. *Mol. Hum. Reprod.* **4**: 439–45.

Vicdan, K., Isik, A. Z. & Delilbasi, L. (2001). Development of blastocyst-stage embryos after round spermatid injection in patients with complete spermiogenesis failure. *J. Assist. Reprod. Genet.* **18**: 78–86.

Wallace, E. M., Aitken, R. J. & Wu, F. C. W. (1992). Residual sperm function in oligozoospermia induced by testosterone enanthate administered as a potential steroid male contraceptive. *Int. J. Androl.* **15**: 416–24.

World Health Organization (1987). *World Health Organization laboratory manual for the examination of human semen and sperm–cervical mucus interaction*, 2nd edn. Cambridge: Cambridge University Press.

World Health Organization (1999). *World Health Organization laboratory manual for the examination of human semen and sperm–cervical mucus interaction*, 4th edn. Cambridge: Cambridge University Press.

Yazawa, H., Yanagida, K. & Sato, A. (2001). Oocyte activation and Ca(2+) oscillation-inducing abilities of mouse round/elongated spermatids and the developmental capacities of embryos from spermatid injection. *Hum. Reprod.* **16**: 1221–8.

Zini, A., Buckspan, M., Jama, L. M. & Jarvi, K. (1999). Effect of varicocelectomy on the abnormal retention of residual cytoplasm by human spermatozoa. *Hum. Reprod.* **14**: 1791–3.

Zini, A., Defreitas, G., Freeman, M., Hechter, S. & Jarvi, K. (2000). Varicocele is associated with abnormal retention of cytoplasmic droplets by human spermatozoa. *Fertil. Steril.* **74**: 461–4.

Zini, A., O'Bryan, M. K., Israel, L. & Schlegel, P. N. (1998). Human sperm NADH and NADPH diaphorase cytochemistry: correlation with sperm motility. *Urology* **51**: 464–8.

4

Donor insemination

Mathew Tomlinson and Chris Barratt

Assisted Conception Unit, Birmingham Women's Hospital, Birmingham, UK

Following the establishment of intracytoplasmic sperm injection (ICSI), the number of donor insemination (DI) treatment cycles performed in the UK has dramatically reduced from 25 623 cycles in 1992/93 to 11 035 in 1998/99 (Human Fertilisation and Embryology Authority, 2000) with an accompanying increased live birth rate (LBR) from median 5% in 1992/93 to 9.9% in 1998/99. Therefore, DI remains a significant fertility treatment option and is likely to remain so until new methods of treating male infertility without recourse to assisted conception are developed. Ideally, all DI centres in the UK should be able to achieve a minimal LBR of 10% but we should continually strive to improve the service to our patients if we are to meet our expectation of improved success rates.

Following the establishment of the Human Fertilisation and Embryology Authority (HFEA), DI has faced many challenges. In this chapter we focus on these challenges and outline methods and lines of investigation that can be used to improve the treatment provided to patients.

Donor recruitment

In the UK, strict adherence to guidelines laid down by the HFEA (www.hfea.gov.uk) has made the recruitment of sperm donors an arduous task. The HFEA strongly recommends that donors should be recruited from a stable heterosexual relationship, preferably with a family of their own, along the lines of the French Centre d'Etude et de Conservation du Sperme Humain (CECOS) system, and that donors provide samples virtually *gratis*, with a low nominated maximum compensation for their time and travel. Only 10 pregnancies per donor are allowed and until recently, multiple pregnancies counted toward this total. In theory therefore, after recruitment and the necessary strict screening and cryopreservation procedures, some donors

Good Clinical Practice in Assisted Reproduction, ed. P. Serhal & C. Overton.
Published by Cambridge University Press. © Cambridge University Press 2004.

are used for only four or five treatment cycles. These restrictions have taken their toll on recruitment in the UK. Previously, infertility clinics would recruit a few donors and supplement any shortfall with samples purchased from large specialist sperm banks. Now the majority of clinics 'buy in' most of their samples as recruitment becomes less cost-effective. With more clinics, buying donor sperm from an increasingly restricted number of suppliers, there has been a marked reduction in donor choice and availability.

Under the current HFEA code of practice it is difficult to know how the number of samples and choice of donor semen available for patient treatment can be increased. One method may be the bulk import of donor semen from donor banks outside the UK. The HFEA is now considering this issue and has granted approval for one UK clinic to import semen on this basis. However, it would appear more appropriate in the long term to modify the practices of donor recruitment within the UK rather than rely on the import of donor semen.

In other countries, the situation is very different. For example, in the USA restrictions vary from state to state and are nowhere near as far-reaching. Donors are rewarded for better quality samples, sometimes being paid per ampoule of frozen sperm produced from a single sample of ejaculate. There appears to be little enforcement of a maximum number of pregnancies per donor and centres offer substantial reward for 'highly fertile' donors of desirable phenotype (e.g. tall, blue-eyed blonde). Therefore, supply of donor sperm is entirely dependent on 'market forces' with prices driven by quality, phenotype, intellect and education. Furthermore, the marketing of donor sperm has shifted towards providing as much information about each donor as possible, with some cryo-banks providing CD recorded interviews or donor photographs.

In France there is an emphasis on 'altruism'. There is no payment other than travelling expenses, and the vast majority of donors recruited have at least one child of their own. Apparently this system works well as centres function under the CECOS umbrella and all CECOS centres operate according to the same guidelines. Providing that donors can be easily recruited this system offers tremendous advantages. Not only does the donor have proven fertility but there is a lowered risk of hereditary disease and a greater willingness to comply with all testing and screening (Le Lannou & Lansac, 1993). With annual evaluation by the CECOS, this collective operation facilitates standardization of methods and analysis of large amounts of data.

In the UK and France, sperm donation is completely anonymous. In the UK, non-identifying information from the HFEA register has not been used effectively, as the majority of recipients opt for secrecy (versus openness) with respect to disclosure of their offspring's genetic origin. In the US, sperm donation is still largely anonymous but clinics work on the premise that supplying an abundance of information on a donor at the time of treatment will satisfy the curiosity of recipients and offspring alike, and reduce the desire to trace the 'biological parent' in the future. In the USA, there is some follow-up by patients and offspring, though not on the same scale as in some European countries like Sweden and Switzerland, where offspring have the legal right to trace their biological origin. Recent European human rights legislation may well force an increase of access to donor information and in the UK this prospect has already added to recruitment problems.

Screening

In DI, the protection of the recipient and potential offspring from sexually transmitted and other inheritable disorders is paramount. It is standard practice to use frozen sperm and to 'quarantine' samples for at least six months to allow for incubation of hepatitis B and C strains and HIV 1 and 2. The American Society of Reproductive Medicine (ASRM, 1998) and the British Andrology Society (BAS, 1999) have published comprehensive guidelines and these should be consulted. Briefly, both recommend the following:
- Clinical assessment (medical history).
- Physical examination (for genital warts, discharge, ulcers).
- STD screening (HIV 1 and 2, hepatitis B and C, syphilis, gonorrhoea, chlamydia)
- CMV (cytomegalovirus) serology.
- Genetic testing and genetic history (minimum of cystic fibrosis, and karyotype).
   CMV testing remains a contentious issue with practical arguments for and against (Curson & Karakosta, 2000; McLaughlin, 2000). However, it is the most common cause of congenital infection occurring in 0.4–2.5% of live births (Liesnard *et al.*, 1998) often with severe consequences and the BAS and ASRM continue to recommend matching donor-recipients for CMV status as standard practice. Sexually transmitted diseases (STD) screening and physical examination should be repeated immediately after the last donation, with final HIV and hepatitis bloods after a further six months.

Sperm cryopreservation

When compared with embryos, the cryopreservation of sperm is usually relatively crude. The majority of clinics use a method first introduced in 1963 (Sherman, 1963), of suspending samples in nitrogen vapour 5–10 cm from the liquid surface. Some have introduced computerised controlled rate freezers (e.g. Planar KR10) and although this method facilitates superior quality control, significantly improved survival rates have not been consistently demonstrated for frozen donor samples (McLaughlin *et al.*, 1990; Morris *et al.*, 1999). However, controlled rate freezers

Component	g/litre
Distilled water	850 ml
Sodium Chloride	5.8
Potassium Chloride	0.4
Calcium Lactate	0.76
Magnesium Sulphate	0.121
Sodium dihydrogen ortho-phosphate	0.005
Sodium bicarbonate	2.6
Hepes	4.76
Glucose	8.59
Fructose	8.59
Glycine	10.0
Kanamycin	0.05
Human Serum Albumin	4
Add Glycerol	150 ml
Filter-sterilize (0.22 μm millipore). Aliquot store at −20 °C	

Figure 4.1. Typical cryoprotectant recipe (adapted from Mahadevan & Trounson, 1983).

appear to provide better survival of poor samples, for example from oncology patients (Ragni *et al.*, 1990).

Ultimately, cryo-survival depends on factors such as intracellular ice formation, extent of dehydration and salt concentrations. In humans the use of an extender or cryoprotectant (usually 10–15% glycerol in combination with a 'slow cooling/rapid freezing') method gives anything up to 50–60% survival. A typical 'home-made' cryoprotectant recipe is shown in Figure 4.1, although some centres prefer commercially available media (e.g. Sperm Freeze, Conception Technologies, USA). Some clinics have suggested that the use of egg-yolk citrate buffer with glycerol improves survival but this is not a widely held view.

More importantly, cryoprotectant should be added to semen extremely slowly to prevent osmotic shock. Some authors advocate serial dilution over a long period or even bringing sperm and cryoprotectant to equilibrium across a dialysis membrane as the most effective method (Storey *et al.*, 1998). The lack of consensus over the most effective methodology is clear and there is much work to be done to optimize sperm cryopreservation conditions and bring survival rates up to the levels observed with embryo cryopreservation.

The concentration of progressively motile sperm must be within acceptable limits to contemplate cryopreservation and storage. With an estimated 50% cryo-survival rate and a rough target of 10 million progressively motile sperm per frozen vial, samples with below 40 million progressively motile sperm per ml are probably not worth freezing. In some centres, any donor producing two successive samples below acceptable standards for cryopreservation are either not used in clinical practice or used only for research. Similarly the French CECOS clinics reject samples with a post-thaw concentration of <8 million per ml (Le Lannou & Lansac, 1993).

Below is an example method for cryopreservation of donor sperm in plastic vials, although this may be adapted for use with 0.25/0.5 ml straws. Rather than suspending samples over liquid nitrogen, we suggest using a 'dry shipper' ready-made nitrogen vapour vessel, e.g. Taylor Wharton CP100 (Taylor-Wharton-Harsco, USA). A suggested program for controlled rate cryopreservation is also described.

Basic cryopreservation protocol (if the sample contains at least 40 x 10^6/ml progressively motile sperm):

1 Carefully label donor vials with a low temperature cryopen.
2 Using a 5 ml syringe or graduated pipette, add cryoprotectant to the semen sample slowly drop-by-drop over 20 min (to reduce osmotic effects on the sperm), to obtain a 1:1 dilution (1 ml semen to 1 ml cryoprotectant).
3 Fill vials to 1 ml. The last vial should contain about 0.25 ml and is used for post-thaw check the following morning. Firmly secure lids on all vials. (Never immerse cryovials completely in liquid nitrogen, unless lids and vials expand and contract at the same rate and a seal can be guaranteed.)
4 Suspend samples for cryopreservation above liquid nitrogen vapour (in the dry shipper) –90 °C for 15 min, then lower to the bottom for a further 30 min.
5 Allocate space in the freezer. Label cryosleeve and cane (using metal tab). Place in freezer canister.
6 The following day, remove post-thaw vial, allow to thaw, and perform concentration and motility analysis.

Computer controlled rate cryopreservation

For example, Planar KR10; Adapted from Morris *et al.* (1999)

1. Start at 24 °C (approximately room temperature)
2. Cooling rate 2 °C per minute to −5 °C
3. Cool at 10 °C per minute from −5 °C to −100 °C
4. Transfer to liquid (−196 °C) or vapour phase (between approx. −150 ° and −190 °C) storage vessel.

Finally, the importance of accurate semen analysis throughout cannot be overstated. Meaningful data from the DI program will only be obtained if standardized methodology is adhered to. Therefore, World Health Organization guidelines for pre-freeze and post-thaw sperm concentration and motility should be followed throughout, with morphology slides prepared for each ejaculate (World Health Organization, 1999).

Safe sperm storage

The majority of sperm banks consist of a series of liquid nitrogen flasks or dewars e.g. Taylor Wharton 35HC. However, following an incident where several patients in the UK contracted hepatitis B from a broken blood bag stored in liquid nitrogen, there have been doubts over the safety of liquid nitrogen (Tedder *et al.*, 1995). The apparent ease with which pathogens may be transmitted in the cryobank led the UK Department of Health to set up an advisory group to develop specific policies for the processing and storage of bone marrow stem cells (NHS Executive, 1997). As a consequence, it is now standard practice for all blood banks in the UK to store in nitrogen vapour instead of liquid.

Although there has been no such incident in a sperm bank, the implications to fertility clinics are clear. In 1998, the HFEA published a consultation document and subsequently established a working group to address the various issues surrounding the safe storage of gametes and embryos (Human Fertilisation and Embryology Authority, 1998). There are certainly serious implications for quarantine in the storage of donor sperm. For example, if one donor sample in a tank of many was found to be seropositive (e.g. for HIV), the entire tank's contents would have to be destroyed due to the risk, however small, of cross-infection to other samples.

With the removal of a vector for microbial transmission and recent evidence suggesting that vapour storage does not reduce sperm or embryo viability, some assisted reproductive technology (ART) clinics are moving toward a vapour system (Figure 4.2) (Clarke, 1999; Tomlinson & Sakkas, 2000). However, as there is no concrete evidence that vapour is inherently safer, a number of measures must be considered for promotion as 'good practice' for sperm storage, possibly to be used alongside storage in the gaseous phase. These are discussed in detail by Clarke (1999).

- Straws or vials should be manufactured from a material that will not shatter after being subjected to ultra-low temperatures. When liquid nitrogen vessels are cleaned it is usual to find broken straws floating in the bottom and these are clearly a potential hazard and source of infection.
- PVA powder, which is in widespread use as a straw sealant is both ineffective and a potential source of contamination. The powder plug is often lost from the straw end after expansion, leaving it susceptible to cross-contamination. New straws are now available with filling and sealing protocols that should reduce the risk of contamination, for example Cryobiosystem (CBS straws^{TM}, I.M.V. Technologies, France).
- Vials should not be used in liquid nitrogen unless with a second skin, e.g. cryoflex, or lids that contract and expand at the same rate.

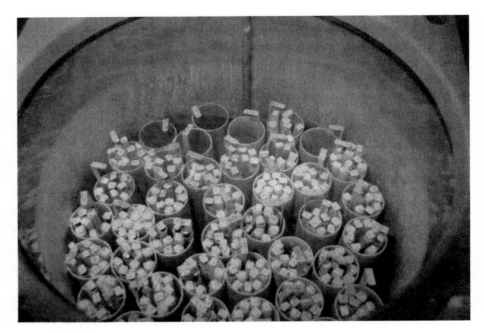

Figure 4.2.   Gaseous phase storage system.

Safety measures can be added to treatment protocols to further reduce any possibility of microbial transmission, e.g. using density gradients and sperm washing techniques to reduce a potential viral load of the sample, either before or after cryopreservation (Kim *et al.*, 1999; Levy *et al.*, 2000). The dilemma is that however small and unquantifiable the risk of cross-infection in a sperm bank, it cannot be ignored and steps must be taken to minimize the risk.

Use of donor sperm and factors influencing outcome

Practical aspects of using frozen sperm

The rate of cryo-survival and perhaps more importantly, the preservation of motility, is highly dependent on sample processing immediately from the time it leaves the freezer up to and including sperm preparation. Conventional semen analysis is ineffective in predicting cryo-survival of a sample. Complex measurements such as membrane fluidity appear to be much more indicative of sperm survival. The sperm able to withstand the movement of cryoprotectant, changes in salt concentrations and changes in temperature, are the sperm that will survive (Giraud *et al.*, 2000).

Although the thaw rate will have some affect on cryo-survival it appears to be less critical in human sperm than in other species. Practically speaking, the rate of thaw depends largely upon the storage material/container, i.e. straws or vials. The 0.25 ml straws thaw rapidly and once the straw ends are cut and placed in a tube, tend to be left at room temperature. Plastic cryo-vials thaw relatively slowly at room temperature and many laboratories speed up the process by incubating at 37 °C (or in a beaker of warm water). Care should be taken when sperm washing with wash buffer/media that it be slowly added in small aliquots 0.1 ml/30 sec, again to reduce osmotic stress (Ford et al., 1992).

Sample preparation

Density gradient centrifugation (DGC) is almost universally accepted as the superior sperm preparation method for assisted reproductive techniques, DI being no exception. The resuspended pellet obtained (see Figure 4.3) provides an inseminate free from contaminating round cells and with a high yield of motile sperm, increased percentage of normal forms and reduced sperm with damaged nuclear DNA (Kelly et al., 1997; Sakkas et al., 2000). Many 'ready to use' DGC media are now commercially available, all providing very acceptable results, e.g.

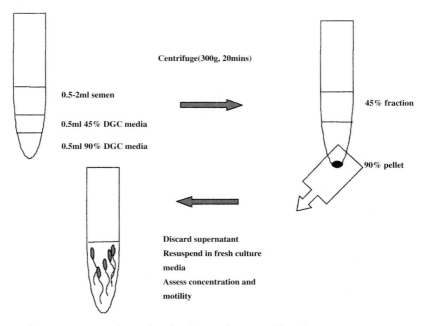

Figure 4.3.   Basic sperm preparation using density gradient centrifugation.

PureSperm (Nidacon, Sweden), Enhance-S-Plus (Conception Technologies USA), IxaPrep (Medicult UK) or Sperm Gradient (Cook IVF, UK). A basic protocol for their use is shown in Figure 4.3 and listed below.

1. Pipette 0.5 ml 90% DGC media into a clean sterile tube.
2. Gently layer 0.5 ml 45% DGC media on top of the 90% layer taking care not to disturb the interface between the two.
3. Layer 0.5–2.0 ml donor sample over the above and centrifuge at 300 g for 20 minutes.
4. Discard supernatant and resuspend 90% pellet in suitable media, e.g. Gamete-100 (Scandinavian IVF, Sweden), Sperm Buffer (Cook IVF, UK).
5. Mix well, wash (×2) in media (300 g, 5 min), resuspend in 0.5 ml.
6. Assess sperm concentration and motility according to WHO guidelines (WHO, 1999).

Intrauterine vs intracervical insemination

The advantages and disadvantages of intrauterine insemination (IUI) versus intracervical insemination (ICI) have been discussed for many years. Whilst ICI is a relatively simple, inexpensive and non-invasive technique, reported pregnancy rates of over 10% per cycle are few. In many centres IUI is considered to be the superior method, although it is more expensive, invasive and technically complex. When donor sperm is scarce IUI is desirable as it has been shown to deliver significantly more sperm to the site of fertilization (Ripps *et al.*, 1994) and many studies have demonstrated improved pregnancy rates when compared to ICI (Byrd *et al.*, 1990; Hurd *et al.*, 1993; Le Lannou *et al.*, 1995; Wainer *et al.*, 1995). However, differences in stimulation, sperm number inseminated and diagnosis in the recipient all contribute to reduce the power of individual findings. For example, Wainer and colleagues (1995) demonstrated a clear superiority of IUI over ICI (19.4% versus 6.75%), in terms of pregnancy rate, reduced use of donor sample and time taken to conceive but they conceded that the increased use of ovarian stimulation in the IUI group had contributed significantly to the result. The French CECOS group also found IUI to be superior. In stimulated patients IUI yielded a 17% pregnancy rate per cycle versus 10% in ICI. However, the type of stimulation used and the dose of sperm inseminated appeared to differ between groups (Le Lannou *et al.*, 1995).

Perhaps the most compelling argument is provided by recent meta-analyses (Goldberg *et al.*, 1999; O'Brien & Vandekerckhove, 2000), which have combined seven and 12 data sets respectively for analysis. Taking into account differences in subject randomization, timing, female diagnosis and ovarian stimulation, both concluded that the evidence for IUI superiority over ICI was overwhelming, particularly where poor pregnancy rates were obtained using ICI (<6%).

Ovarian stimulation, timing and number of inseminations

To some extent the use of ovarian stimulation will govern the method of timing and whether or not to inseminate once or twice. Where patients are 'down regulated' with GnRH (gonadotrophin releasing hormone) and superovulated using gonadotrophins, timing is directed by protocol with usually a single insemination 36–40 h after human chorionic ganadotrophins (HCG) administration (Tomlinson et al., 1996). However, a double insemination protocol for non-down-regulated patients (Ragni et al., 1999) has been recommended. For natural or clomiphene stimulated cycles an array of timing methods have been used (e.g. basal body temperature (BBT), cervical mucus scoring, daily oestradiol, ultrasonography and blood or urinary luteinizing hormone (LH), although there is little agreement over which is the most predictive (Barratt et al., 1989; Grinstead et al., 1989; Lenton, 1993; Brook et al., 1994). Accounting for some of these differences is the subtle variation in methodology, whether methods are used alone or in combination, and whether more than one insemination is performed. Poor pregnancy rates were reported with home LH testing and it is suggested that this was only 72% predictive (Anderson et al., 1996), whereas urinary test kits previously had been found to be 90% and 95% predictive of positive and negative tests respectively (Grinstead et al., 1989). The experience with LH (Clearplan) test kits (Unipath, Bedford, UK) has been favourable. Patients receive one or two inseminations (24 h apart), depending on whether the test is positive from the previous evening's urine and pregnancy rates vary between 11% and 15% for natural and clomiphene stimulated cycles respectively (Lashen et al., 1999)

Factors affecting DI success

As mentioned previously, many factors influence success rates of DI and, as these are discussed at length by Chauhan et al. (1989) and Depyere et al. (1994), they will not be covered in detail in this chapter. However, an example is shown in Figure 4.4, where the influence of female age can be clearly seen. Interestingly, in the early

Age (years)	Under 25	25–29	30–34	35–39	40–44	45 and over
Number of cycles	358	2210	4200	3299	927	41
Live birth rate per cycle	8.7	11.8	11.4	8.4	3.9	2.4

Figure 4.4.   Donor insemination live birth rate by woman's age (Human Fertilisation and Embryology Authority, 2000).

literature there are significantly higher success rates in women with azoospermic partners compared to those with sperm present in the ejaculate, indicating that subtle female factors have an effect on success rates.

DI as a research tool

Donor insemination provides an excellent research model. Several authors have used the system to examine the influence of semen parameters and sperm function testing on success rates (see Holt *et al.*, 1989; Barratt *et al.*, 1998). Such experiments have refined our knowledge on sperm function testing and allow a validated model to be used in the future. For example, it is now almost impossible to carry out long-term follow up studies to determine the in vivo predictive value of semen parameters (Tomlinson *et al.*, 1993) as many patients now require access to immediate treatment. Therefore, donor insemination remains the only tool to examine the predictive value of new assays of sperm function for in vivo as opposed to in vitro conception. This will allow the testing of new simple to use sperm function assays, which are desperately needed in fertility diagnosis.

Donor insemination also provides an excellent tool to examine other factors governing success, e.g. timing of inseminations and subtle female factors as the male gametes are of reasonably standardized quality. By using such a system it should be possible to refine the window of insemination so that improved pregnancy rates can be achieved. We will also be able to test new cryopreservation regimens to examine if their supposed improvements in for example, sperm survival do really translate into improvements in live birth rates.

REFERENCES

American Society for Reproductive Medicine (1998). Guidelines for gamete and embryo donation. *Fertil. Steril.* **70** (3).

Anderson, R. A., Eccles, S. M. & Irvine, D. S. (1996). Home ovulation testing in a donor insemination service. *Hum. Reprod.* **11**: 1674–7.

Barratt, C. L. R., Cooke, S., Chauhan, M. & Cooke, I. D. (1989). A prospective randomized controlled trial comparing urinary LH dipsticks and basal body temperature charts to time donor insemination. *Fertil. Steril.* **52**: 394.

Barratt, C. L., Clements, S. & Kessopoulou, E. (1998). Semen characteristics and fertility tests required for storage of spermatozoa. *Hum. Reprod.* **13**: 8–11.

British Andrology Society (1999). British Andrology Society guidelines for the screening of semen donors for donor insemination. *Hum. Reprod.* 14: 1823–6.

Brook, P. F., Barratt, C. L. & Cooke, I. D. (1994). The more accurate timing of insemination with regard to ovulation does not create a significant improvement in pregnancy rates in a donor insemination program. *Fertil. Steril.* **61**: 308–13.

Byrd, W., Bradshaw, K., Carr, B. *et al.* (1990). A prospective randomized study of pregnancy rates following intrauterine and intracervical insemination using frozen donor sperm. *Fertil. Steril.* **53**: 521–7.

Chauhan, M., Barratt, C. L., Cooke, S. M., & Cooke, I. D. (1989). Differences in the fertility of donor insemination recipients – a study to provide prognostic guidelines as to its success and outcome. *Fertil. Steril.* **51**: 815–19.

Clarke, G. (1999). Sperm cryopreservation: is there a significant risk of cross-contamination? *Hum. Reprod.* **14**: 2941–3.

Curson, R. & Karakosta, C. (2000). Recruitment of only cytomegalovirus (CMV) negative semen donors. *Hum. Reprod.* **15**: 2247–9.

Depyere, H. T., Gordts, S., Campo, R. & Comhaire, F. (1994). Methods to increase the success rate of artificial insemination with donor semen. *Hum. Reprod.* **9**: 661–3.

Ford, W. C., McLaughlin, E. A., Prior, S. M., Rees, J. M., Wardle, P. G. & Hull, M. G. (1992). The yield, motility and performance in the hamster egg test of human spermatozoa prepared from cryopreserved semen by four different methods. *Hum. Reprod.* **7**: 654–9

Giraud, M. N., Motta, C., Boucher, D. & Grizard, G. (2000). Membrane fluidity predicts the outcome of cryopreservation of human spermatozoa. *Hum. Reprod.* **15**: 2160–4.

Goldgerg, J. M., Mascha, E., Falcone, T. & Attaran, M. (1999). Comparison of intra-uterine and intra-cervical insemination with frozen donor sperm: a meta-analysis. *Fertil. Steril.* **72**: 792–5.

Grinsted, J., Jacobsen, J. D., Grinstead, L., Schantz, A., Stenfoss, H. H. & Nielsen, S. P. (1989). Prediction of ovulation. *Fertil. Steril.* **52**: 388–93.

Holt, W. V., Shenfield, F., Leonard, T. *et al.* (1989). The value of sperm swimming speed measurements in assessing the fertility of human frozen semen. *Hum. Reprod.* **4**: 292–7.

Human Fertilisation and Embryology Authority (1998). *Consultation on the Safe Cryopreservation of gametes and embryos.* London: HFEA.

Human Fertilisation and Embryology Authority (2000). *Annual Report.* London: HFEA.

Hurd, W. W., Randolph, J. F., Ansbacher, R. *et al.* (1993). Comparison of intracervical, intrauterine, and intratubal techniques for donor insemination. *Fertil. Steril.* **59**: 339–42.

Kelly, M. P., Corson, S. L., Gocial, B., Batzer, F. R. & Gutmann, J. N. (1997). Discontinuous Percoll gradient preparation for donor insemination: determinants for success. *Hum. Reprod.* **12**: 2682–6.

Kim, L. U., Johnson, M. R., Barton, S. *et al.* (1999). Evaluation of sperm washing as a potential method of reducing HIV transmission in HIV-discordant couples wishing to have children. *AIDS* **16**: 645–51.

Lashen, H., Afnan, M. & Kennefik, A. (1999). Early resort to ovarian stimulation improves the cost-effectiveness of a donor insemination programme. *Hum. Reprod.* **14**: 1983–8.

Le Lannou, D. & Lansac, J. (1993). Artificial procreation with frozen donor semen: the French experience of CECOS. In *Donor Insemination*, ed. C. L. R. Barratt & I. D. Cooke, pp. 152–69. Cambridge: Cambridge University Press.

Le Lannou, D., Gastard, E., Guivarch, A., Laurent, M. C. & Poulain, P. (1995). Strategies in frozen donor semen procreation. *Hum. Reprod.* **7**: 1765–74.

Lenton, E. A. (1993). Ovulation timing. In *Donor Insemination*, ed. C. L. R. Barratt, & I. D. Cooke, pp. 97–110. Cambridge: Cambridge University Press.

Levy, R., Tardy, J. C., Bourlet, T. et al. (2000). Transmission risk of hepatitis C virus in assisted reproductive techniques. *Hum. Reprod.* **15**: 810–16.

Liesnard, C. A., Revelard, P. & Englert, Y. (1998). Is matching between women and donors feasible to avoid cytomegalovirus infection in artificial insemination with donor semen. *Hum. Reprod.* **13**: 25–31.

Mahadevan, M. & Trounson, A. (1983). Effects of CPM and dilution methods on the preservation of human spermatozoa. *Andrologia* **15**: 355–66.

McLaughlin, E. A. (2000). Recruitment of only cytomegalovirus (CMV) negative semen donors. *Hum. Reprod.* **15**: 2247–9.

McLaughlin, E. A., Ford, W. C. L. & Hull, M. G. R. (1990). A comparison of the freezing of human semen in the uncirculated vapor above liquid nitrogen and in a commercial semi-programmable freezer. *Hum. Reprod.* **5**: 734–8.

Morris, G. J., Acton, E. & Avery, S. (1999). A novel approach to sperm cryopreservation. *Hum. Reprod.* **14**: 1013–21.

NHS Executive (1997). *Guidance Notes on the Processing, Storage and Issue of Bone Marrow and Blood Stem Cells.* London: Department of Health.

O'Brien, P. & Vandekerckhove, P. (2000). Intra-uterine versus cervical insemination of donor sperm for subfertility. *Cochrane Database Syst. Rev.* **2**: CD000317.

Ragni, G., Caccamo, A. M., Dalla Serra, A. et al. (1990). Computerized slow-stage freezing of semen from men with testicular tumours or Hodgkin's disease preserves sperm better than standard vapor freezing. *Fertil. Steril.* **53**: 1072–5.

Ragni, G., Maggioni, P., Guermandi, E. et al. (1999). Efficacy of double intrauterine insemination in controlled ovarian hyperstimulation cycles. *Fertil. Steril.* **72**: 619–22.

Ripps, B. A., Minhas, B. S., Carson, S. A. & Buster, J. E. (1994). Intrauterine insemination in fertile women delivers larger number of sperm to the peritoneal fluid than intracervical insemination. *Fertil. Steril.* **61**: 398–400.

Sakkas, D., Manicardi, G. C., Tomlinson, M., et al. (2000). The use of two density gradient centrifugation techniques and the swim-up method to separate spermatozoa with chromatin and nuclear DNA anomalies. *Hum. Reprod.* **15**: 1112–6.

Sherman, J. K. (1963). Improved methods of preservation of human spermatozoa by freezing and freeze-drying. *Fertil. Steril.* **14**: 49–64.

Storey, B. T., Noiles, E. E. & Thompson, K. A. (1998). Comparison of glycerol, other polyols, trehalose, and raffinose to provide a defined cryoprotectant medium for mouse sperm cryo-preservation. *Cryobiology* **37**: 46–58.

Tedder, R. S., Zuckerman, M. A., Goldstone, A. H. et al. (1995). Hepatitis B transmission from contaminated cryopreservation tank. *Lancet* **15**: 137–40.

Tomlinson, M. J., Barratt, C. L. R. & Cooke, I. D. (1993). Prospective study of leukocytes and leukocyte subpopulations in semen suggests they are not a cause of male infertility. *Fertil Steril.* **60**: 1069–75.

Tomlinson, M. J., Amissah-Arthur, J. B., Thompson, K. A., Kasraie, J. & Bentick, B. (1996). Prognostic indicators for IUI: Statistical model for IUI success. *Hum. Reprod.* **11**: 1892–6.

Tomlinson, M. J. & Sakkas, D. (2000). Safe and effective cryopreservation – should sperm banks and fertility centres move toward storage in nitrogen vapour. *Hum. Reprod.* **15**: 2460–3.

Wainer, R., Merlet, F., Ducot, B., Bailly, M., Tribalat, S. & Lombroso, R. (1995). Prospective randomized comparison of intrauterine and intracervical insemination with donor spermatozoa. *Hum. Reprod.* **10**: 2919–22.

World Health Organization (1999). *WHO Laboratory Manual for the Examination of Human Semen and Sperm–Cervical Mucus Interaction.* Cambridge: University of Cambridge.

5

Treatment options prior to IVF

Roger Hart[1] and Melanie Davies[2]

[1]UWA School of Women's and Infant's Health, Subiaco, Australia
[2]Reproductive Medicine Unit, Elizabeth Garrett Anderson Hospital and Obstetric Hospital, London, UK

Introduction

The treatment options that face a couple prior to IVF essentially depend upon the cause of their infertility. The surgical techniques to treat mild or moderate endometriosis will not be discussed here neither will we enter the debate of surgery (open or laparoscopic) versus IVF for distal tubal disease. This chapter will discuss the role of controlled ovarian hyperstimulation and intrauterine insemination (COH-IUI) in the management of mild male factor subfertility, endometriosis and ovulation induction in anovulatory infertility, and will concentrate on the management of unexplained subfertility.

Male factor subfertility

Severe male factor subfertility is treated by intracytoplasmic sperm injection (ICSI) after excluding carrier status for cystic fibrosis and performing a karyotype. However, the point at which a physician should advise a trial of COH-IUI prior to embarking on the more 'medicalized' procedure of IVF-ICSI is controversial. A meta-analysis of couples with male factor infertility suggested that the chance of conception with male factor subfertility is half that of other couples with other causes of subfertility after IUI – odds ratio 0.48 after stepwise logistic regression (Hughes *et al.*, 1997). In contrast a prospective randomized trial concluded that COH-IUI was equally effective in couples with male factor infertility and unexplained infertility (Goverde *et al.*, 2000). It is therefore important to define the degree of male factor subfertility because inevitably the cycle fecundity will vary according to the degree of oligoasthenozoospermia. In the prospective study of Goverde *et al.* (2000), male factor subfertility was defined in couples where three out of five semen analyses showed a total motile sperm count of less than 20 million progressively moving sperm in the ejaculate. Male factor subfertility is further

Good Clinical Practice in Assisted Reproduction, ed. P. Serhal & C. Overton.
Published by Cambridge University Press. © Cambridge University Press 2004.

confirmed if the remainder of the infertility investigations reveal no additional abnormalities and, after centrifugation and processing by Percoll gradient, a minimum of 1 million motile sperm result at least once.

To clarify the definition of male factor subfertility to produce a pragmatic approach to treatment, Van Voorhis *et al.* (2001) published a study that correlates the effect of the total motile sperm count with the outcome of assisted reproduction. In this study a logistic regression analysis was performed to elicit the significant prognostic factors in women undergoing COH-IUI who had at least one patent fallopian tube, were ovulatory and some motile sperm were present in the male partner's ejaculate. Female age, gravidity and COH were all independent factors in predicting pregnancy after IUI. The average total motile sperm count in the ejaculate was also significant with a threshold of 10 million. The woman's diagnosis of anovulation, endometriosis or tubal disease made no significant difference to the pregnancy rate. Of note was the higher pregnancy rate in cycles stimulated with human menopausal gonadotrophins (HMG) as compared to clomiphene. This study demonstrated in an American model that with a total motile sperm count of less than 10 million, IVF with ICSI is more cost effective than COH-IUI. Although with a threshold sperm count greater than 10 million that natural cycle IUI and COH-IUI with clomiphene citrate was more cost effective than IVF or COH-IUI with hMG.

This advice is in contrast to the opinion of the Cochrane Collaboration that COH-IUI with gonadotrophins should be the treatment of choice with an average total motile sperm concentration greater than 10 million. Couples with a severe male factor subfertility (at least 1 million motile sperm after preparation) should be offered natural cycle IUI Cohlen *et al.*, 2001). The Cochrane Collaboration have also reviewed the use of anti-oestrogens, tamoxifen and clomiphene citrate, for idiopathic oligo/asthenospermia and did not find enough evidence to support their use in male factor subfertility (Vandekerckhove *et al.*, 2001).

A frequent finding in a semen analysis is the presence of antisperm antibodies, usually IgA or IgG immunoglobulins, with reports of a prevalence of 10–15% in men undergoing evaluation as part of subfertility investigations (Mazumdar *et al.*, 1998). The most frequently performed investigation for the presence of antisperm antibodies is the mixed antiglobulin reaction (MAR) test. Most studies demonstrate a clear association between antisperm antibodies and male fertility potential (Ombelet *et al.*, 1997). Methods to reduce the effect of antisperm antibodies consist of the use of high doses of systemic steroids or sperm washing. The former is potentially dangerous and has a poor success rate (Mazumdar *et al.*, 1998). A cost benefit analyses performed in Belgium found that after sperm washing, 64.3% of patients conceived after up to three cycles of COH-IUI, which led the authors to suggest that this should be performed prior to IVF/ ICSI (Ombelet *et al.*, 1997).

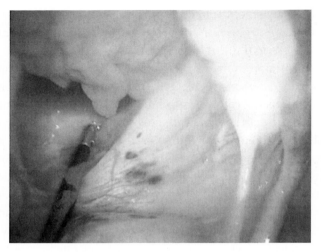

Figure 5.1.   Deposits of endometriosis on the uterosacral ligament. (See colour plate)

Endometriosis associated subfertility

Despite demonstration of tubal patency, by hysterosalpingography or by hystero-contrast-sonography, a diagnosis of unexplained infertility cannot be made without a laparoscopy to exclude the presence of pelvic adhesions or endometriosis (Figure 5.1). There is evidence that in couples with otherwise unexplained infertility, the fecundity of women with minimal and mild endometriosis is improved by laparoscopic ablation of the endometriotic deposits (Marcoux *et al.*, 1997). After treatment for endometriosis it would be reasonable to wait six months prior to further assisted reproduction techniques, which is usually COH-IUI in women under 38 years of age and IVF in women aged 38 years and above. Also women with more extensive endometriosis should be advised that the most effective treatment for them is IVF.

Prior to embarking on IVF, any endometriomas should be drained laparoscopically (Figure 5.2) and the cyst wall should be either stripped or ablated as the endometriomas may limit the response of the ovary to ovarian hyperstimulation and risk infection if punctured during oocyte retrieval (Donnez, 2001). The procedure of stripping or ablation of the endometrioma does not reduce the response to ovarian hyperstimulation (Canis *et al.*, 2001; Donnez, 2001).

COH-IUI for endometriosis should be undertaken if the patient has not conceived six months after treatment to the endometriotic deposits. Unfortunately the success rates of COH-IUI in women with endometriosis is less than in women with

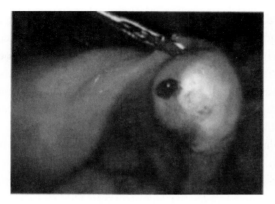

Figure 5.2.   Endometrioma rupturing. (See colour plate)

unexplained infertility. Indeed two studies, each using logistic regression analysis, demonstrate a halving of COH-IUI success rates when compared to women with unexplained infertility (Hughes, 1997; Nuojua-Huttunen *et al.*, 1999). This information must be passed onto the couple, because if they only have a 1 in 15 chance of the treatment working (Nuojua-Huttunen *et al.*, 1999) they may well be best served by early recourse to IVF treatment.

Anovulatory subfertility

The management of anovulatory infertility will not be discussed at great length here as this is not the focus of this chapter. Essentially the aim of induction of ovulation is entirely different to that of the treatment of superovulation and intrauterine insemination. In the former the purpose of treatment is to induce monofollicular ovulation in a couple with no other cause of infertility to enable a spontaneous conception, which is achievable in the majority (Messinis & Milingos, 1997). However, superovulation and IUI is performed in couples who have another cause of infertility, and where the woman is ovulating, to increase the chance of one of the oocytes being fertilized. In this situation, depending on the age of the female partner and the duration and cause of subfertility, the aim is to try to generate three or more follicles to maximize the chance of conception.

The commonest cause of anovulatory infertility is polycystic ovarian syndrome (PCOS). The other main causes are anovulation due to poor ovarian reserve and the perimenopause (this will be addressed in Chapter 6) and anovulation due to idiopathic hypogonadotrophic hypogonadism or partially recovered weight-related amenorrhoea. Idiopathic hypogonadotrophic hypogonadism or partially recovered weight-related amenorrhoea is managed initially by controlled induction of monofollicular ovulation using the GnRH pump using the subcutaneous route. This treatment starts with 15 μg per pulse every 90 minutes and monitoring the patient's progress by serial ultrasound scanning and taking measurements of serum gonadotrophin and oestradiol concentrations. If the patient does not respond, the next step is to add clomiphene citrate to the treatment, if this is unsuccessful then superovulation and IUI is commenced (Shoham et al., 1990).

A rationale for the treatment of anovulatory subfertility due to PCOS is outlined below. Initial induction of ovulation may be performed with an anti-oestrogen, such as clomiphene citrate or tamoxifen, which displaces oestrogen from pituitary receptors preventing negative feedback control over FSH (follicle stimulating hormone) production. Consequently there is an initial surge in FSH at a critical time of follicular recruitment leading to follicular maturation. Women undergoing clomiphene induction of ovulation should have ultrasound follicular tracking done to ensure that a response is being achieved and also to ensure that ovarian hyperstimulation has not occurred. To ensure follicular rupture, clomiphene induction of ovulation can be combined with human chorionic gonadotrophin (HCG) administration. Ovulation induction can also be combined with IUI after HCG administration. Clomiphene induction of ovulation is normally started at a dose of 50 mg beginning on the second and continuing through to the sixth day of the menstrual cycle. Subsequent doses may be increased to 150 mg per day. However, a woman who fails to ovulate on increasing doses of clomiphene is referred to as 'clomiphene resistant'. Overall success in achieving ovulation is approximately 80%, with pregnancy rates of approximately 35% (Tan et al., 2001). The usual second line of treatment is to progress to the use of gonadotrophins. However, the recent use of insulin sensitizing agents in hyperinsulinaemic women has provided another therapeutic strategy in the management of women with PCOS (Velazquez et al., 1994). Indeed the combination of metformin with clomiphene in women with an impaired glucose tolerance test who were clomiphene resistant led to ovulation in 90% of women compared to 8% of a control group of clomiphene-resistant women with impaired glucose tolerance who received only clomiphene (Nestler et al., 1998).

Women who fail to ovulate with clomiphene can be treated with gonadotrophins. Due to the risk of multiple follicular development in women with PCOS, ovarian hyperstimulation syndrome stimulation should commence with a low dose of FSH and careful ultrasound follicular tracking should be performed. A Cochrane review of the use of urinary FSH compared with human menopausal gonadotrophin (HMG) demonstrated no difference in the pregnancy rates in women with PCOS (Hughes et al., 2001). This is despite the theoretical advantage of the absence of LH in the urinary FSH preparation.

If a woman with PCOS is resistant to induction of ovulation with gonadotrophins then she may well be advised to undergo ovarian drilling, either by electrosurgical diathermy, laser or by ultrasound guided follicular aspiration (Hart & Magos, 1997). The aim of all these therapeutic strategies is to cause a degree of damage to the ovarian stroma. Balen & Jacobs (1994) suggested that the damage corrects an abnormal ovarian–pituitary feedback by a cascade of local growth factors that interact with FSH, resulting in stimulation of follicular growth and production of a 'gonadotrophin surge attenuating or inhibiting factor' leading to a fall in LH. The success rate of ovarian drilling at inducing ovulation is between 70% and 90%, with a 60% chance of conception without the necessity for intensive monitoring and the risk of a multiple pregnancy (Hart & Magos, 1997; Tan *et al.*, 2001). However, it should be borne in mind that that the procedure of ovarian drilling may potentially cause periovarian adhesions, up to 35% in one series, which could limit oocyte pick-up (Naether, 1995).

Cervical factor subfertility

Natural cycle IUI, or superovulation and IUI, can be used in women to overcome a suspected cervical cause of infertility. This diagnosis can be made after a post-coital test, however this is a test that is now infrequently performed as a routine investigation and indeed is not recommended by The Royal College of Obstetricians and Gynaecologists (RCOG) in their protocol for investigation of the subfertile couple (RCOG, 1998).

Unexplained infertility

Unexplained infertility is a diagnosis of exclusion, which is reported to occur in up to 60% of couples (Templeton & Penney, 1982), but with the application of stricter diagnostic criteria it is usually quoted to have a prevalence of around 25%. To lead to a diagnosis of unexplained infertility, the male partner's semen analysis must fulfil the WHO criteria of at least 20 million/ml, with a forward motility of 30% and normal morphology in 50% (WHO, 1992), although many units impose their own reference ranges. The female partner must have at least two midluteal phase progesterone measurements consistent with ovulation. However, the level at which ovulation can be inferred is disputed. Most units take a progesterone reading of at least 25 nmol/litre as indicative of ovulation. If this is combined with follicular tracking demonstrating a corpus luteum then ovulation is confirmed. Although a woman may be ovulating on a regular basis, her oocyte quality may be poor as expressed by her 'ovarian reserve'. A woman with an impaired ovarian reserve, whether expressed by a high follicular phase FSH, or a poor response to a clomiphene challenge test (Bukman & Heineman, 2001) or 'G-test' (Ranieri *et al.*, 2001) may well be best served by early referral for IVF or GIFT (gamete intrafallopian transfer) treatment rather than proceeding to superovulation and IUI treatment where the results in these women are very poor. To exclude a tubal factor as the aetiology of the couple's subfertility, a test of the patency of the fallopian tubes is mandatory. This can be performed either by hysterosalpingography or by hystero-contrast-sonography but is best performed at the time of a diagnostic laparoscopy by dye hydrotubation. The reason for performing a pelvic assessment by laparoscopy is to exclude any periovarian adhesions which may impair oocyte pick-up, and to exclude the presence of endometriosis which may not have been apparent on initial history or examination. The division of adhesions and the treatment of minor degrees of endometriosis will improve fecundity, as discussed previously. At the time of laparoscopy it is usual to perform a hysteroscopy to exclude the presence of an intrauterine lesion, polyp, submucous fibroid or intrauterine adhesions, all of which may reduce a couples chance to conceive. These lesions can also be identified by hysterosalpingography or hystero-contrast-sonography.

Once the diagnosis of unexplained infertility has been reached then a pragmatic approach to the management of the couple should be instituted. A woman of 40 years or older should undoubtedly be referred for IVF treatment as the chance of success per cycle of superovulation and IUI is so poor, around 5–7% (Sahakyan *et al.*, 1999; Goverde *et al.*, 2000) (Figures 5.3 and 5.4). Indeed many clinicians would advocate IVF as the more pragmatic option as compared to superovulation and IUI in a couple where the female partner is aged 38 years or over.

Many couples with unexplained infertility will each month enquire as to their chance of conceiving, as they optimistically expect that as no obvious cause for their infertility has been determined then they have a reasonable chance of spontaneous conception. However, the evidence is to the contrary; in a meta-analysis of the literature Guzick *et al.* (1998) produced a figure between 1.3 % and 4.1% for cycle fecundity by expectant management in a couple with at least one year of unexplained infertility. Collins *et al.* (1991) also observed the cycle fecundity in couples without intervention and found that couples with unexplained infertility have a cumulative three-year live birth rate without treatment of 33.3%. However, if a couple have been attempting to conceive for over three years with unexplained infertility and are over 30 years of age, their chance of conceiving spontaneously in the next year is only 14.3%. Consequently, to maximize the chance of a couple conceiving, superovulation and IUI is performed. Collins analysed the effect of IUI alone at improving fecundity but the relative risk of conception was 1.1 when compared to expectant management alone suggesting that it is the combination of superovulation with IUI that is important (Collins *et al.*, 1991, 1995).

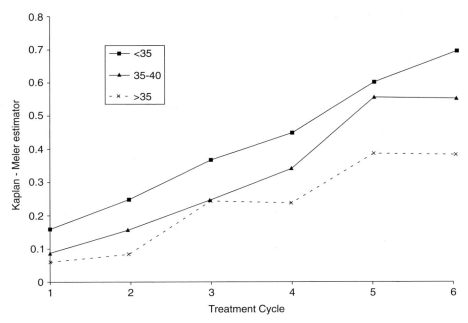

Figure 5.3.   Influence of age on pregnancy rates with gonadotropin-induced controlled ovarian hyper-stimulation and intrauterine insemination (Sahakyan *et al.*, 1999). (Reproduced with kind permission of Elsevier Science Inc, USA. Copyright © 1999 American Society for Reproductive Medicine.)

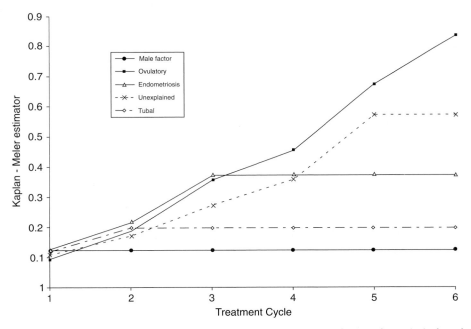

Figure 5.4.   Influence of diagnosis and cycle number on pregnancy rates with gonadotropin-induced controlled ovarian hyperstimulation and intrauterine insemination (Sahakyan *et al.*, 1999). (Reproduced with kind permission of Elsevier Science Inc, USA. Copyright © 1999 American Society for Reproductive Medicine.)

Controlled superovulation and IUI

The aim of this treatment is to generate three follicles by ovarian stimulation and to trigger the release of the follicles by HCG and to perform intrauterine insemination 36 hours later with washed prepared semen. There is evidence that performing two inseminations increases the likelihood of conception (Ragni *et al.*, 1999). It is imperative that treatment is monitored by serial vaginal ultrasound examination to ensure that an ovarian response is achieved and that multiple follicular development has not occurred with the consequent risk of multiple pregnancy and ovarian hyperstimulation syndrome.

The simplest, least invasive and cheapest regime for superovulation and IUI is the use of clomiphene citrate. In a meta-analysis of randomized controlled trials of the use of clomiphene citrate as opposed to no intervention in women with unexplained infertility the odds ratio for clinical pregnancy per cycle was 2.5 (Hughes *et al.*, 2001). Zayed & Abu-Heja (1999) reviewed the use of clomiphene citrate and IUI in couples with unexplained subfertility and derived a cycle fecundity rate of about 10%. The reported side-effects of clomiphene consist of vasomotor flushes in 10% of women and rarely, visual disturbances are reported. The risk of a multiple gestation is approximately 10% overall.

Another potential drug that can be used for ovulation induction and super-ovulation is letrazole, an aromatase inhibitor which reduces the conversion of androgens to oestogens, consequently diminishing the negative feedback on the pituitary and hypothalamus. This leads to an increase in FSH production without the anti-oestrogenic effects on the endometrium of clomiphene leading to follicular development. Sammour *et al.* (2001) and Mitwally & Casper (2002) suggest that letrazole is a promising new therapeutic option with results at least as good as that achieved with clomiphene with a trend towards an increased pregnancy rate.

The next therapeutic option is to use gonadotrophins. It is more expensive than clomiphene citrate, with a greater risk of multiple gestation and ovarian hyperstim-ulation syndrome. Gonadotrophins are usually used in conjunction with HCG and IUI. A meta-analysis of 45 studies demonstrated that the addition of the IUI leads to a significant increase in the pregnancy rate and is also more cost effective after unsuccessful attempts with clomiphene and IUI (Guzick *et al.*, 1998). There are many different regimes used to effect superovulation. All aim to commence ovar-ian stimulation in a woman between the second and fourth day of her menstrual cycle after exclusion of any residual ovarian cysts. Stimulation continues either on a daily or alternate day regime with serial vaginal ultrasound examination to exclude multifollicular development. When three follicles are greater than 18 mm in size, HCG is injected to initiate ovulation. As mentioned previously IUI should ideally be performed on two occasions subsequent to HCG injection after 12 and 36 hours.

One of the largest series of COH-IUI was reported by Stone *et al.* (1999), which included 9963 consecutive cycles. This series included all diagnoses of subfertility, COH was performed by either clomiphene or gonadotrophins with IUI performed the day following a positive LH test kit had suggested that ovulation had occurred. The patient's age was the single most significant determinant of the likelihood of pregnancy in this study. Pregnancy rates begin to decline after the age of 37 years, once one or two follicles are obtained, pregnancy rates tend to plateau. Therefore, once at least two follicles are obtained, further increase in drug dose does not seem to be indicated (Stone *et al.*, 1999).

REFERENCES

Balen, A. H. & Jacobs, H. S. (1994). A prospective study comparing unilateral and bilateral laparoscopic ovarian diathermy in women with polycystic ovary syndrome. *Fertil. Steril.* **62**: 921–5.

Bukman, A. & Heineman, M. J. (2001). Ovarian reserve testing and the use of prognostic models in patients with subfertility. *Hum. Reprod. Update* **7**: 581–90.

Canis, M., Pouly, J. L., Tamburro, S., Mage, G., Wattiez, A. & Bruhat, M. A. (2001). Ovarian response during IVF–embryo transfer cycles after laparoscopic ovarian cystectomy for endometriotic cysts of >3 cm in diameter. *Hum. Reprod.* **16**: 2583–6.

Cohlen, B. J., Vandekerckhove, P., te Velde, E. R. & Habbema, J. D. F. (2001). Timed intercourse versus intra-uterine insemination with or without ovarian hyperstimulation for subfertility in men (Cochrane Review). In *The Cochrane Library*, vol. 4. Oxford: Update Software.

Collins, J., Burrows, E. A. & Willan, A. R. (1995). The prognosis for livebirth among untreated infertile couples. *Fertil. Steril.* **64**: 22–8.

Collins, J. A., Milner, R. A. & Rowe, T. C. (1991). The effect of treatment on pregnancy among couples with unexplained infertility. *Int. J. Fertil.* **36**: 140–52.

Donnez, J., Wyns, C. & Nisolle, M. (2001). Does ovarian surgery for endometriomas impair the ovarian response to gonadotropin? *Fertil. Steril.* **76**: 662–5.

Goverde, A. J., McDonnell, J., Vermeiden, J. P. W., Schats, R., Rutten, F. F. H., & Schoemaker, J. (2000). Intrauterine insemination or in-vitro fertilisation in idiopathic subfertility and male subfertility: a randomised trial and cost-effectiveness analysis. *Lancet* **355**: 12–18.

Guzick, D. S., Sullivan, M. W., Adamson, G. D., Cedars, M. I., Falk, R. J., Peterson, E. P. & Steinkampf, M. P. (1998). Efficacy of treatment for unexplained infertility. *Fertil. Steril.* **70**: 207–31.

Hart, R. & Magos, A. (1997). The ovary. *Semin. Laparosc. Surg.* **4**: 210–18.

Hughes, E. G. (1997). The effectiveness of ovulation induction and intrauterine insemination in the treatment of persistent infertility: meta-analysis. *Hum. Reprod.* **12**: 1865–72.

Hughes, E., Collins, J. & Vandekerckhove, P. (2001). Clomiphene citrate for unexplained subfertility in women (Cochrane review). In *The Cochrane Library*, vol. 4. Oxford: Update Software.

Marcoux, S., Maheux, R., Berube, S. & Canadian Collaborative Group on Endometriosis (1997). Laparoscopic surgery in infertile women with minimal or mild endometriosis. *N. Engl. J. Med.* **337**: 217–22.

Mazumdar, S. & Levine, A. S. (1998). Antisperm antibodies: etiology, pathogenesis, diagnosis, and treatment. *Fertil. Steril.* **70**: 799–810.

Messinis, I. E., Milingos, S. D. (1997). Current and future status of ovulation induction in polycystic ovarian syndrome. *Hum. Reprod. Update* **3**: 235–53.

Mitawally, M. F. & Casper, R. F. (2002). Armatase inhibition for ovarian stimulation: future avenues for infertility management. *Curr. Opin. Obstet. Gynecol.* **14**: 255–63.

Naether, O. G. F. (1995). Significant reduction in incidence of adnexal adhesions following ovarian electrocautery by lavage and artificial ascites. *Gynaecol. Endosc.* **4**: 17–19.

Nestler, J., Jakubowicz, D. J., Evans, W. S. & Pasquali, R. (1998). Effects of metformin on spontaneous and clomiphene-induced ovulation in the polycystic ovary syndrome. *N. Engl. J. Med.* **338**: 1876–80.

Nuojua-Huttunen, S., Tomas, C., Bloigu, R., Tuomivaara, L., Martikainen H. (1999). *Hum. Reprod.* **14**: 698–703.

Ombelet, W., Vandeput, H., Janssen, M., Cox, A., Vossen, C., Pollet, H., Steeno O. & Bosmans, E. (1997). Treatment of male infertility due to sperm surface antibodies: IUI or IVF. *Hum. Reprod.* **12**: 1165–70.

Ragni, G., Maggioni, P., Guermandi, E., Testa, A., Baroni, E., Colombo, M. & Crosignani, P. G. (1999). Efficacy of double intrauterine insemination in controlled ovarian hyperstimulation cycles. *Fertil. Steril.* **72**: 619–22.

Ranieri, D. M., Phophong, P., Khadum, I., Meo, F., Davis, C. & Serhal, P. (2001). Simultaneous evaluation of basal FSH and oestradiol response to GnRH analogue (F-G-test) allows effective drug regimen selection for IVF. *Hum. Reprod.* **16**: 673–5.

Royal College of Obstetricians and Gynaecologists (1998). *Evidence Based Guidelines. The Investigation and Management of the Infertile Couple.* London: RGOG Press.

Sahakyan, M., Harlow, B. L. & Hornstein, M. D. (1991). Influence of age, diagnosis, and cycle number on pregnancy rates with gonadotrophin-induced controlled ovarian hyperstimulation and intrauterine insemination. *Fertil. Steril.* **72**: 500–4.

Sammour, A., Biljan, M. M., Tan, S. L. & Tulandi, T. (2001). Prospective randomized trial comparing the effects of letrazole (LE) and clomiphene citrate (CC) on follicular development, endometrial thickness and pregnancy rate in patients undergoing super-ovulation prior to intrauterine insemination (IUI). *Fertil. Steril.* **76** (Suppl 1): S110.

Shoham, Z., Homburg, R. & Jacobs, H. S. (1990). Induction of ovulation with pulsatile GnRH. *Baillières Clin. Obstet. Gynaecol.* **4**: 589–608.

Stone, B. A., Vargas, J. M., Ringler, G. E., Stein, A. L. & Marrs, R. P. (1999). Determinants of the outcome of intrauterine insemination: Analysis of outcomes of 9963 consecutive cycles. *Am. J. Obstet. Gynecol.* **180**: 1522–34.

Tan, W. C., Yap, C. & Tan, A. S. A. (2001). Clinical management of PCOS. *Acta Obstet. Gynecol. Scand.* **80**: 689–96.

Templeton, A. A. & Penney, G. C. (1982). The incidence, characteristics, and prognosis of patients whose infertility is unexplained. *Fertil. Steril.* **37**: 175–82.

Vandekerckhove, P., Lilford, R., Vail, A. & Hughes, E. (2001). Clomiphene or tamoxifen for idiopathic oligo/asthenospermia (Cochrane Review). In *The Cochrane Library*, vol. 4. Oxford: Update Software.

Van Voorhis, B.J., Barnett, M.R., Sparks, A.E.T., Syrop, C.H., Rosenthal, G. & Dawson, J. (2001). Effect of the total motile sperm count on the efficacy and cost-effectiveness of intrauterine insemination and in vitro fertilization. *Fertil. Steril.* **75**: 661–8.

Velazquez, E. M., Mendoza, S., Hamer, T., Sosa, F. & Glueck, C. J. (1994). Metformin therapy in polycystic ovary syndrome reduces hyperinsulinemia, insulin resistance, hyperandrogenemia, and systolic blood pressure, while facilitating normal menses and pregnancy. *Metabolism* **43**: 647–54.

World Health Organization (1992). Collection and examination of human sperm. In *WHO Laboratory Manual for the Examination of Human Semen and Sperm–Cervical Mucus Interaction*, 3rd ed., pp. 3–20. Cambridge: Cambridge University Press.

Zayed, F. & Abu-Heja, A. (1999). The management of unexplained infertility. *Obstet. Gynecol. Surv.* **54**: 263–72.

6

Strategies for superovulation for IVF

Adam Balen

Department of Reproductive Medicine, Leeds General Infirmary, Leeds, UK

Introduction

The primary aim of an IVF treatment cycle is the creation of two 'good quality' pre-embryos for transfer, with a secondary aim of additional embryos for cryo-preservation. Because of the need for sufficient oocytes for fertilization, and embryos for selection, it is necessary to stimulate sufficient follicles to generate an adequate number of mature oocytes. Recent advances towards the transfer of one or two blastocysts for transfer, sometimes after blastomere biopsy and aneuploidy screening, also requires a sufficient number of oocytes for fertilization.

Primordial follicle recruitment is determined by factors that are still to be fully determined and is independent of follicle stimulating hormone (FSH) stimulation. In a given cycle an individual woman has a certain number of follicles that will be sensitive to FSH – the main determinants being a combination of her chronological age and ovarian age ('ovarian reserve'). There are a number of tests of ovarian reserve, which may be used singly or in combination to predict ovarian response and gonadotrophin dosage: baseline serum concentrations (FSH, inhibin, oestradiol), ovarian stimulation/challenge tests and ultrasonography (ovarian volume, primordial follicle number and blood flow).

There are a large number of regimens for superovulation in IVF protocols. The evolution of superovulation strategies has encompassed the development of new classes of drugs and has lead to improved efficiency of the treatment cycle. This chapter will outline the current options, concentrating on evidence for clinical effectiveness. Complications of treatment, such as ovarian hyperstimulation syndrome (OHSS), are dealt with elsewhere in this book.

Good Clinical Practice in Assisted Reproduction, ed. P. Serhal & C. Overton.
Published by Cambridge University Press. © Cambridge University Press 2004.

Overview of superovulation regimens

The first regimens used gonadotrophins either alone or combined with clomiphene citrate (CC) – this required careful monitoring in order to predict and prevent the occurrence of an endogenous preovulatory LH (luteinizing hormone) surge. There was a cancellation rate of 15–20% as oocyte retrieval has to be performed 26–28 hours after the detection of the endogenous surge and this often meant that oocyte collections were performed at night and at weekends. The use of gonadotrophin releasing hormone (GnRH) agonists with gonadotrophins has resulted in greater ease of planning the superovulation stimulation. When GnRH agonists are used the oocyte retrieval can be precisely timed to occur 34–38 hours after the administration of human chorionic gonadotrophins (HCG). This acts as a surrogate for the normal mid-cycle LH surge and causes resumption of meiosis within the oocytes and their preparation for fertilization. Furthermore, there is good evidence that the oocytes do not become overmature within follicles that are considered to be ready for collection and so the administration of HCG can be delayed to avoid oocyte collection at weekends. This is advantageous for the clinic staff and does not seem to affect success rates, which, if anything, appear to be better when GnRH agonists are used. Furthermore, the rates of miscarriage, especially in patients with polycystic ovaries, are reduced when GnRH agonists are used.

A disadvantage of the use of GnRH agonists is the two weeks or more lead in to the therapy during which pituitary desensitization ('downregulation') is achieved before stimulation with gonadotrophins can be commenced. Furthermore, some clinics use the combined oral contraceptive pill prior to the GnRH agonist to help further with the programming of the cycle. Pituitary desensitization is assessed by a combination of endometrial shedding and low serum concentrations of oestradiol and LH (although ultrasound confirmation of a thin endometrium and quiescent ovaries is probably adequate). The side effects experienced during desensitization are those of oestrogen deficiency.

The GnRH agonists can be administered intranasally, subcutaneously or intramuscularly (by depot in some instances). The shorter acting preparations can be used to induce a 'flare' response, being commenced on day 1 of the cycle, with gonadotrophin stimulation starting the following day. The agonist is then either continued through to the day of HCG administration (the 'short protocol') (Tan *et al.*, 1992) or given for three days only (the 'ultrashort protocol') (Macnamee *et al.*, 1989). The flare response can be used in those patients who have had a poor response in the past in order to try to maximize the response to stimulation – this it does to varying degrees and there is a paucity of supportive data for this approach. It is, in fact, difficult to predict an individual's response to stimulation: young women and those with polycystic ovaries tend to respond well, whilst older patients and those with elevated baseline serum concentrations of FSH (>10 iu/l on most assays) respond less well.

The advent of the third-generation GnRH *antagonists* now allows us to dispense with pituitary desensitization and commence ovarian stimulation on day 2, with the administration of the antagonist from about days 6–7, which will prevent an endogenous LH surge and allow oocyte retrieval at the desired time. The use of GnRH antagonists may also reduce the total requirements for gonadotrophins and negate any need for luteal support.

Gonadotrophin therapy for the stimulation of superovulation can be with either human menopausal gonadotrophins (HMG), which contain urinary-derived FSH and LH in differing proportions depending on the preparation, or with urinary-derived FSH alone, which is available for administration subcutaneously because of its higher purity. The advent of the recombinantly derived gonadotrophins has resulted in a nonhuman source, which aesthetically is more acceptable with current concerns about prion diseases (although transmission in human urine has not been demonstrated), and also the suggestion of greater 'potency' – although the debate about cost effectiveness continues. The use of recombinant LH will provide a more physiological surrogate for the LH surge and, with a shorter half-life than HCG, should theoretically reduce the risk of OHSS.

Monitoring therapy

Monitoring of the ovarian response to superovulation can be achieved by ultra-sonography alone. From about day 8 of stimulation, the dimensions of the growing follicles are plotted either daily or every other day, together with a measurement of endometrial thickness. The daily measurement of serum oestradiol concentrations is little help in the prediction of either success or the OHSS. Furthermore, serum oestradiol concentrations appear to be proportional to the amount of LH in the gonadotrophin preparation used in the stimulation regimen. When FSH alone is used to stimulate the ovaries, the serum oestradiol concentration is approximately half of the level found when HMG is used in the 'long protocol'. The preovulatory HCG 'trigger' is usually administered when the leading follicle is at least 17–18 mm in mean diameter and there are at least three follicles >16 mm.

Evolution of the use of GnRH agonists

The move towards pituitary desensitization with a GnRH agonist (Porter *et al.*, 1984) has become almost universal in assisted conception clinics. The reversible hypogonadotrophic hypogonadism so produced permits unimpeded control over follicular development (Fleming *et al.*, 1985). As with many aspects of current

Table 6.1. Gonadotrophin releasing hormone agonist preparations

	Trade name	Structure	Relative potency	Route
Native GnRH	–	Glu.His.Trp.Ser.Tyr.Gly.Leu.Arg.Pro.Gly.NH	1	
Buserelin	Suprecur	Glu.His.Trp.Ser.Tyr.**D-Ser9.t(But)**.Leu.Arg.Pro.**EA**	100	nasal spray subcutaneous
	Suprefact		100	
Nafarelin	Synarel	Glu.His.Trp.Ser.Tyr.**D-Nal(2)**.Leu.Arg.Pro.Gly.NH	100	nasal spray
Triptorelin	Decapeptyl	Glu.His.Trp.Ser.Tyr.**D.Trp**.Leu.Arg.Pro.Gly.NH	100	i.m. depot
Goserelin	Zoladex	Glu.His.Trp.Ser.Tyr**D.Ser.(+But)**.Leu.Arg.Pro.**Aza**.Gly.NH	50	s.c. depot
Leuprorelin	Prostap	Glu.His.Trp.Ser.Tyr.**D.Leu**.Leu.Arg.Pro.**EA**	50	s.c./i.m. depot

clinical practice, the evidence on which our therapy is based relies upon data from small trials. Furthermore, different preparations, criteria for treatment and protocols have been used making the comparison of studies difficult. This has lead to the use of meta-analysis of studies in order to provide firmer conclusions. An early meta-analysis indicated that cycle cancellation rates had decreased and clinical pregnancy rates increased since the introduction of the 'long' protocol of pituitary desensitization (Hughes *et al.*, 1992). Ten studies were included in this analysis, with 914 agonist/gonadotrophin cycles compared against 722 with clomiphene citrate and gonadotrophins. The clinical pregnancy rates per cycle started were significantly greater with agonist treatment with an odds ratio for IVF of 1.8 (95% CI, 1.33–2.44) and for gamete intrafallopian transfer (GIFT) 2.37 (95% CI, 1.24–4.51). There were fewer cancelled cycles (odds ratio 0.33, 95% CI, 0.25–0.44) and more oocytes collected (odds ratio 1.5, 95% CI, 1.18–1.87). There was also a greater gonadotrophin requirement by approximately 12 ampoules per cycle (in the days when an ampoule was universally 75 iu) and a trend towards a higher rate of ovarian hyperstimulation syndrome with agonist use (Hughes *et al.*, 1992). A more recent analysis of the different types of agonist regimen has been published in the Cochrane database in which 26 trials met the inclusion criteria (Daya, 1999), data from which will be discussed below.

The different GnRH agonist preparations (Table 6.1) differ in their formulation, potency and route of administration. Once pituitary desensitization has been achieved the dose can be reduced during the period of gonadotrophin stimulation. The longer acting preparations produce a more profound desensitization and therefore require a greater dose of ovarian stimulation (Hazout *et al.*, 1993). The choice of preparation should be based on ease and frequency of administration, cost and clinical efficacy. A comparative study of buserelin, triptorelin and leuprorelin indicated that there were similar numbers of oocytes collected and similar pregnancy rates with the three preparations (Tarlatzis *et al.*, 1994). Nafarelin has been found to achieve pituitary desensitization more quickly and require a lower dose of ovarian stimulation than leuprorelin, triptorelin (Tanos *et al.*, 1995) and buserelin (Lockwood *et al.*, 1995) respectively.

Short and long protocols

The short and ultrashort protocols have already been discussed earlier.

However, the 'long' protocol relies upon pituitary desensitization, which usually takes between 10 and 14 days to achieve. The GnRH agonist is commenced in either the mid-luteal or follicular phase of the cycle and continued through to the day of HCG. After pituitary desensitization has been achieved the dose of agonist can be reduced and the gonadotrophin stimulation commenced concurrently. The long protocol has the advantage of suppressing serum LH levels during the IVF cycle and allows the greatest flexibility with respect to throughput of patients through the clinic and timing of oocyte collections. The disadvantages are the time taken to achieve desensitization, which increases the length of the treatment cycle, the potential for profound desensitization requiring an increased dose of stimulation and the possibility of ovarian cyst formation.

Luteal versus follicular phase start

Comparisons have been performed between a follicular and luteal phase for a long protocol. The beginning of the follicular phase is easier to define for the patient and clinic, and there is virtually no risk that the patient is pregnant. The flare effect might, however, result in development of a 'functional' cyst and has been thought by some to have a detrimental effect on endometrial development. It has been suggested that a luteal phase start allows gonadotrophin stimulation to commence after the ensuing menstrual bleed and subsequent endometrial development might be more synchronous. A day 21, or mid-luteal start, also carries the risk of rescuing a corpus luteum and subsequent cyst formation. Functional ovarian cysts have been encountered with GnRH agonist use in at least 5% of IVF cycles; their incidence is higher if the agonist is commenced in the follicular phase compared with the luteal phase of the menstrual cycle (Jenkins 1996). The pre-treatment administration of either a progesterone preparation or the oral contraceptive pill helps to reduce the development of agonist-induced cysts. There is also the possibility of exposure of an early pregnancy to the agonist when started in the luteal phase. Whilst there is no evidence that this causes harm in humans (Fleming *et al.*, 1996) such a situation was observed in almost 4% of cases in one study (Ron-El et al., 1990) and in 2.5% of cycles of another (Gonen et al., 1996).

There have been a number of comparative studies of the timing of the 'long' protocol. It has been shown in one, small study that initiation of agonist administration in the *early* luteal phase results in the development of significantly fewer follicles than in the follicular or mid-luteal to late luteal phases (Pellicer et al., 1989). Larger studies have failed to demonstrate such a difference and usually use a mid-luteal start compared with a follicular start. No significant differences were reported in the study of Kondaveeti et al. (1996). Whilst in another two studies the mid-luteal start was favoured with a quicker time to desensitization (Ron-El et al., 1990) and in the largest study to date a greater pregnancy rate (37% versus 14% per embryo transfer, $P = 0.004$) (Urbancsek & Witthaus, 1996).

Comparison of the long and short protocols

In a study that used life-table analysis to calculate cumulative conception rates (CCR) and cumulative livebirth rates (CLBR) in relation to ovarian stimulation regimen in 2893 women, we found that the long protocol was significantly better (Tan et al., 1994). After three cycles of treatment the CCR and CLBR with the long regimen were 59% and 55% respectively, compared with the use of HMG or FSH $\pm$ CC in which they were 39% and 29% respectively ($P = 0.001$ and $P = 0.0001$). The miscarriage rates were also lower with the long protocol (22.4% compared with 33.3%, $P = 0.03$). A multiple logistic regression analysis was used to account for possible confounding factors. The long protocol was also significantly better than the ultrashort and short regimens, although in the absence of prospective randomization it is not possible to draw firm conclusions about efficacy as the 'flare' regimens tended to be selected for patients expected to be 'poor responders' (Tan et al., 1994).

Twenty-six trials met the inclusion criteria for the Cochrane meta-analysis (Daya, 1999). In four trials, the ultrashort agonist protocol was compared with the long protocol (Check et al., 1992; Chen et al., 1992; Kingsland et al., 1992; Marcus et al., 1993). The remaining 22 trials compared the short and long GnRH agonist protocols. There were six trials using the long follicular regimen (Foulot et al., 1988; Frydman et al., 1988; Hedon et al., 1988; Acharya et al., 1992; Tan et al., 1992; Hazout et al., 1993) and 14 trials in which the long luteal regimen was used (Fenichel et al., 1988; Loumaye et al., 1989; Remorgida et al., 1989 (the only trial using GIFT); Berg van de-Helder et al., 1990; Maroulis et al., 1991; Padilla et al., 1991; DePlacido et al., 1991; San Roman et al., 1992, Buvat et al., 1991; Zaki et al., 1994; Tasdemir et al., 1995; Suganuma et al., 1996). In two trials (Dirnfield et al., 1991; Yang et al., 1996) the short protocol was compared with the long protocol, which included follicular phase administration of GnRH agonist in some patients and luteal phase administration in others.

The common odds ratio for clinical pregnancy *per cycle started* was 1.32 (95% CI, 1.10–1.57) in favour of the long GnRH agonist protocol. The studies were subgrouped, depending on whether, in the long protocol, the agonist was commenced in the follicular phase (eight trials) or luteal phase (16 trials). The respective odds ratios were 1.54 (95% CI, 1.11–2.13) and 1.21 (95% CI, 0.98–1.51). After excluding the four trials using the ultrashort protocol, the odds ratio for long versus short protocols (22 trials) was 1.27 (95% CI, 1.04–1.56). A comparison of long versus ultrashort protocols (four trials) produced an odds ratio of 1.47 (95% CI, 1.02–2.12). Thus on the basis of clinical pregnancy rate per cycle started, the meta-analysis demonstrated the superiority of the long protocol over the short and ultrashort protocols for GnRH agonist use in IVF and GIFT cycles (Daya, 1999). With respect to clinical pregnancy per oocyte retrieval the overall odds ratio was 1.32 (95% CI, 1.09–1.60) and similarly per embryo transfer the overall odds ratio was 1.31 (95% CI, 1.03–1.67) in favour of the long protocol over the short and ultrashort protocols.

Daya (1999) states that except for the trials of Hedon *et al.* (1988) and Tasdemir *et al.*, (1995), the individual trials showed no statistically significant differences between the long and short or ultrashort protocols. In general, the direction of the treatment effect was in favour of the long protocol, except in seven trials (Fenichel *et al.*, 1988; Foulot *et al.*, 1988; Berg van de-Helder *et al.*, 1990; Maroulis *et al.*, 1991; Buvat *et al.*, 1991; Suganuma *et al.*, 1996; Yang *et al.*, 1996), in which the short protocol was favoured. The sample size varied across the trials from 18 in the smallest trial to 320 in the largest, with a median sample size of 91. It is important to note that to detect with 80% power an improvement in clinical pregnancy of 5% from a control rate of 20%, with a probability level of 0.05, a sample size of 2188 would be required. Thus, none of the trials were designed to test adequately the null hypothesis of no difference in pregnancy rates between the different protocols.

Data of the average number of ampoules of gonadotrophin used were available in 20 trials. The weighted mean difference in the amount of gonadotrophin used was 8.1 (95% CI, 7.4–8.9) ampoules more for the long protocol compared with the short and ultrashort protocols. This difference might have been expected as the 'flare' effect in the short protocols uses endogenous FSH to aid in the stimulation of the ovaries.

The benefits of the long protocols suggests that the environment in which follicular development is taking place is suboptimal during short protocols, either because of inadequate suppression of LH (Filicori *et al.*, 1996), or of other pituitary or ovarian factors. This may be of particular relevance for patients with polycystic ovaries, even if they do not have the polycystic ovary syndrome per se. The use of the 'flare' effect in short protocols has been advocated for 'poor responders', older patients or those with elevated baseline FSH concentrations (Dirnfield *et al.*, 1991; Acharya *et al.*, 1992). Whilst short protocols may have a role to play in this group of patients there is still no consensus on the best approach for the 'poor responder'.

In summary, the use of a GnRH agonist to achieve pituitary desensitization has become popular in IVF clinics because of the flexibility in programming oocyte recovery. There has been debate as to whether the improved pregnancy rates observed by some clinics are seen consistently, although the meta-analysis of Hughes *et al.* (1992) does provide strong evidence of benefit. Of the different agonist regimens, those that achieve pituitary desensitization produce the best pregnancy rates (Daya, 1999). The luteal phase commencement of GnRH agonist is probably more advantageous than starting in the follicular phase.

Gonadotrophin antagonists

Modifications of the GnRH decapeptide have enabled the development of competitive inhibitors of gonadotrophin secretion, which enable a significant shortening of the stimulation regimen. Thus the protocol is not only free of the side effects of hypo-oestrogenism but is also completed within 10 days to hCG. Stimulation with gonadotrophins commences on day 2 with the antagonist being started on day 6 of stimulation, or when the leading follicle has reached a mean diameter of 14 mm (before which an LH surge is extremely unlikely to occur) (Ganirelix Dose-Finding Study Group, 1998).

Gonadotrophin preparations

The purification of post-menopausal urine, which was pioneered in Italy in the late 1940s, resulted in the production of HMG, which for many years was the sole gonadotrophin product available for ovarian stimulation. Up to 20–30 l of post-menopausal urine are required to treat one patient with one cycle of HMG. Through the 1960s the extraction process to remove non-specific co-purified proteins became more sophisticated such that activity was increased tenfold over the early preparations to 100–150 iu FSH/mg protein.

The clinical importance of the relative amounts of the two pituitary gonadotrophins was appreciated as early as 1932, but it was not until 1966 that LH was successfully removed from HMG. The eluate was more than 99% devoid of LH activity but still contained high levels of non-specific urinary proteins. The FSH activity was equivalent to HMG at 100–150 iu FSH/mg protein. Despite the vastly increased purity of HMG (menotropin) and uFSH (urofollitropin) compared with the original preparations, their active ingredients only make up 1–2% of the final product. These products contain large amounts of urinary protein (including cytokines, growth factors, transferrins and other proteins), which made uniform standardization very difficult and occasionally led to local reactions at the injection sites. The advent of monoclonal antibodies in the 1980s enabled further purification to be achieved by specifically selecting FSH out from the bulk HMG. The extract was 95% pure with a several hundredfold enhancement of specific gonadotrophin bioactivity and known as 'highly purified urinary FSH' (u-hFSH HP). Extended clinical trials comparing urofollitropin and highly purified FSH demonstrated equivalent ovulation and pregnancy rates. Much reduced hypersensitivity was reported such that the subcutaneous route could be adopted for administration.

FSH belongs to the family of glycoproteins that are heterodimers consisting of two noncovalently linked alpha and beta subunits. These are encoded by separate genes. Post-translational modification in the form of glycosylation of FSH occurs in the rough endoplasmic reticulum and Golgi apparatus of the mammalian cell. The FSH isolated from the human pituitary consists of many structural variants, or isoforms that differ not in their primary structure but in the modifications that result from glycosylation. Each subunit of FSH possesses two carbohydrate side chains that can vary in composition, branching and sialic acid residue capping. These accessories affect the biological activity of the molecule. This is appreciated when the elimination of glycoprotein molecules is clarified. The hepatic and renal plasma membrane contain a receptor that isolates asialoglycoproteins from the circulation such that the more basic isoforms have a shorter half-life. Heavily sialylated isoforms with more acidic caps escape for a longer period of in vivo biological activity but have lower receptor binding affinity and lower in vitro biological activity. Menopausal urine comprises predominantly acidic isoforms. Post-translational modification requires eukaryotic organelles and therefore the well-established Chinese hamster ovary cell line was chosen for protein synthesis.

Advantages and disadvantages of recombinant FSH (rFSH)

There are a number of immediately apparent advantages of rFSH over its urinary predecessors. Aside from the improved logistics of the pharmaceutical process, controlled manufacture has undoubtedly led to a more homogeneous product with much reduced inter-batch variability (Loumaye *et al.*, 1995) compared with the purification of enormous quantities of heterogeneous urine. The supply is potentially unlimited and shortages should no longer be a threat to clinical practice. There is no risk of infection or contamination with drugs or their metabolites as there is, in theory, with products from a human source, despite the precautions that are taken. The purity of the products has certainly enhanced their administration which is effective, safe and much less traumatic when the subcutaneous route is adopted. The vast majority of patients now elect to self-inject after appropriate instruction. The specific activity of rFSH is estimated at 10 000 iu/mg protein, some one hundredfold greater than HMG or uFSH.

Assays of hormonal activity

Two companies currently have a licence to produce recombinant gonadotrophins for the human pharmaceutical market. Ares-Serono produce follitropin alpha (Gonal-F®) and NV Organon produce follitropin beta (Puregon®). Research has been focused on comparing one or the other with urinary preparations and to date they have not been compared with each other directly. Any differences that might exist between them are likely to be subtle.

The measurement of gonadotrophin function is an extremely controversial area and remains far from standardized. Studies referring to specific aspects of function need to be assessed carefully. A number of different assays exist that determine aspects of pharmacokinetic and pharmacodynamic behaviour. Immunoassays measure structural features (usually specific protein epitopes) and generally indicate the amount of hormone present. Receptor-binding assays assess whether the hormonal conformation matches its receptor. Bioassays are functional and determine whether the expected effect occurs: they can be in vitro measures of biological action such as second messenger engagement (e.g. the induction of aromatase activity in immature rat Sertoli cells by FSH), or in vivo determinations of the overall effect of all the component elements. The gold standard in vivo bioassay for FSH has been the rat Steelman–Pohley assay in which an increase in ovarian weight is correlated with FSH dose (Steelman & Pohley, 1953), although an inherent variation of $\pm20\%$ is quoted for this assay (Bergh et al., 1997).

Recominant FSH (rFSH) in clinical practice in superovulation for IVF

Clinical evidence followed in therapeutic trials for IVF suggesting that r-hFSH yields more oocytes, embryos and on-going pregnancies with a smaller dose for a shorter time than uFSH (Out et al., 1995, 1996; Bergh et al., 1997). These end points were chosen as they are the most direct reflections of gonadotrophin effect in vivo, and the least subject to bias in large multicentre trials involving many uncontrollable variables such as more than one sonographer assessing follicular growth. Frozen-thawed embryos were included in the figures as they resulted from the stimulation cycle involving the gonadotrophin in question. Ongoing pregnancy rates (at 12 weeks' gestation) were consistently higher in the rFSH groups but not significantly so. Embryo quality appeared to be improved and having a surplus of embryos from which to choose the best to transfer, increased the number available to be frozen. Explanations for increased potency include a higher composition of basic isohormones, differences in pharmaceutical formulation, and FSH-inhibiting contaminants in uFSH. That a difference does exist is undeniable.

In the study of Bergh *et al.* (1997), patients undergoing intracytoplasmic sperm injection (ICSI) were included, where oocyte maturation is assessed prior to injection. There was no significant difference in oocyte maturity in the two groups. The clinical pregnancy rate for those patients who reached embryo transfer was similar for both groups suggesting no difference in embryo quality. This is interesting because pregnancy rates tend to be greater if there is a larger embryo pool from which to select for transfer. However, differences may become evident when frozen embryo transfer cycles using embryos from the same stimulated fresh cycle are taken into account. Lambert *et al.* (1998) have attempted to explain these effects by claiming that the greater the FSH receptor activation, the less acidic (rFSH) species is capable of, which is more important than an increased metabolic clearance rate.

Very few studies have been performed comparing rFSH with menotropin, HMG which contains urinary contaminants and high levels of LH. However, a first meta-analysis of urinary FSH with HMG has demonstrated that a significantly higher clinical pregnancy rate appears to be achieved with uFSH (Daya *et al.*, 1995). This study implied that an adequate level of endogenous LH exists to achieve follicular and endometrial maturation, despite down-regulation of the pituitary with a GnRH analogue. Moreover, it has been suggested that exogenous LH supplementation in the form of HMG may be detrimental to the chances of achieving a pregnancy (Loumaye *et al.*, 1996). Conversely, a subsequent meta-analysis (Agrawal *et al.*, 2000), which included additional studies, came out with a counter view: namely, that there was no advantage to using rFSH. Furthermore, a recent series of publications have demonstrated improved fertilization and ongoing pregnancy rates in women who have serum LH concentrations >0.5 iu/l on the day of HCG compared with those whose LH concentrations are <0.5 iu/l (Westergaard *et al.*, 2000). Overall it does appear that a low but critical level of LH is required throughout and towards the end of the follicular phase of the cycle and during superovulation regimens. The required LH need not necessarily be contained within the gonadotrophin preparation that is administered, provided that the level of pituitary desensitization is not too profound. (Cautionary note: in assessing this debate it is essential to be aware of the interests of the pharmaceutical companies that manufacture gonadotrophin preparations and to examine both authorship and sponsorship of the published studies.)

The half-life of FSH after subcutaneous injection is approximately 37 h which has enabled current treatment schedules to remain unchanged and for rFSH to be administered in parallel with uFSH. In the future it is not unreasonable to foresee modifications to the molecular structure that lead to an extension of the half-life and in vivo bioactivity – such preparations are currently undergoing phase 3 studies. This could enable the frequency of injections to be reduced, perhaps to once every seven days.

The response of the polycystic ovary to stimulation for IVF

Particular consideration needs to be given to superovulation when polycystic ovaries are present – either in women with polycystic ovary syndrome (PCOS) requiring IVF for whatever reason or when polycystic ovaries have been noted as an incidental finding at the time of the baseline ultrasound scan. Polycystic ovaries have twice as many FSH sensitive follicles as normal ovaries and are therefore prone to over-respond. Furthermore, after a period of quiescence there may be an 'explosive' ovarian response. In some cases, this may result in OHSS, to which patients with polycystic ovaries are particularly prone.

There are two additional factors to be considered. The first is that many women with PCOS, particularly those who are obese, have compensatory hypersecretion of insulin in response to the insulin resistance specifically related to the PCOS and that caused by obesity. Since the ovary is spared the insulin resistance, it is stimulated by insulin, acting, as it were, as a co-gonadotrophin. Insulin both augments theca cell production of androgens in response to stimulation by LH and granulosa cell production of oestrogen in response to stimulation by FSH. Insulin sensitizing agents, such as metformin, have recently been used with success in improving ovarian response for women with PCOS and anovulatory infertility – preliminary work indicates that they may also be beneficial to those with polycystic ovaries undergoing superovulation induction.

The second factor to be considered relates to the widespread expression of vascular endothelial growth factor (VEGF) in the polycystic ovary. VEGF is an endothelial cell mitogen that stimulates vascular permeability and is responsible there for invasion of the relatively avascular Graafian follicle by blood vessels after ovulation. The increase of LH at mid-cycle leads to expression of VEGF, which has recently been shown to be an obligatory intermediate in the formation of the corpus luteum Recent studies (Agrawal et al., 1998) have shown that, compared with women with normal ovaries, women with polycystic ovaries and PCOS have increased serum VEGF, which may contribute both to hypervascularity and the pathophysiology of ovarian hyperstimulation syndrome. Thus when polycystic ovarian morphology is identified on baseline ultrasound (whether or not the patient has polycystic ovary *syndrome*) it is important to induce superovulation with low doses of gonadotrophins and to ensure extra vigilance in monitoring the patient's response (for review see Balen et al., 1999).

Conclusions

Regimens for superovulation have become simplified over recent years in order to streamline therapy and improve throughput in the IVF clinic. Recent attention has been directed toward the use of recombinant FSH preparations and the GnRH antagonists. Together these preparations provide an opportunity to administer 'pure' products subcutaneously over a much shorter period of time than required with the long protocol, which has been routinely used over the last 10 years. It is still not possible to predict response precisely not only regarding follicular development but also regarding those patients who are more susceptible to profound pituitary suppression – in whom too low a circulating level of LH would be undesirable.

REFERENCES

Acharya, U., Small, J., Randall, J., Hamilton, M. & Templeton, A. (1992). Prospective study of short and long regimens of gonadotropin-releasing hormone agonist in in vitro fertilization program. *Fertil. Steril.* **57**: 815–18.

Agrawal, R., Sladkevicius, P., Engman, L., Conway, G. S., Payne, N. N., Bekir, J., Tan, S. L., Campbell, S. & Jacobs, H. S. (1998). Serum vascular endothelial growth factor concentrations and ovarian stromal blood flow are increased in women with polycystic ovaries. *Hum. Reprod.* **13**: 651–5.

Agrawal, R., Holmes, J. & Jacobs, H. S. (2000). Follicle stimulating hormone or human menopausal gonadotrophin for ovarian stimulation in in vitro fertilization cycles: a meta-analysis. *Fertil. Steril.* **73**: 338–43.

Balen, A. H., MacDougal, J. & Jacobs, H. S. (1999). Polycystic ovaries and assisted conception. In *Bourn Hall Textbook of IVF*, ed. P. Brinsden, pp. 109–130. Carnforth: Parthenon Press.

Bergh, C., Howles, C. M., Borg, K., Hamberger, L., Josefsson, B., Nilsson, L. & Wickland, M. (1997). Recombinant human follicle stimulating hormone (r-hFSH; Gonal-F®): results of a randomized comparative study in women undergoing assisted reproductive techniques *Hum. Reprod.* **12**: 2133–9.

Berg van de-Helder, A., Helmerhorst, F. M., Blankhart, A., Brand, R., Waegemaekers, C. & Naaktgeboren, N. (1990). Comparison of ovarian stimulation regimens for in vitro fertilization (IVF) with and without a gonadotropin-releasing hormone (GnRH) agonist: results of a randomized study. *J. In Vitro Fert. Embryo Transfer* **7**: 358–62.

Buvat, J., Marcolin, G., Guittard, C., Louvet, A. L., Couplet, G. & Renouard, O. (1991). Randomized comparison of 2 long and short protocols of ovarian stimulation with LHRH-agonist for IVF including 342 cycles in 175 women. *Hum. Reprod.* and *Abstract Book, 7th Annual Meeting of the ESHRE and 7th World Congress on IVF and Assisted Reproduction, Paris*, pp. 335–6.

Check, J. H., Nowroozi, K. & Chase, J. S. (1992). Comparison of short versus long-term leuprolide acetate – human menopausal gonadotrophin hyperstimulation in in-vitro fertilization patients. *Hum. Reprod.* **7**: 31–34.

Chen, S. U., Yang, Y. S., Ho, H. N., Hwang, J. L., Lien, Y. R., Lin, H. R., Hsieh, C. Y. & Lee, T. Y. (1992). Comparison of long-term versus three-day leuprolide acetate for ovarian stimulation in human in vitro fertilization program. *J. Reprod. Infertil.* **1**: 9–16.

Daya, S. (1999). Long versus short gonadotropin releasing hormone agonist protocols for pituitary desensitization in assisted reproduction cycles (Cochrane Review). In *The Cochrane Library*, vol. 4. Oxford: Update Software.

Daya, S., Gunby, J., Hughes, E. G, Collins, J. A. & Sagle, M. A. (1995). Follicle-stimulating hormone versus human menopausal gonadotropin for in vitro fertilisation cycles: a meta-analysis. *Fertil. Steril.* **64**: 347–54.

De Placido, G., Zullo, F., Colacurci, N., Perrone, D., Carravetta, C. & Montemagno, U. (1991). Long acting versus daily administration GnRH analogs in IVF. *Abstracts of the 7th Annual Meeting of the ESHRE and the 7th World Congress on IVF and Assisted Procreations*, Abstract No. P482.

Dirnfeld, M., Gonen, Y., Lissak, A., Goldman, S., Koifman, M., Sorokin, Y. & Abramovici, H. (1991). A randomized prospective study on the effect of short and long buserelin treatment in women with repeated unsuccessful in vitro fertilization (IVF) cycles due to inadequate ovarian response. *J. In Vitro Fert. Embryo Transfer* **8**: 339–43.

Fenichel, P., Grimaldi, M., Hieronimus, S., Olivero, J. F., Donzeau, A., Benoit, B., Fiorentini, M., Tran, D. K., Harter, M. & Gillet, J. Y. (1988). Inhibition systématique de l'hormone lutéinisante par un analogue de la gonadolibérine, la triptoréline, au cours de la stimulation ovarienne pour fécondation in vitro: choix du protocole (Luteinizing hormone inhibition with an LH-RH analogue, triptorelin, in ovarian stimulation for in vitro fertilization: choice of the therapeutic regimen). *Presse Méd.* **17**: 719–22.

Filicori, M., Flamigni, C., Cognigni, G. E., Falbo, A., Arnone, R., Capelli, M., Pavani, A., Mandini, M., Calderoni, P. & Brondelli, L. (1996). Different gonadotropin and leuprorelin ovulation induction regimens markedly affect follicular fluid hormone levels and folliculogenesis. *Fertil. Steril.* **65**: 387–93.

Fleming, R., Haxton, M. J., Hamilton, M. P. R., McCune, G. S., Black, W. P., McNaughton, M. C. & Coutts, J. R. T. (1985). Successful treatment of infertile women with oligomenorrhoea using a combination of an luteinising hormone releasing hormone agonist and exogenous gonadotrophins. *Br. J. Obstet. Gynaecol.* **92**: 369–74.

Fleming, R., Abu-Heija, A. T., Yates, R. W. S. & Coutts, J. R.T. (1996). Pregnancy outcome after exposure to gonadotropin releasing hormone analog during implantation. *Gynecol. Endocrinol.* **10** (Suppl. 1): 78 (Abstract No. 155).

Foulot, H., Dubuisson, J. B., Ranoux, C., Aubriot, F. X. & Poirot, C. (1988). Etude randomisée entre protocole court et protocole long de bvsereline concernant 100 cycles de fécondation in vitro. *Contr. Fertil. Sex* **16**: 628–9.

Frydman, R., Belaisch-Allart, J., Parneix, I., Forman, R., Hazout, A. & Testart, J. (1988). Comparison between flare up and down regulation of luteinising hormone releasing hormone agonists in an in-vitro fertilisation programme. *Fertil. Steril.* **50**: 471–5.

Ganirelix Dose-Finding Study Group (1998). A double-blind, ransomized, dose-finding study to assess the efficacy of the gonadotrophin-releasing hormone antagonist, Ganirelix (Org 37462) to prevent premature luteinising hormone surges in women undergoing ovarian stimulation with recombinant follicle stimulating hormone (Puregon). *Hum. Reprod.* **13**: 3023–31.

Gonen, Y., Dirnfeld, M., Calderon, I. & Abramovici, H. (1996). Outcome of pregnancies inadvertently exposed to GnRH-a in early gestation. *Gynecol. Endocrinol.* **10** (Suppl. 1): 78 (Abstract No. 156).

Hazout, A., de Ziegler, D., Cornel, C., Fernandez, H., Lelaidier, C. & Frydman, R. (1993). Comparison of short 7-day and prolonged treatment with gonadotropin-releasing hormone agonist desensitization for controlled ovarian hyperstimulation. *Fertil. Steril.* **59**: 596–600.

Hedon, B., Arnal, F., Badoc, E., Boulot, P., Huet, J. M., Fries, N., Deschamps, F., Cristol, P. & Humeau, C. (1988). Comparaison randomisée protocole long – protocole court dans les stimulations de l'ovaire en association avec un agoniste de la GnRH en vue de fécondation in vitro. *Contr. Fertil. Sex* **16**: 624–7.

Hughes, E. G., Fedorkow, D. M., Daya, S, Sagle, M. A., Van de Koppel, P. & Collins, J. A. (1992). The routine use of gonadotropin-releasing hormone agonists prior to in vitro fertilization and gamete intrafallopian transfer: a meta-analysis of randomized trials. *Fertil. Steril.* **58**: 888–96.

Jenkins, J. M. (1996). The influence, development and management of functional ovarian cysts during IVF cycles. *J. Br. Fertil. Soc.* **1**: 132–6.

Kingsland, C., Tan, S. L., Bickerton, N., Mason, B. A. & Campbell, S. (1992). The routine use of gonadotrophin releasing hormone agonists for all patients undergoing in vitro fertilisation. Is there any medical advantage? A prospective randomised study. *Fertil. Steril.* **57**: 804–9.

Kondaveeti-Gordon, U., Harrison, R. F., Barry-Kinsella, C., Gordon, A. C., Drudy, L. & Cottell, E. (1996). A randomized prospective study of early follicular or midluteal initiation of long protocol gonadotrophin releasing hormone in an ivf program. *Fertil. Steril.* **66**: 582–6.

Lambert, A., Talbot, J. A., Anobile, C. J. & Robertson, W. R. (1998). Gonadotrophin heterogeneity and biopotency: implications for assisted reproduction. *Mol. Hum. Reprod.* **4**: 619–29.

Lockwood, G. M., Pinkerton, S. M. & Barlow, D. H. (1995). A prospective randomised single-blind comparative trial of nafarelin acetate with buserelin in long-protocol gonadotrophin releasing hormone analogue controlled ivf cycles. *Hum. Reprod.* **10**: 293–8.

Loumaye, E., Vankrieken, L., Depreester, S., Psalti, I., de Cooman, S. & Thomas, K. (1989). Hormonal changes induced by short-term administration of a gonadotrophin releasing hormone agonist during ovarian hyperstimulation for in-vitro fertilisation and their consequences for embryo development. *Fertil. Steril.* **51**: 105–11.

Loumaye, E., Campbell, R. & Salat-Baroux, J. (1995). Human follicle stimulating hormone produced by recombinant DNA technology: a review for clinicians. *Hum. Reprod. Update* **1**: 188–99.

Loumaye, E., Martineau, I., Piazzi, A. *et al.* (1996). Clinical assessment of human gonadotrophins produced by recombinant DNA technology. *Hum. Reprod.* **11**: 95–107.

Macnamee, M. C., Howles, C. M., Edwards, R. G., Taylor, P. J. & Elder, K. T. (1989). Short-term luteinising hormone releasing hormone agonist treatment: prospective trial of a novel ovarian stimulation regimen for in-vitro fertilisation. *Fertil. Steril.* **52**: 264–9.

Marcus, S. F., Brinsden, P. R., Macnamee, M., Rainsbury, P. A., Elder, K. T. & Edwards, R. G. (1993). Comparative trial between an ultra-short and long protocol of luteinizing hormone-releasing hormone agonist for ovarian stimulation in in-vitro fertilization. *Hum. Reprod.* **8**: 238–43.

Maroulis, G. B., Emery, M., Verkauf, B. S., Saphier, A., Bernhisel, M. & Yeko, T. R. (1991). Prospective randomized study of human menotropin versus a follicular and a luteal phase gonadotropin-releasing hormone analog-human menotropin stimulation protocols for in vitro fertilization. *Fertil. Steril.* **55**: 1157–64.

Out, H. J., Mannerts, B. M. J. L., Driessen, S. G. A. J. & Coelingh Benninck, H. J. T. (1995). A prospective randomised assessor-blind, multicentre study comparing recombinant and urinary follicle stimulating hormone (Puregon vs. Metrodin) in in-vitro fertilisation. *Hum. Reprod.* **10**: 2534–40.

Out, H. J., Mannaerts, B. M. J. L., Driessen, S. G. A. J. & Coelingh Benninck, H. J. T. (1996). Recombinant follicle stimulating hormone (rFSH; Puregon) in assisted reproduction: More oocytes, more pregnancies. Results from five comparative studies. *Hum. Reprod. Update* **2**: 162–71.

Padilla, S. L., Smith, R. D. & Garcia, J. E. (1991). The Lupron screening test: tailoring the use of leuprolide acetate in ovarian stimulation for in vitro fertilization. *Fertil. Steril.* **56**: 79–83.

Pellicer, A., Simon, C., Miró, F., Castellví, R. M., Ruiz, A., Ruiz, M., Pérez, M. & Bonilla-Musoles, F. (1989). Ovarian response and outcome of in-vitro fertilization in patients treated with gonadotrophin-releasing hormone analogues in different phases of the menstrual cycle. *Hum. Reprod.* **4**: 285–9.

Porter, R. N., Smith, W., Craft, I. L., Abdulwahid, N. A. & Jacobs, H. S. (1984). Induction of ovulation for in-vitro fertilisation using buserelin and gonadotrophins. *Lancet* **2**: 1284–5.

Remorgida, V., Anserini, P., Croce, S., Costa, M., Ferraiolo, A., Centonze, A., Gaggero, G. & Capitanio, G. L. (1989). The duration of pituitary suppression by means of intranasal gonadotropin hormone-releasing hormone analogue administration does not influence the ovarian response to gonadotropin stimulation and success rate in a gamete intrafallopian transfer (GIFT) program. *J. In Vitro Fert. Embryo Transfer* **6**: 76–80.

Ron-El, R., Herman, A., Golan, A., van der Ven, H., Caspi, E. & Diedrich, K. (1990). The comparison of early follicular and midluteal administration of long-acting gonadotrophin releasing hormone agonist. *Fertil. Steril.* **54**: 233–7.

San Roman, G. A., Surrey, E. S., Judd, H. L. & Kerin, J. F. (1992). A prospective randomized comparison of luteal phase versus concurrent follicular phase initiation of gonadotropin-releasing hormone agonist for in vitro fertilization. *Fertil. Steril.* **58**: 744–9.

Steelman, S. L. & Pohley, F. M. (1953). Assay of the follicle stimulating hormone based on the augmentation with human chorionic gonadotrophin. *Endocrinology* **53**: 604–16.

Suganuma, N., Tsukahara, S. I., Kitagawa, T., Furuhashi, M., Asada, Y. & Kondo, I. (1996). A controlled ovarian hyperstimulation regimen involving intermittent gonadotropin administration with a 'short' protocol of gonadotropin releasing hormone agonist for in vitro fertilization. *J. Assist. Reprod. Genet.* **13**: 43–8.

Tan, S. L., Kingsland, C., Campbell, S., Mills, C., Bradfield, J., Alexander, N., Yovich, J. & Jacobs, H. S. (1992). The long protocol of administration of gonadotrophin releasing hormone agonist is superior to the short protocol for ovarian stimulation for in vitro fertilisation. *Fertil. Steril.* **57**: 810–14.

Tan, S. L., Maconochie, N., Doyle, P., Campbell, S., Balen, A. H., Bekir, J., Brinsden, P., Edwards, R. G. & Jacobs, H. S. (1994). Cumulative conception and livebirth rates after IVF, with and without, pituitary desensitization with the gonadotropin-releasing hormone agonist, buserelin. *Am. J. Obstet. Gynecol.* **171**: 513–20.

Tanos, V., Friedler, S., Shushan, A., Strausss, N., Hetsroni, I. & Lewin, A. (1995). Comparison between nafaraelin acetate and D-Trp6-LHRH for temporary pituitary suppression in ivf patients: a prospective crossover study. *J. Assist. Reprod. Genet.* **12**: 715–19.

Tarlatzis, B. C., Bili, H., Bontis, J., Lagos, S., Vatev, I. & Mantalenakis, S. (1994). Follicle cyst formation after administration of different gonadotrophin releasing hormone analogues for assisted reproduction. *Hum. Reprod.* **9**: 1983–6.

Tasdemir, M., Tasdemir, I., Kodama, H. & Higuchi, M. (1995). Is long-protocol gonadotropin releasing hormone agonist administration superior to the short protocol in ovarian stimulation for in vitro fertilization? *Int. J. Fertil.* **40**: 25–8.

Urbanczek, J. & Witthaus, E. (1996). Midluteal buserelin is superior to early follicular phase buserelin in combined gonadotrophin releasing hormone analog and gonadotropin stimulation in ivf. *Fertil. Steril.* **65**: 966–71.

Westergaard, L. G., Laursen, S. B. & Andersen, C. Y. (2000). Increased risk of early pregnancy loss by profound suppression of luteinising hormone during ovarian stimulation in normo-gonadotrophic women undergoing assisted reproduction. *Hum. Reprod.* **15**: 1003–8.

Yang, T. S., Tsan, S. H., Wang, B. C., Chang, S. P. & Ng, H. T. (1996). The evaluation of a new 7-day gonadotropin-releasing hormone agonist protocol in the controlled ovarian hyperstimulation for in vitro fertilization. *J. Obstet. Gynaecol. Res.* **22**: 133–7.

Zaki, S. M., Hakam, A. & Shawki, H. (1994). Comparison of short versus long protocol of LHRHa-HMG stimulation in IVF. *Hum. Reprod.* **9** (Suppl. 4): 120 (Abstract No. 311).

7

Techniques for IVF

Tim J. Child, Imran R. Pirwany and Seang Lin Tan

Women's Centre, John Radcliffe Hospital, Oxford, UK
McGill Reproductive Centre, Royal Victoria Hospital, Montreal, Quebec, Canada

Much recent research in IVF treatment has concentrated on ovarian stimulation drugs, regimens, improving the laboratory techniques of oocyte fertilization and embryo culture. However, efficient and effective oocyte recovery and embryo transfer techniques may have been neglected. This is unfortunate, as efforts to maximize ovarian stimulation and the work of embryologists in producing high quality embryos and blastocysts may be squandered if suboptimal oocyte retrieval and embryo transfer techniques are used. In this chapter we describe an evidence-based approach to oocyte retrieval and embryo transfer and briefly review the ongoing debate on the number of embryos transferred.

Oocyte retrieval

The early years of IVF were characterized by laparoscopic oocyte retrieval from unstimulated ovaries during the natural menstrual cycle. The disadvantages of laparoscopic oocyte retrieval include the need for general anaesthesia, the small but finite risk of damage to abdominal organs and blood vessels, and the greater overall cost and inconvenience to the patient of an IVF treatment cycle. Since most women will require repeated IVF treatment cycles, laparoscopy is not satisfactory as a routine method of oocyte retrieval.

By the early 1980s ultrasound technology had developed to such an extent that the first cases of transvesical oocyte recovery under transabdominal ultrasound guidance were reported (Lenz *et al.*, 1981). This was a major advance over the laparoscopic approach. By the late 1980s the development of high frequency vaginal probe ultrasound transducers allowed direct transvaginal ultrasound directed oocyte retrieval (TUDOR). A number of randomized trials testify to the advantages of this method over alternative approaches and TUDOR remains the method of choice (Tan *et al.*, 1990).

Good Clinical Practice in Assisted Reproduction, ed. P. Serhal & C. Overton.
Published by Cambridge University Press. © Cambridge University Press 2004.

Recently, follicular aspiration under three-dimensional ultrasound control has been reported (Feichtinger, 1998). On very rare occasions, laparoscopy may be considered for oocyte retrieval if the ovaries are high in the pelvis due to adhesions or surgery, or hidden due to an enlarged uterus and not accessible from the vagina.

Timing of oocyte retrieval

When an appropriate follicular response to gonadotrophin stimulation has been achieved the patient receives a subcutaneous injection of 5000 or 10 000 iu of human chorionic gonadotrophin (HCG) to commence the final stage of oocyte maturation (Abdalla *et al.*, 1987). Follicular tracking is performed with vaginal ultrasonography, with or without measurements of serum oestradiol concentrations. Various thresholds of the number and sizes of ovarian follicles required for HCG administration have been advocated. The maturity and implantation potential of an oocyte is related to the volume (and hence diameter) of its follicle (Scott *et al.*, 1989). Continuing ovarian stimulation and follicular growth for too long before HCG administration risks oocyte post-maturity, ovulation prior to oocyte recovery or ovarian hyperstimulation syndrome (OHSS).

Ovarian stimulation may be continued until at least three follicles of ≥ 18 mm average diameter are present. In a prospective study where patients were randomized to receive HCG when there was one follicle of ≥ 18 mm and at least two > 14 mm, or one or two days afterwards, no differences were found in the rates of oocyte retrieval, fertilization, embryo cleavage or pregnancy (Tan *et al.*, 1992a). This suggests a window of at least three days during which HCG can be administered with equally good results and has implications for the timing of oocyte retrievals to reduce weekend clinic workloads.

Studies using colour Doppler ultrasound during stimulation for IVF suggest further parameters for the timing of administration of HCG to optimize oocyte recovery rates and endometrial receptivity for implantation. The proportion of follicles demonstrating pulsatile vascularity (the follicular vascularity index), is positively correlated with the oocyte retrieval rate (Colour Plate 3) (Oyesanya *et al.*, 1996). If the follicular vascularity index is poor, perhaps the administration of HCG could be delayed until improved flow is present. Colour Doppler analysis of the uterine artery and subendometrial blood flow on the day of HCG administration during IVF has been correlated with the receptivity of the uterus to embryo implantation (Zaidi *et al.*, 1995, 1996). We suggested that, if on the day of planned HCG administration the uterine artery pulsatility index is >3 and there is no subendometrial blood flow, delaying HCG administration by a day or two to await improved blood flow parameters may be beneficial. However, to date no studies of the prospective use of Doppler ultrasound of follicular, uterine artery or subendometrial blood flow to select the day of HCG administration have been reported.

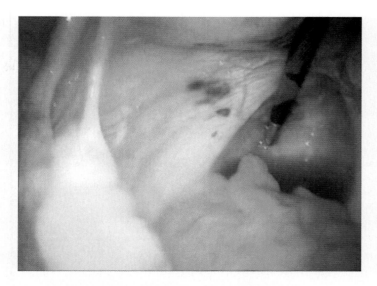

Plate 1   (See also Fig. 5.1) Deposits of endometriosis on the uterosacral ligament.

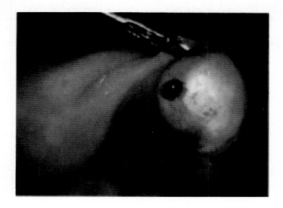

Plate 2   (See also Fig. 5.2) Endometrioma rupturing.

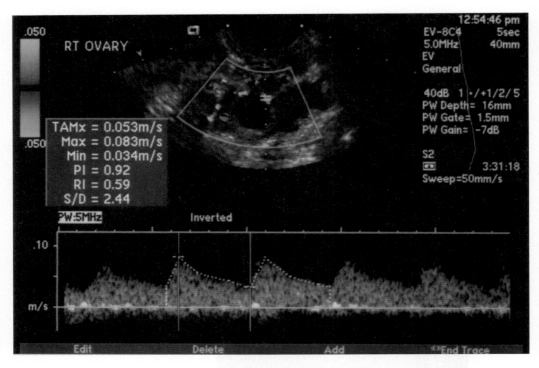

Plate 3   Ovarian perifollicular blood flow demonstrated with transvaginal colour Doppler ultrasound.

Randomized trials suggest no difference in outcome for HCG to oocyte retrieval intervals of 34 to 38 hours (Mansour *et al.*, 1994; Bjercke *et al.*, 2000). However, after 38 hours the risk of ovulation will increase and an interval of 36 hours is preferred. If due to oversight no HCG has been administered, very few or no oocytes can be retrieved. However, if the oocyte retrieval procedure is postponed and HCG administered, oocyte recovery may be successful 34 hours later (Esposito & Patrizio, 2000).

If oocyte collection is delayed beyond 39–40 hours it is advisable to scan the woman before sedation to ensure that the follicles are still intact. In cases where ovulation has started, as evidenced by a number of collapsed follicles and free fluid in the Pouch of Douglas oocyte, collection can still be undertaken in addition to aspiration of the fluid in the Pouch of Douglas.

Analgesia

Many women require more than one IVF cycle and oocyte retrieval can be a painful procedure. Therefore, adequate sedation and analgesia is important for oocyte retrieval. The three main anaesthetic options include general anaesthesia, spinal anaesthesia or intravenous sedation and analgesia. The latter is the most commonly used and may be combined with a local anaesthetic paracervical block. For example, midazolam 1–2 mg and fentanyl 100–150 μg intravenously, along with a local anaesthetic paracervical block. Prior to oocyte retrieval the patient must be adequately reviewed for drug allergies, previous anaesthetic problems or risk factors, and an anaesthetist should be consulted if there are concerns or contraindications.

During anaesthesia the oxygen saturation, blood pressure and heart rate of the patient must be monitored. Both local and intravenous anaesthetics collect in the follicular fluid during oocyte retrieval, though no effect on fertilization, cleavage or pregnancy rates has been demonstrated in humans (Bailey-Pridham *et al.*, 1990; Christiaens *et al.*, 1998). However, it is sensible to perform the retrieval quickly and safely to minimize discomfort to the patient and exposure of the oocytes to the drugs used.

Recovery room arrangements and patient preparation

Ideally the oocyte retrieval room should be located adjacent to the embryology laboratory, so that the follicular fluid contained in a test tube can be passed without delay directly from the warming block to the embryologist and direct communication facilitated between the embryologist and physician during examination of the follicular aspirate.

In preparation for treatment the patient should place herself in the lithotomy position. Cardio-respiratory monitoring devices should then be attached to the patient, intravenous access gained, a saline drip commenced and anaesthesia

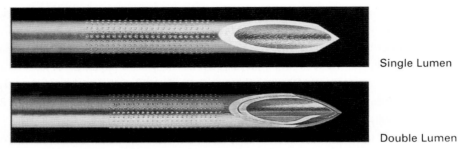

Single Lumen

Double Lumen

Figure 7.1.   Single and double lumen aspiration needles. Note the etching that increases ultrasound echogenicity and visibility within the ovary. (Courtesy of Cook Ob/Gyn, Spencer, Indiana, USA.)

administered. The vaginal vault is then cleansed with saline to remove mucus and pathogenic contamination and, if necessary, up to 10 ml of 1.5% lidocaine injected at the 4 and 8 o'clock positions to a depth of 1.5 cm below the vaginal mucosa (Ng *et al.*, 1999, 2000). Coupling gel is placed on the end of the vaginal ultrasound probe and a latex condom and needle guide fitted. The ultrasound probe is inserted into the vagina and a brief survey made of the uterus and ovaries. The aspiration needle is placed within the guide and advanced to the vaginal skin. The functioning of the aspiration and flushing mechanism must be checked prior to needle insertion. The ultrasound probe needs to be pushed firmly against the vaginal fornix with one hand to stabilize the ovary. The patient is asked to inhale deeply and hold her breath after which the needle is advanced to the centre of the selected follicle with a short firm stabbing motion. Negative aspiration pressure should be applied prior to needle entry into the follicle. This is because there is slight positive pressure within the follicle, which may lead to leakage of follicular fluid around the needle entry site as the needle enters the follicle. The tip of the needle is then kept at the centre of the collapsing follicle as fluid is aspirated. The ultrasound probe is then rotated from side to side, upward and downward (thereby scraping the sides of the follicle gently) until every drop of follicular fluid has been aspirated. This is important as an equal proportion of oocytes are found in the dead space of the needle as are found in the aspirated fluid within the test tube, implying that most oocytes are found in the terminal portion of the follicular aspirate (el Hussein *et al.*, 1992). Aspiration needles have etched areas at the needle tip to increase ultrasound echogenicity and visibility within the ovary (Figure 7.1). If flushing is to be performed it is done at this stage (see below). Negative pressure should be maintained as the aspiration needle is withdrawn from the emptied follicle, otherwise some fluid (perhaps with the oocyte) may inadvertently flow back into the follicle as pressure equilibrates. The remaining follicles are then drained in turn. Before advancing the needle into a follicle, care must be exercised to ensure that what appears to be a follicle is not one of the iliac vessels pictured in cross-section. Rotation of the ultrasound probe will elongate the 'follicle' into a tubular blood vessel. Usually, one needle entry into each ovary is sufficient to drain all follicles. This may not be the case if the ovary is hyperstimulated with numerous follicles or if the needle must be navigated around endometriomas. In these situations there may be less discomfort for the patient if the needle is removed and reintroduced rather than forcing it laterally across the ovary. The ovary is sometimes very mobile and in these circumstances it may help to tilt the woman head up. If the ovary is seen to be located behind the uterus, it is usually easy to move the ovary into an accessible position using the transvaginal probe. If the ovary is fixed behind the uterus a transmyometrial oocyte collection will need to be undertaken.

When all follicles have been drained from one ovary, the needle is withdrawn and a little fluid aspirated from a test tube to clear the dead-space of the needle. After the follicles in the contralateral ovary have also been drained a speculum is inserted to check for bleeding from the needle puncture points in the vaginal fornices. Firm pressure for a few minutes with a swab will usually stop the bleeding. If not, a suture may be required but this is rarely the case. The patient should then be moved to a recovery area and her vital signs are monitored for two to three hours until she is well enough to be escorted home.

The aspiration needle and vacuum system

The vacuum pressure for follicular aspiration should be <150 mmHg, since at pressures above this the rate of oocyte injury increases. The negative pressure at the needle tip will always be less than at the machine and will vary according to the distance between the two points. Therefore, the length of tubing in the system should be minimized and this will also serve to reduce oocyte cooling between the follicle and the test tube. Aspiration needles vary in gauge, length, bevel angle, stiffness and in single or double lumen design. Randomized studies demonstrate that increased needle gauge is associated with higher pain scores by the patient without differences in oocyte retrieval rate, fertilization rate, the proportion of oocytes with fractured zonae, implantation and pregnancy rate (Awonuga *et al.*, 1996). With a double lumen needle, aspiration is performed through the inner lumen whilst flushing fluid passes through the needle via the outer lumen (Figures 7.1 and 7.2). In this way, movement of flushing and follicular fluid is unidirectional. When a single lumen needle is used, flushing will push the last part of the follicular aspirate from the dead space of the needle back into the follicle before it is subsequently aspirated back into the needle. Therefore, a double lumen needle should be used if flushing is undertaken.

OVUM ASPIRATION

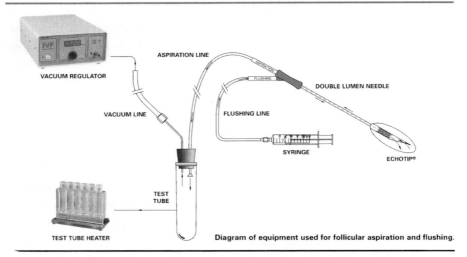

ASPIRATION LINE

VACUUM REGULATOR

DOUBLE LUMEN NEEDLE

VACUUM LINE

FLUSHING LINE

SYRINGE

ECHOTIP®

TEST TUBE

TEST TUBE HEATER

Diagram of equipment used for follicular aspiration and flushing.

Figure 7.2.   Diagram of equipment used for follicular aspiration and flushing. (Courtesy of Cook Ob/Gyn, Spencer, Indiana, USA.)

Follicular flushing

Randomized controlled trials demonstrate that follicular flushing after aspiration does not significantly increase the number of oocytes retrieved or the pregnancy rate. However, flushing significantly prolongs the oocyte retrieval procedure and also increases the amount of analgesia the patient requires (Tan *et al.*, 1992b). If oocyte retrieval is performed carefully, in the manner described above, follicular flushing is not necessary. However, if very few follicles are present then follicular flushing may be warranted to maximize the chances of retrieving oocytes. A randomized trial has shown that heparinized saline is equally effective as a flushing fluid compared with heparinized embryo culture medium (Biljan *et al.*, 1997).

Endometriomas and hydrosalpinges

During oocyte retrieval the aspiration needle should avoid endometriomas. If an endometrioma is punctured the contents may leak into the pelvic cavity causing chemical peritonitis and infection. Also, endometriotic fluid is embryotoxic and the aspirating system should be flushed well, once contaminated. Occasionally, it is not possible to aspirate follicles without passing through an endometrioma. In this situation an intravenous bolus dose of a broad spectrum antibiotic, such as a cephalosporin, should be given after the oocyte retrieval.

Hydrosalpinges visible on ultrasound are associated with reduced implantation and pregnancy rates in IVF (Camus *et al.*, 1999; Strandell *et al.*, 1999). This may be due to the embryotoxic effect of fluid leakage from the Fallopian tube into the uterine cavity interfering with implantation. Data suggest that in these patients salpingectomy increases success rates (Johnson *et al.*, 2002). It is unclear whether transvaginal needle aspiration of hydrosalpingeal fluid at the time of oocyte retrieval improves outcome, particularly since fluid often re-accumulates by the time of embryo transfer.

Risks of oocyte retrieval

The major risks of transvaginal oocyte retrieval are infection and bleeding. There is no evidence that routine antibiotics reduce the risk of infection though it is wise to give an intravenous bolus of antibiotics post-retrieval to women with a history of severe pelvic infection or if endometriomas are traversed. In a review of 2670 oocyte retrievals, pelvic infection occurred post-operatively in 0.6% of cases (Bennett *et al.*, 1993). The other important risk is that of haemorrhage from needle injury to pelvic blood vessels. If a vessel is punctured the needle should be carefully withdrawn and pressure exerted to the vaginal fornix with the vaginal probe. The incidence of bleeding >100 ml during oocyte retrieval has been estimated at 0.8% (Bennett *et al.*, 1993).

Immature oocyte recovery

There is increasing interest in the retrieval and in vitro maturation of immature oocytes from unstimulated ovaries (Chian *et al.*, 1999, 2000; Child *et al.*, 2001). Advantages include increased simplicity and safety of treatment and reduced cost, since no gonadotrophins for ovarian stimulation are required. Immature oocytes are retrieved transvaginally under ultrasound guidance from the small 2–8 mm ovarian antral follicles. The retrieval is performed in a similar manner to that described above for IVF oocyte retrieval. A specially designed 17-gauge single-channel aspirating needle is used (K-OPS-1235-Wood, Cook, Australia). The needle is stiffer and shorter, with a shorter bevel than those used for IVF. No flushing is performed since the follicles contain too small a volume of fluid. As it passes through the thickened ovarian stroma, the needle tends to block frequently. Therefore, a multiple puncture technique is used. On average, immature oocyte retrievals take longer and require more analgesia than standard retrievals. After initially using spinal anaesthesia, intravenous sedation combined with a paracervical local anaesthetic block has been found to have similar effectiveness to a regional technique (Child *et al.*, 2001).

Embryo transfer

The technique for embryo transfer has changed little since the first successful transfer in the early days of IVF (Steptoe & Edwards, 1978), but this critical step is an important determinant of the final outcome of treatment and the experience of the operator plays an important role (Barber *et al.*, 1996). Generally, transfer is carried out 48–72 hours after oocyte retrieval, when the embryos are usually in the 2- to 8-cell stage of cleavage, although with improvements in culture media there is an increasing tendency to replace embryos at a later stage of development.

Prior to the procedure the patient's identity should be confirmed, the number of embryos to be transferred agreed between the physician and the patient, and the patient consent checked. The patient and her partner may be given an opportunity to see the embryos on the television monitor in the operating theatre linked to the embryologist's microscope.

Procedure

The patient is placed in a lithotomy position. A Cusco vaginal speculum lubricated with saline is introduced and the cervix is visualized. The vagina is cleaned with warm saline and cervical secretions are gently removed with cotton tipped buds.

In the laboratory, the embryologist identifies the embryos and those to be transferred are placed into a drop of culture medium. Soft catheters are preferred and the end of a Wallace (Sims Portex, Hythe, Kent, UK) soft embryo replacement catheter fitted with a 1 ml insulin syringe (Norm-Jet, GMBH, Germany), pre-flushed with medium, is placed carefully into the medium droplet and the embryos to be replaced are aspirated into the transfer catheter in the following way: 10 µl air gap followed by 10 µl of IVF Science® culture medium (Scandinavia IVF Science, Gothenburg, Sweden) containing the embryos and finally another 5 µl air gap is aspirated at the end. The catheter is passed to the waiting surgeon.

With the hubs locked in position, the catheter is advanced so that the inner cannula is introduced into the external os and advanced gently through the cervical canal and the internal os into the mid-uterine cavity. It is often necessary to twist the catheter in the cervical canal to aid negotiation through the internal os. Occasionally, resistance to the easy passage of the inner cannula is encountered, usually at the level of the internal os. When this occurs, the stiffer Teflon outer sheath is released from the catheter hub so that only the tip of the inner cannula is visible, ensuring that a smooth surface presents. The outer sheath may be shaped to correspond to the long axis of the uterus (in 20% of cases the uterus is retroverted and retroflexed), and advanced in the cervical canal, thus freeing the inner cannula and assisting its passage through the canal. The outer sheath should never be advanced further than the level of the internal os. Once the inner cannula is felt to pass through the internal os, the outer sheath is withdrawn and the hubs are once again locked in position. In exceptional cases, where difficulty is encountered, the cervix is grasped by a single toothed tenaculum, and gentle traction applied to straighten the cervical canal and correct the uterine position. However, the application of the tenaculum is associated with uterine junctional zonal contractions (Lesny *et al.*, 1999a), which may cause expulsion of the embryos and affect successful outcome. With the tip of the catheter approximately 1cm from the uterine fundus, the embryos are expelled slowly and gently into the mid-uterine cavity. Time is allowed for equilibration of the fluid with the uterine environment, and the catheter is then slowly withdrawn in its entirety by a rotational movement, and handed to the waiting embryologist to ensure the complete expulsion of the embryos. The speculum is removed and the patient is transferred to the recovery area and allowed to rest for 20 minutes before being allowed home. It is now well recognized that prolonged bed rest following embryo transfer is not necessary and does not influence the outcome of treatment (Botta & Grudzinskas, 1997). Luteal support may be provided by progesterone pessary 200 mg *tid*. In the event of pregnancy this can be continued until 4–12 weeks' gestation.

Variables affecting successful embryo transfer

Among the factors known to influence outcome of IVF treatment following embryo transfer are: the choice of catheter; the stage of embryo transfer; the difficulty of the transfer; and the number of embryos transferred.

Choice of catheter

Repeated attempts at embryo transfer may have adverse effects on treatment outcome (Visser *et al.*, 1993). Therefore, the initial choice of transfer catheter is an important decision. The use of stiff catheters with a rigid outer sheath makes catheter placement easier, may facilitate the negotiation of anatomical difficulties and prevents entry of cervical mucus into the endometrial cavity (Craft *et al.*, 1981). However, they result in more bleeding, trauma, mucus plugging, and stimulation of uterine contractions. Given that the aim of embryo replacement is to deliver the embryos atraumatically to the uterine cavity, soft catheters are preferred as they are less likely to induce cervical and endometrial lacerations and to provoke uterine contractions. Clinical pregnancy rates appear to be significantly higher with the use of soft catheters (Wallace or Frydman – Figure 7.3; Wood *et al.*, 2000). However, soft catheters are often difficult to pass, and are associated with the highest rate of difficult embryo transfers (Mansour *et al.*, 1990). Studies comparing the Wallace and Frydman catheters have suggested that the inner stiff stylet of the Frydman catheter is liable to cause trauma though no difference in pregnancy or embryo expulsion rates have been demonstrated (al Shawaf *et al.*, 1993). Therefore, the choice of soft catheters remains controversial. Interestingly, the straightening of the utero-cervical junction by the filled bladder (Sundstrom *et al.*, 1984) may favour easy entry into the endometrial cavity (especially in the acutely anteflexed uterus), but this has not been evaluated in a randomized controlled trial.

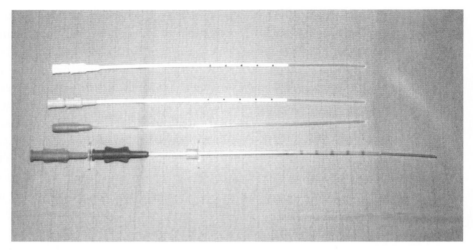

Figure 7.3.   Embryo transfer catheters. From top to bottom: Trial Wallace (no lumen), Wallace, stylet for Frydman, Frydman catheter. (Photograph courtesy of Simon Phillips.)

Ultrasound guided embryo transfer

Despite the improvement in catheter technology, embryo transfer remains a blind procedure that is operator dependent. It is difficult to judge accurately the direction of passage of the soft catheters and it is not uncommon for the catheter tip to abut the uterine fundus (Lesny *et al.*, 1998) or inadvertently be directed posteriorly. Endometrial wave-like contractions are apparent in 36.4% of transfers. Although sub-endometrial myometrial contractions in a cervico-fundal direction are thought to have a beneficial effect on implantation rate (Woolcott & Stanger, 1997), fundo-cervical contractions that are apparent in other cases may favour embryo expulsion and the dysperistalsis may also favour ectopic pregnancy. The unreliability of tactile assessment of embryo transfer would support the use of embryo replacements under transabdominal ultrasound guidance to ensure correct positioning of the transfer catheter. However, the matter is controversial, with some studies reporting an improved pregnancy rate (Wood *et al.*, 2000), while others failing to demonstrate a significant improvement in treatment outcome (Lesny *et al.*, 1999b). Recent meta-analyses suggest, however, higher pregnancy rates using ultrasound guided embryo transfer (Buckett, 2003; Sallam & Sadek, 2003).

Catheter contamination

Mucus plugging of the catheter tip can cause retained embryos, damage to the embryos and improper embryo placement, and a consequently lower pregnancy rate (Nabi *et al.*, 1997). Cervical aspiration has been advocated to minimize contact with blood, fibrin and endocervical organisms that may have an adverse affect on pregnancy outcome (Awonuga *et al.*, 1998; Egbase *et al.*, 1996). However, based on current evidence cervical lavage is not routinely recommended.

Trial transfer

Difficult embryo transfers are associated with a significantly lower pregnancy rate. To avoid or minimize difficult embryo transfers, the use of mock embryo transfer immediately prior to transfer has been advocated (Sharif, 1996) and has become routine practice in some centres. This allows the direction of the cervix and uterus to be mapped, whilst facilitating treatment and minimizing the disruption to the patient schedule that a precycle mock transfer entails (Mansour *et al.*, 1990). The procedure involves the use of the close-ended catheter tip that is replaced with the inner (open ended) Wallace embryo transfer catheter, while keeping the outer sleeve in position immediately prior to transfer.

Alternatively mock embryo transfer can be carried out in the month prior to treatment. If the cervix is found to be stenotic the woman will benefit from cervical dilatation just before starting gonadotrophin stimulation.

Stage of embryo transfer

Traditionally, embryos are transferred two to three days after oocyte retrieval, after confirming fertilization and cleavage to the 4- and 8-cell stage of development. Recent improvements in embryo culture media have permitted extended incubation of embryos to the blastocyst stage of development (days 5–6). Delaying embryo transfer until the blastocyst stage provides a longer opportunity to observe the embryos, thus permitting self-selection of those embryos that may have a greater implantation potential (Schoolcraft *et al.*, 1999). However, given that 50% of the embryos do not develop to the blastocyst stage (Dean *et al.*, 2000), not all embryos are suitable for blastocyst culture. Although the criteria for blastocyst transfer (quality and number) have not been defined, a general policy for patients under the age of 35 years who have at least five good quality embryos on day 3 is to continue embryo culture with a view to replacing a maximum of two blastocysts.

Number of embryos transferred

The question of the optimum number of embryos to be transferred has been fiercely debated. Multiple pregnancy is unarguably the most serious complication of assisted reproductive technique (ART) and approximately 30% of all pregnancies following ART are twin and higher order multiple pregnancies (World Collaborative Report on In Vitro Fertilization, 1997). The figure is even higher in the US, where it is believed that 75% of all multiple pregnancies are the result of ART treatment (Assisted Reproductive Technology in the United States and Canada, 1998). Given the 10-fold increased risk of perinatal death and morbidity, even in twin pregnancy

(Bergh *et al.*, 1999), a 47-fold higher incidence of cerebral palsy in babies resulting from triplet and higher-order multiple pregnancies (Jonas & Lumley, 1993), and the resulting financial drain on the health care system (Callahan *et al.*, 1994), every effort should be made to minimize this frequent complication of ART.

Multiple pregnancies in ART can be avoided, first by the judicious use of ovulatory agents, secondly by reducing the number of embryos transferred, thirdly by improving the quality selection criteria of embryos and fourthly by improving in vitro embryo culture, cryopreservation and thawing techniques.

The use of ovulatory agents has been discussed elsewhere (Child & Barlow, 1998). Maternal age is of paramount importance in determining the success of IVF treatment (Tan *et al.*, 1992c). Advancing maternal age may have a detrimental affect on ovarian responsiveness, oocyte and embryo quality, and uterine receptivity, accounting for the lower rate of implantation and increased rates of miscarriage, perinatal morbidity and mortality. Therefore, it is not uncommon for some clinics to transfer a greater number of embryos in older women to compensate for their poorer quality and implantation potential. This is particularly so when IVF treatment is self-financed. In the UK, by law the Human Fertilisation and Embryology Authority (HFEA) limits the number of embryos to be replaced (three per cycle regardless of the procedure used) and in 1999 the Royal College of Obstetricians and Gynaecologists recommended the replacement of no more than two embryos where four or more embryos are available for transfer. Recent studies have demonstrated that for women aged <35 years who have three or more good quality embryos, replacement of more than two embryos is not associated with an increased pregnancy rate (Dean *et al.*, 2000). Strictly limiting the number of embryos is criticized because it restricts clinical freedom and does not allow for individual variation according to individual patient circumstances. In the US, where it is common practice in some centres to replace more embryos, the American Society for Reproductive Medicine (ASRM, 1999) recommends the transfer of up to five embryos depending upon an assessment of prognosis for successful outcome based on the maternal age, embryo quantity, number of attempts at IVF treatment and quality based on morphological assessment.

Embryo quality has an important correlation with the outcome of IVF treatment (Steer *et al.*, 1992; Roseboom *et al.*, 1995). However, it remains subjective and to date we do not have unequivocal clinical and technological means to identify individual patients whose embryos may have an enhanced implantation potential.

Replacement of cryopreserved embryos results in a lower pregnancy rate (World Collaborative Report on In Vitro Fertilization, 1997). However, if embryo cryopreservation rates could be improved it would be possible to replace fewer embryos per transfer. Indeed, there are indications that transferring one embryo per cycle may not affect pregnancy rates adversely (Gerris & Van Royen, 2000).

Embryo transfer procedures applicable in special circumstances

Transmyometrial embryo transfer

Transmyometrial embryo transfer may be necessary when the transcervical approach is not possible. The 18-gauge needle with its stylet is passed transvaginally under ultrasound guidance though the myometrium of the anterior uterine wall to the junction with the endometrium, without puncturing the latter. The stylet is then removed, the preloaded 'Towako' embryo transfer catheter (Cook, Queensland, Australia) passed through the needle, and the embryos injected. Successful transfer is heralded by echogenic brightness at the injection site. Success rates of the procedure are conflicting (Groutz *et al.*, 1997; Kato *et al.*, 1993).

Zygote intrafallopian transfer (ZIFT)

Current indications for ZIFT include cervical stenosis, cervical hypoplasia and replacement of embryos after assisted hatching. The procedure involves intratubal replacement of 1- to 2-day-old embryos under laparoscopic guidance, transcervically by blind tactile assessment, or under ultrasound guidance. Prospective studies have not demonstrated an advantage over IVF and the procedure cannot be recommended as a routine treatment (Scholtes *et al.*, 1994).

Peritoneal oocyte sperm transfer (POST)

The strongest indication for POST is where more than four oocytes are generated following ovulation induction during the course of intrauterine insemination (IUI) treatment, but with attendant high risk of multiple pregnancy. The procedure involves replacement of up to four oocytes retrieved by conventional transvaginal ultrasound guidance, meticulous aspiration of the Pouch of Douglas (POD) of all blood, and injection of four oocytes and 4×10^6 sperms through a long transfer catheter into the POD through the aspiration needle that is left in place after flushing of the posterior cul de sac. The procedure avoids the laboratory costs associated with IVF-ET and pregnancy rates of 3–20% per cycle have been reported (Tan *et al.*, 1992d).

Conclusion

The goal of the final, and perhaps most important step in the IVF process, is to replace embryos atraumatically into the uterine cavity. This is best performed using soft embryo transfer catheters, probably inserted under ultrasound guidance. In women with a good prognosis, no more than two embryos should be replaced. Delaying the transfer until the blastocyst stage of development may have a beneficial effect on the pregnancy rate. However, the optimal number of blastocysts to replace is not currently known. Improvements in embryo cryo-preservation will allow fewer embryos to be transferred, decreasing the incidence of multiple pregnancies, which is the most important complication of ART treatment.

REFERENCES

Abdalla, H. I., Ah-Moye, M., Brinsden, P. *et al.* (1987). The effect of the dose of human chorionic gonadotropin and the type of gonadotropin stimulation on oocyte recovery rates in an in vitro fertilization program. *Fertil. Steril.* **48**: 958–63.

al Shawaf, T., Dave, R., Harper, J. *et al.* (1993). Transfer of embryos into the uterus: how much do technical factors affect pregnancy rates? *J. Assist. Reprod. Genet.* **10**: 31–6.

American Society for Reproductive Medicine (1999). *Guidelines on number of embryos transferred; a Practice Committee Report.* Birmingham, AL: American Society for Reproductive Medicine.

Assisted Reproductive Technology in the United States and Canada (1998). 1995 results generated from the American Society for Reproductive Medicine/Society for Assisted Reproductive Technology Registry. *Fertil. Steril.* **69**: 389–98.

Awonuga, A., Waterstone, J., Oyesanya, O. *et al.* (1996). A prospective randomized study comparing needles of different diameters for transvaginal ultrasound-directed follicle aspiration. *Fertil. Steril.* **65**: 109–13.

Awonuga, A., Nabi, A., Govindbhai, J. *et al.* (1998). Contamination of embryo transfer catheter and treatment outcome in in vitro fertilization. *J. Assist. Reprod. Genet.* **15**: 198–201.

Bailey-Pridham, D. D., Reshef, E., Drury, K. *et al.* (1990). Follicular fluid Lidocaine levels during transvaginal oocyte retrieval. *Fertil. Steril.* **53**: 171–3.

Barber, D., Egan, D., Ross, C. *et al.* (1996). Nurses performing embryo transfer: successful outcome of in-vitro fertilization. *Hum. Reprod.* **11**: 105–8.

Bennett, S. J., Waterstone, J. J., Cheng, W. C. *et al.* (1993). Complications of transvaginal ultrasound-directed follicle aspiration: a review of 2670 consecutive procedures. *J. Assist. Reprod. Genet.* **10**: 72–7.

Bergh, T., Ericson, A., Hillensjo, T. *et al.* (1999). Deliveries and children born after in-vitro fertilisation in Sweden 1982–95: a retrospective cohort study. *Lancet* **354**: 1579–85.

Biljan, M. M., Dean, N., Hemmings, R. *et al.* (1997). Prospective randomized trial of the effect of two flushing media on oocyte retrieval and fertilization rates after in vitro fertilization. *Fertil. Steril.* **68**: 1132–4.

Bjercke, S., Tanbo, T., Dale, P. O. *et al.* (2000). Comparison between two hCG-to-oocyte aspiration intervals on the outcome of in vitro fertilization. *J. Assist. Reprod. Genet.* **17**: 319–22.

Botta, G. & Grudzinskas, G. (1997). Is a prolonged bed rest following embryo transfer useful? *Hum. Reprod.* **12**: 2489–92.

Buckett, W. M. (2003). A meta-analysis of ultrasound-guided versus clinical touch embryo transfer. *Fertil. Steril.* **80**: 1037–41.

Callahan, T. L., Hall, J. E., Ettner, S. L. *et al.* (1994). The economic impact of multiple-gestation pregnancies and the contribution of assisted-reproduction techniques to their incidence. *N. Engl. J. Med.* **331**: 244–9.

Camus, E., Poncelet, C., Goffinet, F. *et al.* (1999). Pregnancy rates after in-vitro fertilization in cases of tubal infertility with and without hydrosalpinx: a meta-analysis of published comparative studies. *Hum. Reprod.* **14**: 1243–9.

Chian, R. C., Gulekli, B., Buckett, W. M. *et al.* (1999). Priming with human chorionic gonadotropin before retrieval of immature oocytes in women with infertility due to the polycystic ovary syndrome. *N. Engl. J. Med.* **341**: 1624–6.

Chian, R. C., Buckett, W. M., Tulandi, T. *et al.* (2000). Prospective randomized study of human chorionic gonadotrophin priming before immature oocyte retrieval from unstimulated women with polycystic ovarian syndrome. *Hum. Reprod.* **15**: 165–70.

Child, T. J. & Barlow, D. H. (1998). Strategies to prevent multiple pregnancies in assisted conception programmes. *Baillières Clin. Obstet. Gynaecol.* **12**: 131–46.

Child, T. J., Abdul-Jalil, A. K., Gulekli, B. & Tan, S. L. (2001). In vitro maturation and fertilization from unstimulated normal ovaries, polycystic ovaries, and women with polycystic ovary syndrome. *Fertil. Steril.* **76**: 936–42.

Christiaens, F., Janssenswillen, C., Van Steirteghem, A. C. *et al.* (1998). Comparison of assisted reproductive technology performance after oocyte retrieval under general anaesthesia (propofol) versus paracervical local anaesthetic block: a case-controlled study. *Hum. Reprod.* **13**: 2456–60.

Craft, I., McLeod, F. & Edmonds, K. (1981). Human embryo transfer technique. *Lancet* **2**: 1104–5.

Dean, N. L., Phillips, S. J., Buckett, W. M. *et al.* (2000). Impact of reducing the number of embryos transferred from three to two in women under the age of 35 who produced three or more high-quality embryos. *Fertil. Steril.* **74**: 820–3.

Egbase, P. E., al Sharhan, M., al Othman, S. *et al.* (1996). Incidence of microbial growth from the tip of the embryo transfer catheter after embryo transfer in relation to clinical pregnancy rate following in-vitro fertilization and embryo transfer. *Hum. Reprod.* **11**: 1687–9.

el Hussein, E., Balen, A. H. & Tan, S. L. (1992). A prospective study comparing the outcome of oocytes retrieved in the aspirate with those retrieved in the flush during transvaginal ultrasound directed oocyte recovery for in-vitro fertilization. *Br. J. Obstet. Gynaecol.* **99**: 841–4.

Esposito, M. A. & Patrizio, P. (2000). Partial follicular aspiration for salvaging an IVF cycle after improper hCG administration. A case report. *J. Reprod. Med.* **45**: 511–14.

Feichtinger, W. (1998). Follicle aspiration with interactive three-dimensional digital imaging (Voluson): a step toward real-time puncturing under three-dimensional ultrasound control. *Fertil. Steril.* **70**: 374–7.

Gerris, J. & Van Royen, E. (2000). Avoiding multiple pregnancies in ART: a plea for single embryo transfer. *Hum. Reprod.* **15**: 1884–8.

Groutz, A., Lessing, J. B., Wolf, Y. *et al.* (1997). Comparison of transmyometrial and transcervical embryo transfer in patients with previously failed in vitro fertilization-embryo transfer cycles and/or cervical stenosis. *Fertil. Steril.* **67**: 1073–6.

Johnson, N. P., Mak, W. & Sowter, M. C. (2002). Laparoscopic salpingectomy for women with hydrosalpinges enhances the success of IVF: a cochrane review. *Hum. Reprod.* **17**: 543–8.

Jonas, H. A. & Lumley, J. (1993). Triplets and quadruplets born in Victoria between 1982 and 1990. The impact of IVF and GIFT on rising birthrates. *Med. J. Aust.* **158**: 659–63.

Kato, O., Takatsuka, R. & Asch, R. H. (1993). Transvaginal-transmyometrial embryo transfer: the Towako method; experiences of 104 cases. *Fertil. Steril.* **59**: 51–3.

Lenz, S., Lauritsen, J. G. & Kjellow, M. (1981). Collection of human oocytes for in vitro fertilisation by ultrasonically guided follicular puncture. *Lancet* **i**: 1163–4.

Lesny, P., Killick, S. R., Tetlow, R. L. *et al.* (1998). Embryo transfer – can we learn anything new from the observation of junctional zone contractions? *Hum. Reprod.* **13**: 1540–6.

Lesny, P., Killick, S. R., Robinson, J. *et al.* (1999a). Junctional zone contractions and embryo transfer: is it safe to use a tenaculum? *Hum. Reprod.* **14**: 2367–70.

Lesny, P., Killick, S. R., Robinson, J. *et al.* (1999b). Ectopic pregnancy after transmyometrial embryo transfer: case report. *Fertil. Steril.* **72**: 357–9.

Mansour, R., Aboulghar, M. & Serour, G. (1990). Dummy embryo transfer: a technique that minimizes the problems of embryo transfer and improves the pregnancy rate in human in vitro fertilization. *Fertil. Steril.* **54**: 678–81.

Mansour, R. T., Aboulghar, M. A. & Serour, G. I. (1994). Study of the optimum time for human chorionic gonadotropin-ovum pickup interval in in vitro fertilization. *J. Assist. Reprod. Genet.* **11**: 478–81.

Nabi, A., Awonuga, A., Birch, H. *et al.* (1997). Multiple attempts at embryo transfer: does this affect in-vitro fertilization treatment outcome? *Hum. Reprod.* **12**: 1188–90.

Ng, E. H., Tang, O. S., Chui, D. K. *et al.* (1999). A prospective, randomized, double-blind and placebo-controlled study to assess the efficacy of paracervical block in the pain relief during egg collection in IVF. *Hum. Reprod.* **14**: 2783–7.

Ng, E. H., Tang, O. S., Chui, D. K. *et al.* (2000). Comparison of two different doses of lignocaine used in paracervical block during oocyte collection in an IVF programme. *Hum. Reprod.* **15**: 2148–51.

Oyesanya, O. A., Parsons, J. H., Collins, W. P. *et al.* (1996). Prediction of oocyte recovery rate by transvaginal ultrasonography and color Doppler imaging before human chorionic gonadotropin administration in in vitro fertilization cycles. *Fertil. Steril.* **65**: 806–9.

Roseboom, T. J., Vermeiden, J. P., Schoute, E. *et al.* (1995). The probability of pregnancy after embryo transfer is affected by the age of the patient, cause of infertility, number of embryos transferred and the average morphology score, as revealed by multiple logistic regression analysis. *Hum. Reprod.* **10**: 3035–41.

Sallam, H. N. & Sadek, S. S. (2003). Ultrasound-guided embryo transfer: a meta-analysis of randomized controlled trials. *Fertil. Steril.* **80**: 1042–6.

Scholtes, M. C., Roozenburg, B. J., Verhoeff, A. *et al.* (1994). A randomized study of transcervical intrafallopian transfer of pronucleate embryos controlled by ultrasound versus intrauterine transfer of four- to eight-cell embryos. *Fertil. Steril.* **61**: 102–4.

Schoolcraft, W. B., Gardner, D. K., Lane, M. *et al.* (1999). Blastocyst culture and transfer: analysis of results and parameters affecting outcome in two in vitro fertilization programs [see comments]. *Fertil. Steril.* **72**: 604–9.

Scott, R. T., Hofmann, G. E., Muasher, S. J. *et al.* (1989). Correlation of follicular diameter with oocyte recovery and maturity at the time of transvaginal follicular aspiration. *J. In Vitro Fert. Embryo Transf.* **6**: 73–5.

Sharif, K., Afnan, M., Lenton, W. *et al.* (1996). Transmyometrial embryo transfer after difficult immediate mock transcervical transfer. *Fertil. Steril.* **65**: 1071–4.

Steer, C. V., Mills, C. L., Tan, S. L. *et al.* (1992). The cumulative embryo score: a predictive embryo scoring technique to select the optimal number of embryos to transfer in an in-vitro fertilization and embryo transfer programme. *Hum. Reprod.* **7**: 117–19.

Steptoe, P. C. & Edwards, R. G. (1978). Birth after the reimplantation of a human embryo. *Lancet* **2**: 366.

Strandell, A., Lindhard, A., Waldenstrom, U. *et al.* (1999). Hydrosalpinx and IVF outcome: a prospective, randomized multicentre trial in Scandinavia on salpingectomy prior to IVF. *Hum. Reprod.* **14**: 2762–9.

Sundstrom, P., Wramsby, H., Persson, P. H. *et al.* (1984). Filled bladder simplifies human embryo transfer. *Br. J. Obstet. Gynaecol.* **91**: 506–7.

Tan, S. L., Bennett, S. & Parsons, J. (1990). Surgical techniques of oocyte collection and embryo transfer. *Br. Med. Bull.* **46**: 628–42.

Tan, S. L., Balen, A., el Hussein, E. *et al.* (1992a). A prospective randomized study of the optimum timing of human chorionic gonadotropin administration after pituitary desensitization in in vitro fertilization. *Fertil. Steril.* **57**: 1259–64.

Tan, S. L., Waterstone, J., Wren, M. *et al.* (1992b). A prospective randomized study comparing aspiration only with aspiration and flushing for transvaginal ultrasound-directed oocyte recovery. *Fertil. Steril.* **58**: 356–60.

Tan, S L., Pampiglione, J., Steer, C. *et al.* (1992c). Transvaginal peritoneal oocyte and sperm transfer for the treatment of nontubal infertility. *Fertil. Steril.* **57**: 850–3.

Tan, S. L., Royston, P., Campbell, S. *et al.* (1992d). Cumulative conception and livebirth rates after in-vitro fertilisation. *Lancet* **339**: 1390–4.

Visser, D. S., Fourie, F. L. & Kruger, H. F. (1993). Multiple attempts at embryo transfer: effect on pregnancy outcome in an in vitro fertilization and embryo transfer program. *J. Assist. Reprod. Genet.* **10**: 37–43.

Wood, E. G., Batzer, F. R., Go, K. J. *et al.* (2000). Ultrasound-guided soft catheter embryo transfers will improve pregnancy rates in in-vitro fertilization. *Hum. Reprod.* **15**: 107–12.

Woolcott, R. & Stanger, J. (1997). Potentially important variables identified by transvaginal ultrasound-guided embryo transfer. *Hum. Reprod.* **12**: 963–6.

World Collaborative Report on In Vitro Fertilization (1997). Preliminary Data for 1995. *J. Assist. Reprod. Genet.* **14**: 251S–65S.

Zaidi, J., Campbell, S., Pittrof, R. *et al.* (1995). Endometrial thickness, morphology, vascular penetration and velocimetry in predicting implantation in an in vitro fertilization program. *Ultrasound Obstet. Gynecol.* **6**: 191–8.

Zaidi, J., Pittrof, R., Shaker, A. *et al.* (1996). Assessment of uterine artery blood flow on the day of human chorionic gonadotropin administration by transvaginal color Doppler ultrasound in an in vitro fertilization program. *Fertil. Steril.* **65**: 377–81.

8

Ovarian hyperstimulation syndrome

Botros Rizk and Mary George Nawar

Department of Obstetrics and Gynecology, University of South Alabama College of Medicine, Alabama, USA

Introduction

Ovarian hyperstimulation syndrome (OHSS) is a serious and life-threatening complication of induction of ovulation or superovulation. The syndrome is characterized by ovarian enlargement and a shift of fluid from the intravascular to the extravascular space. This leads to accumulation of fluid in the peritoneal, pleural and, rarely, the pericardial cavities, resulting in intravascular fluid depletion and haemoconcentration.

Any woman undergoing ovarian stimulation is at risk, although OHSS occurs more frequently in women with polycystic ovaries. Women with high oestradiol levels and/or a large number of follicles during ovulation induction have an increased risk of OHSS. The incidence of OHSS is between 0.25% and 4%, and severe hyperstimulation is seen in about one in 200 patients.

During the last 10 years the pathophysiology of the syndrome has been extensively investigated. Vascular endothelial growth factor (VEGF) plays a central role in the cascade of events leading to OHSS. The renin–angiotensin–aldosterone system, luteinizing hormone (LH), histamine, prostaglandins or ovarian prorenin may also have a role in the development of OHSS.

Complications are more frequent when conception does occur and a protracted course may evolve.

Classification of ovarian hyperstimulation syndrome

Mild OHSS:
- Abdominal distension.
- Mild pain.
- Ovarian size usually <8cm.

Good Clinical Practice in Assisted Reproduction, ed. P. Serhal & C. Overton.
Published by Cambridge University Press. © Cambridge University Press 2004.

Moderate OHSS:
- Features of mild OHSS and ultrasonic evidence of ascites.
- Nausea, vomiting and diarrhoea.
- Ovarian size usually 8–12 cm.

Severe OHSS:
- Clinical ascites and/or hydrothorax.
- Haemoconcentration (haematocrit >45%, wbc >15 000/ml).
- Coagulation and/or electrolyte disturbances.
- Hypovolaemia.
- Oliguria with elevated serum creatinine.
- Renal failure.
- Thromboembolic phenomena.
- Ovarian enlargement >12 cm.

A modification of this classification was proposed by Rizk and Aboulghar in 1999, allowing the identification of those women who require immediate hospitalization and differentiates between severe and life-threatening OHSS. It also allows a simple comparison between different series reported in the literature. The mild degree of OHSS is omitted because it is so common after ovarian stimulation for assisted reproductive technology (ART) and does not require medical intervention. Ultrasound evidence of ascites is maintained as part of moderate OHSS. The presence of any abnormality in hepatic or renal functions would indicate Grade B severe OHSS. Grade C includes women with respiratory syndrome, venous thromboembolism or renal shutdown – all medical emergencies that require intensive medical care.

Pathophysiology of ovarian hyperstimulation syndrome

OHSS is characterized by massive bilateral cystic ovarian enlargement and a shift of fluid from the intravascular to the extravascular space. The ovarian stroma is oedematous with multiple theca lutein and follicular cysts. The shift of fluid results in ascites and pleural effusions. The current hypothesis is that human chorionic gonadotrophin (HCG) stimulates VEGF, resulting in increased capillary permeability and fluid leakage, leading to ascites and haemoconcentration.

Vascular endothelial growth factor

This is one of a family of heparin binding proteins that act directly on endothelial cells to induce proliferation and angiogenesis. In vivo, VEGF is a powerful mediator of vessel permeability. McClure *et al.* (1994) studied the evidence for VEGF in the pathogenesis of OHSS in rats. They demonstrated that VEGF was responsible for ascites in more than 70% of OHSS cases and could be prevented by anti-VEGF serum. VEGF (mRNA) expression in the rat ovary increased after the LH surge.

Treatment with gonadotrophin releasing hormone agonist (GnRHa) and luteal phase progesterone supplementation decreased VEGF.

Significantly higher VEGF levels are present in the serum, peritoneal and follicular fluid of patients considered at risk for OHSS (Krasnow *et al.*, 1996). Plasma VEGF levels were followed from the time of admission until clinical resolution (Abramov *et al.*, 1996). High levels were detected in the plasma of all women admitted for severe OHSS compared with controls. These levels fell significantly with clinical improvement and were at a minimum after complete resolution.

Angiogenin

Aboulghar *et al.* (1998) investigated the role of angiogenin in the pathogenesis of OHSS. On the day of admission, the mean serum and peritoneal fluid angiogenin levels were significantly higher in OHSS patients compared to control patients after oocyte retrieval. Angiogenin may play a role in neovascularization leading to the development of OHSS.

Complications

Vascular complications

The combination of a hypercoagulable state and haemoconcentration may result in arterial and venous thrombosis. Severe OHSS is associated with thromboembolism and cerebrovascular thrombosis resulting in either hemiparesis or death. Severe cerebrovascular accidents have been reported with only moderate OHSS.

Liver dysfunction

Sueldo *et al.* (1988) reported the first case of liver dysfunction in OHSS. Although the liver function tests were markedly abnormal, liver biopsy showed significant abnormalities only at the ultrastructural level.

Renal complications

The shift in fluid from the intravascular to the extravascular space results in a decreased circulating volume, with reduced blood pressure, central venous pressure and renal perfusion, together with increased vascular stasis. The diminished circulating blood volume stimulates secretion of antidiuretic hormone and activates the renin–angiotensin–aldosterone system. Fluid retention causes hyponatraemia and impaired renal excretion leads to hyperkalaemia and acidosis. A case of pre-renal failure after treatment with indomethacin has been reported (Balasch *et al.*, 1990). Prostaglandin synthetase inhibitors should be avoided in renal compromise.

Respiratory complications

Pleural effusion may be the sole presentation of OHSS. Adult respiratory distress syndrome is a rare but life-threatening complication. The severe hypoxaemia associated with adult respiratory distress syndrome may lead to cardiorespiratory arrest and requires intensive medical treatment.

Gastrointestinal complications

The first presentation of OHSS may be gastrointestinal symptoms of nausea and vomiting.

Management of ovarian hyperstimulation syndrome

Current management of OHSS relies on the prediction and active prevention. Any patient undergoing ovarian stimulation is at risk of OHSS but it appears to be more frequent in younger women (aged <35 years) and women with polycystic ovarian syndrome (PCOS), and is increased with exogenous HCG administration in the luteal phase or in conception cycles. The majority of cases can be predicted by the combined use of ultrasound and endocrine monitoring.

Prediction of OHSS:

- Young women (<35 years).
- PCOS.
- High and rapid rise of serum oestradiol.
- Ultrasonography.
- Polycystic ovarian syndrome (PCOS) pattern of response to GnRHa before human menopausal gonadotrophin (HMG).
- Large number of follicles with a high portion of small and intermediate follicles.
- Conception cycles, particularly multiple pregnancies.
- OHSS in a previous cycle.
- GnRH-agonist.
- Luteal phase supplementation with HCG.
- Multiple pregnancy.

Oestradiol monitoring of ovulation

The oestradiol level above which different authors have recommended withholding HCG, has gradually increased. There is general agreement that permissible levels are higher in ART cycles compared to in vivo conception. Generally, the higher the serum oestradiol and the quicker the rise, the higher the chance of OHSS. Asch *et al.* (1991) found that in women who had >30 oocytes retrieved, the chance of OHSS was 23%. In cases where oestradiol was >6000 pg/ml (approx. 20 000 pmol/l) on the day of HCG administration and with both these risk factors, there was an 80%

chance of developing severe OHSS. There is general consensus that the chances of OHSS are minimal if oestradiol is <1500 pg/ml.

Levy *et al.* (1996) reported severe OHSS in women with hypogonadotrophic hypogonadism during ovulation induction with urinary human FSH (follicle stimulating hormone) and HCG in the presence of low oestradiol. The development of severe OHSS in the presence of low oestradiol levels is the exception rather than the rule. However, it does demonstrate that oestradiol is not the mediator of increased capillary permeability.

Ultrasonographic monitoring of OHSS

Blankstein *et al.* (1987) reported a correlation between the number and size of periovulatory follicles observed on transvaginal ultrasonography and the development of OHSS. The follicles were classified as small (5–8 mm), medium (9–15 mm) and large (16–25 mm). A decrease in the fraction of mature follicles and an increase in the fraction of the very small follicles were associated with an increased risk of OHSS.

Prevention of ovarian hyperstimulation syndrome

There are numerous strategies for reducing the risk of OHSS, and the list is ever increasing:
1. Withholding HCG.
2. Reducing the ovulatory dose of HCG.
3. Delaying HCG/coasting.
4. Using high dose GnRH-antagonists after coasting.
5. Use of GnRH-agonists to trigger ovulation.
6. Recombinant LH to trigger ovulation.
7. Cryopreservation and replacement of frozen–thawed embryos on another cycle.
8. Follicular and luteal cyst aspiration.
9. Selective oocyte retrieval in subsequent cycle.
10. Progesterone for luteal phase support.
11. Laparoscopic ovarian drilling prior to IVF.
12. Low dose step up protocol in PCOS patients.
13. Intravenous albumin administration at the time of retrieval.

Withholding human chorionic gonadotrophin

Withholding HCG and cancellation of the IVF cycle has been the classic approach to reduce the risk of severe OHSS. This creates a frustrating situation for both the physician and patient.

Reducing the dose of human chorionic gonadotrophin

There are very few data comparing the dose of HCG and the incidence of OHSS. Abdalla *et al.* (1987) compared three doses of HCG to trigger ovulation (2000 iu; 5000 iu; 10 000 iu). The number of oocytes was significantly lower when 2000 iu were used. A similar oocyte retrieval rate was achieved with 5000 and 10 000 iu with significantly less OHSS when 5000 iu was used.

Delaying human chorionic gonadotrophin

Coasting or delaying HCG has been used successfully to reduce the severity of OHSS. Rabinovici *et al.* (1987) studied 12 'overstimulated' women where OHSS was completely avoided by delaying HCG. HMG was withheld for several days and HCG was administered when oestradiol was ≤1700 pg/ml and the leading follicles were 17–22 mm diameter. During the withholding phase, follicular growth continued in all women, while oestradiol levels declined in all but three and these three women conceived. Ovulation was observed in six additional women. Urman *et al.* (1992) reported the results of 40 IVF cycles in 32 women with PCOS. The women were considered at risk of OHSS when estradiol levels were >1500 pg/ml. Coasting significantly reduced the severity of OHSS. The clinical pregnancy rate was 20% and multiple pregnancy rate 50%, with severe OHSS in 2.5%. Sher *et al.* (1993) reported 17 women whose oestradiol level rose above 6000 pg/ml and developed more than 30 follicles during controlled ovarian hyperstimulation for IVF. Coasting was continued for four to nine days until oestradiol levels dropped to <3000 pg/ml. None of the women developed severe OHSS and 16 conceived.

GnRH-agonists to trigger ovulation in gonadotrophin cycles

In a prospective randomized study, Segal & Casper (1992) studied 179 women undergoing IVF. Leuprorelide acetate 500 μg or HCG 5000 IU was administered 34–36 hours before oocyte retrieval, with similar pregnancy rates in both groups. Luteal phase oestradiol and progesterone levels were significantly lower in the GnRHa group compared with the HCG group, and it was suggested that this may be beneficial in preventing OHSS. Revel & Casper (2001) reviewed the use of GnRH-agonists to trigger ovulation in cycles where HMG/FSH or CC/FSH/HMG were used (Table 8.1). The effectiveness of GnRH-agonist to trigger ovulation has been studied in both uncontrolled and controlled studies. In uncontrolled studies, the GnRH-agonist was successful in triggering ovulation in 88% of the cases resulting in a 29% pregnancy rate (Table 8.2). In controlled studies, GnRH-agonist resulted in LH surge in 99% of cases compared to 98% with HCG and the pregnancy rate was 22% versus 17% (P <0.05) (Table 8.3). In uncontrolled studies where GnRH-agonist was used to trigger ovulation, the incidence of OHSS was 0.9% (3/334). In

Table 8.1. Uncontrolled studies to determine the effectiveness of GnRH-agonists for triggering ovulation

Study	Criteria	Number	LH Surge (%)	Pregnancy rate per ET(%)
Lanzone *et al.*, 1989		8	8(100)	–
Emperaire & Ruffie, 1991	E2 > 1200 pg/ml	126	–	27(22)
Imoedemhe *et al.*, 1991	E2 > 4000 pg/ml	27	–	11(29)
Itskovitz *et al.*, 1991	–	12	12(100)	4(29)
Tulchinsky *et al.*, 1991	Pilot study	13	11(85)	4(36)
van der Meer *et al.*, 1993	Pilot study	48	44(92)	10(23)
Balasch *et al.*, 1994	Cycles that would otherwise have been cancelled	23	17(74)	4(17)
Shalev *et al.*, 1994	E2 > 3500 pg/ml	12	–	6(50)
All	–	269	88%	29%

Note: LH: luteinizing hormone; ET: embryo transfer; E2: 17-beta-estradiol.
From: Revel & Casper (2001).

Table 8.2. Uncontrolled studies to determine whether GnRH-agonists for triggering ovulation would prevent OHSS

Study	Criteria	Number of cycles	Number with OHSS	Comments
Emperaire & Ruffie, 1991	E2 >1200 pg/ml or > 3 follicles of 17mm	37	0	
Imoedemhe *et al.*, 1991	E2 > 4000 pg/ml	38	0	
Itskovitch *et al.*, 1991	E2 5000–13 000 pg/ml	8	0	
Van der Meer *et al.*, 1993	–	48	3	Mild to moderate
Balasch *et al.*, 1994	Cycles to be cancelled owing to high risk	23	0	
Balasch *et al.*, 1995		30	0	
Lanzone *et al.*, 1994	PCOS	40	0	Some GnRH agonist Some hCG
Lewit *et al.*, 1995	High risk?	80	0	
Shalev *et al.*, 1994	E2 >3500 pg/ml Number of follicles >20	12	0	Not IVF
Total	–	316	3(0.9%)	

Note: E2, 17-beta oestradiol; OHSS, ovarian hyperstimulation syndrome; PCOS, polycystic ovary syndrome; HCG, human chorionic gonadotrophin; IVF, in vitro fertilization.

Table 8.3. Effectiveness of GnRH-agonist versus HCG in controlled studies

Study	Stimulation	hCG n	LH surge (%)	Pregnancies (%)	GnRH agonist n	LH surge (%)	Pregnancies (%)	P
Gonen et al., 1990	CC-HMG	9	9(100)	0	9	9	3(33)	NS
Segal & Casper, 1992	CC-HMG	95	–	19(19)	84	–	18(20)	NS
Scott et al., 1994	CC	21	21(100)	–	21	21(100)	–	–
Kulikowski et al., 1995	CC-HMG	34	–	3(9)	32	–	4(13)	NS
Gerris et al., 1995	HMG	10	10	–	19	19	–	–
Schmidt-Sarosi et al., 1995	CC	15	8(53)	2(13)	11	11(100)	3(27)	<0.01
Shalev et al., 1995a	CC	106	–	14(13)	104	–	12(12)	NS
Shalev et al., 1995b	HMG	68	–	18(27)	72	–	11(15)	NS
Romeu et al., 1997	FSH	416	413(99)	71(17)	345	342(99)	93(27)	= 0.0007
All		774	461/471(98)	127/734(17)	697	402/405(99)	144/657(22)	<0.05

Note: GnRH, gonadotrophin releasing hormone; HCG, human chorionic gonadotropin; LH, luteinizing hormone; CC, clomiphene citrate; HMG, human menopausal gonadotropin; FSH, follicle stimulating hormone; NS, not significant.

controlled studies comparing GnRH-agonist with HCG, the incidence of OHSS was 1.5% (12/780) in the HCG group compared to 0.7% (5/716) in the GnRH-agonist group ($P = 0.047$). Therefore, it appears that GnRH-agonist is as effective as HCG in triggering ovulation in gonadotrophin only cycles with almost half the incidence of severe OHSS (Table 8.4).

GnRH-agonist to trigger ovulation in GnRH-antagonist/gonadotrophin cycles

The recent introduction of GnRH-antagonists into clinical practice avoids the need for pituitary desensitization and enables the use of GnRH-agonists to trigger ovulation. GnRH-antagonist decreases serum LH and FSH levels within hours. GnRH-agonists have a much higher receptor affinity than the antagonist so that the pituitary gland remains responsive to the GnRH stimulus.

A variety of agents have been successfully used to induce the final stages of oocyte meiotic maturation after GnRH-antagonist. These include GnRH-agonist, native GnRH, recombinant LH, HCG and withdrawal of GnRH-antagonist. GnRH-agonist has been shown to be successful in inducing the final stages of oocyte meiotic maturation in monkeys and in humans. Chillik *et al.* (1987) demonstrated in monkeys that although tonic gonadotrophins remained suppressed under GnRH-antagonist treatment, acute LH release can be stimulated in a GnRH challenge test. In humans the pituitary response was preserved during treatment with the GnRH-antagonist, cetrorelix, confirming that ovulation could be triggered by GnRH-agonist following GnRH-antagonist suppression (Felberbaum *et al.*, 1995). Olivennes *et al.* (1996) demonstrated that ovulation can be triggered by GnRH-agonist after GnRH-antagonist treatment in stimulation cycles for intrauterine insemination.

Itskovitz-Eldor *et al.* (2000) reported on the use of a single bolus of GnRH-agonist (decapeptyl 0.2 mg) to trigger ovulation in women who underwent controlled ovarian hyperstimulation with recombinant FSH and concomitant treatment with the GnRH-antagonist ganirelix for the prevention of a premature LH surge. All women were considered to have an increased risk for OHSS with a serum oestradiol >3000 pg/ml and 20 follicles. None developed any signs or symptoms of OHSS and four conceived.

Bracero *et al.* (2001) studied 19 women who underwent controlled ovarian hyperstimulation for IVF using a combination of gonadotrophins and GnRH-antagonist (ganirelix) 0.25 mg per day. The women were considered at risk for OHSS if the serum oestradiol was >3000 pg/ml or with 20 or more follicles >15mm diameter. Group A consisted of eight women who received two doses of leuprorelide acetate 1 mg subcutaneously 12 hours apart. Group B consisted of 11 women who received HCG 10 000 IU followed by oocyte retrieval 36 hours later. None of the women in Group A had signs or symptoms of OHSS but two women in Group B

Table 8.4. Controlled studies to determine whether GnRH-agonist for triggering ovulation prevent OHSS

Gonen et al., 1990		9	0	9	0	
Segal & Casper, 1992	Randomized	84	0	95	0	
Gerris et al., 1995	Controlled	28	1	10	0	On native GnRH
Kulikowski et al., 1995	Nonrandomized	48	0	34	4	Moderate OHSS
Shalev et al., 1995b	Randomized	72	4	84	8	Not significant
Shalev et al., 1995a	Randomized	104	0	106	0	Clomiphene cycles
Romeu et al., 1997	Prospective Non randomized	345	0	416	0	FSH, IUI Two doses of HCG & LA
Penarrubia et al., 1998	Prospecive Non randomized	26	0	26	0	
All		716	5(0.7%)	780	12(1.5%)	$P = 0.047$ (z test)

Note: OHSS, ovarian hypestimulation syndrome; HCG, human chorionic gonadotrophin; FSH, follicle stimulating hormone; IUI, intrauterine insemination; LA, leuprorelide acetate, GnRH, gonadotrophin releasing hormone.

developed mild OHSS ($P = 0.05$). The authors concluded that triggering ovulation with leuprorelide acetate instead of HCG after the use of antagonist may prevent OHSS. The study had insufficient power to show a statistically significant difference.

High dose GnRH-antagonist to prevent OHSS

De Jong et al. (1998) reported a case where severe OHSS was prevented by using a high-dose GnRH-antagonist. A 33-year-old, ovulatory woman received recombinant FSH 150 IU from cycle day 2 together with GnRH-antagonist (ganirelix) 0.125 mg from cycle day 7 onwards. On cycle day 10 the serum oestradiol was 16 500 pmol/l and on ultrasound four pre-ovulatory follicles (>16mm) and nine intermediate sized (10–16 mm) follicles were present. Recombinant FSH was discontinued, HCG withheld and ganirelix increased to 2 mg per day. Oestradiol rapidly decreased and severe OHSS was avoided.

Laparoscopic ovarian drilling prior to ART

Laparoscopic ovarian drilling to trigger ovulation in patients with PCOS is more widely used in Europe and Australia than the USA. Laser vaporization of the ovarian surface in PCOS has resulted in reduction of OHSS rate and improvement in pregnancy rates (Fukaya et al., 1995). Rimington et al. (1997) designed a prospective randomized study including 50 women with PCOS undergoing IVF for reasons other than anovulation. In the first group, 25 women were treated by long protocol pituitary desensitization followed by gonadotrophin stimulation and IVF. In the second group, 25 women underwent laparoscopic diathermy after pituitary desensitization followed by gonadotrophin stimulation and IVF. The incidence of OHSS was significantly lower in the second group compared to the first and significantly fewer cancelled cycles because of threatened OHSS.

Unilateral ovarian diathermy prior to IVF may also be effective in the prevention of OHSS. Egbase *et al.* (1998) reported three patients who underwent unilateral ovarian diathermy followed by IVF. All had PCOS and had previously been hospitalized for severe OHSS. After the ovarian diathermy, two conceived and none developed OHSS. In a retrospective study Tozer *et al.* (2001) compared 15 women who underwent 22 cycles of IVF preceded by laparoscopic ovarian diathermy (Group A) and 16 women who underwent 24 cycles of IVF (Group B). The incidence of severe OHSS was higher in Group B compared to Group A (4.2% versus 0%).

Cryopreservation of embryos and subsequent replacement

Cryopreservation has enabled the replacement of embryos in a subsequent cycle in order to avoid OHSS. Amso *et al.* (1990) reported the first four cases in which cryopreservation and subsequent replacement achieved successful pregnancies while avoiding OHSS. This protocol was used at Bourn Hall, Cambridge, UK between 1989 and 1990 achieving a 37% clinical pregnancy rate with no case of severe OHSS (Rizk, 1993). Wada *et al.* (1993) compared the incidence of OHSS before and after the introduction of embryo cryopreservation for patients at high risk of OHSS and this occurred in 10/105 (9.5%) and 12/136 (8.8%) cycles in the two phases. The incidence of severe OHSS was 6% in the cryopreserved group compared to 60% in the other group ($P < 0.05$). The authors concluded that cryopreservation reduces the severity but not the incidence of OHSS.

Selective oocyte retrieval

Belaisch-Allart (1988) used selective oocyte retrieval in spontaneous conception by puncture of the majority of the ovarian follicles 35 hours after HCG administration. The remaining intact follicles may result in singleton or twin pregnancy thereby completely avoiding OHSS and multiple pregnancies. Selective oocyte retrieval is no longer clinically useful, as it has been superceded by cryopreservation.

Intravenous albumin

Administration of albumin during oocyte retrieval has been postulated to bind and inactivate vasoactive substances in patients with severe OHSS. The oncotic properties of albumin may also serve to maintain intravascular volume and prevent the development of oocytes. Asch *et al.* (1993) reported 36 women undergoing ART who were at significant risk of developing severe OHSS, with no cases of severe OHSS after intravenous albumin at 5% in Ringers lactate in doses of 500 ml during oocyte retrieval and 500 ml in the recovery room immediately after. However,

Morris & Paulson (1994) criticized the study as uncontrolled with a small sample size and low embryo transfer rate.

Shoham *et al.* (1994) performed a prospective randomized placebo controlled study in 31 women at high risk of developing severe OHSS. The women were randomized to receive either 50 g of human albumin diluted in 500 ml of sodium chloride 0.9% or 500 ml of sodium chloride 0.9% intravenously at the time of oocyte retrieval. None of the women who received human albumin developed severe OHSS, while four in the control group were hospitalized for severe OHSS. Mukherjee *et al.* (1995) reported two cases of severe OHSS despite the administration of 50 g of albumin at the time of oocyte retrieval and in a cohort study Ng *et al.* (1995) found the administration of two infusions of 5% human albumin did not prevent severe OHSS.

Intravenous hydroxyaethyl starch infusion

Graf *et al.* (1997) studied the administration of intravenous hydroxyaethyl starch (HAES) infusion at the time of oocyte retrieval. One hundred women received HAES and were compared to 82 controls. Severe OHSS occurred in two of the HAES group compared to seven in the control group and moderate OHSS occurred in 10 compared to 32 patients respectively.

Follicular aspiration

It has been postulated that severe OHSS after ART is lower than in vivo cycles, because the follicles are aspirated. Studies have failed to show any impact of follicular aspiration on the incidence of OHSS.

Luteal phase support

The use of HCG for luteal phase support significantly increases the incidence of OHSS (Rizk & Smitz, 1992). Progesterone should be used for all patients at risk of OHSS.

VEGF receptor blockade

Gomez and colleagues (2001) in a prize winning presentation addressed the production and release of VEGF by the human granulosa and luteal cells in experimental animals who developed OHSS. In a second series of experiments, they investigated whether VEGF receptor-2 (VEGFR-2) blockade would prevent ovarian hyperstimulation.

In their experiment, they divided immature 22-day-old Wistar rats into four groups. Group I (OHSS): pregnant mare's serum gonadotrophin (PMSG) was given for four consecutive days followed by HCG on the fifth day to induce OHSS. Group II (VEGFR-2): PMSG was given for four days followed by HCG on the fifth day. On the following 2 days a specific VEGFR-2 inhibitor was injected. Group III (stimulated group): PMSG was given and HCG was given in a dosage similar to a routine ovarian stimulation. Group IV (control group): saline was injected from day 22 to day 26. In the first series, time course experiments were done in Group I and IV and vascular permeability was measured after HCG or saline. Peritoneum, mesentery and ovarian biopsies were frozen for VEGF expression analysis at each time point. Vascular permeability was measured 48 hours after HCG or saline in all four groups.

Time course experiments demonstrated increased vascular permeability in Group I reaching maximum levels 48 hours after HCG as compared to Group IV. In the second series of experiments, VEGFR-2 blockade in Group II significantly reduced vascular permeability. Group I also had higher vascular permeability than Groups III or IV. Similarly, VEGF expression in Group 1 ovaries peaked 48 hours after HCG administration and was 4 to 6 times higher than Group IV. No difference was detected in VEGF expression in the mesentery at any time or Group. Only VEGF-121 or 164 isoforms were detected in the ovary, whereas all the other tissues expressed VEGF isoforms.

The authors concluded that the ovary is the main source of VEGF in hyperstimulated animals. The isoforms VEGF-121 and 164 are differentially expressed. They may increase vascular permeability through the VEGF receptor-2 since its specific inhibition prevents increased vascular permeability.

Treatment of ovarian hyperstimulation syndrome

Women with mild and moderate OHSS should be followed up as outpatients with regular visits. The woman should be advised to report to the hospital should they develop shortness of breath or decrease in the volume of urine passed. Women with severe OHSS require hospital admission. The aim of treatment is to be supportive whilst waiting for the condition to resolve spontaneously:

- Provide reassurance and symptomatic relief.
- Avoid haemoconcentration.
- Prevent thromboembolism.
- Maintain cardiorespiratory and renal function.

Serious complications can suddenly occur in all grades and extreme caution should be exercised.

Management of severe OHSS: in-hospital monitoring

Check on examination:

1. General state of hydration:
2. Chest: pleural or pericardial effusion.
3. Abdomen: degree of distension, ascites.
4. Evidence of thrombosis.

Investigations:
1. Ultrasound scan of ovaries (dimensions), abdomen (ascites), chest (pleural or pericardial effusion).
2. FBC and haematocrit.
3. Urea and electrolytes.
4. Albumin and liver function tests.
5. Clotting screen.
6. Chest X-ray if dyspnoeic.

Nursing observations:
1. BP, pulse and temperature four-hourly.
2. Weight and abdominal girth daily.
3. Strict fluid input/output chart.
4. Consider urinary catheterization.
5. Pulse oximeter if dyspnoeic.

Basic treatment

- Rehydration: encourage oral fluid intake if not vomiting.
- Analgesia: as required. Preferred drugs; paracetamol, codeine and paracetamol, pethidine. Try to avoid non-steroidal anti-inflammatory drugs.
- Anti-emetics: as required – metoclopramide or stemetil (PR or im).
- Thromboprophylaxis: full length thromboembolic compression stockings to reduce the risk of venous thrombosis. Consider subcutaneous heparin therapy.
- Luteal support: stop HCG support if being given and change to progesterone pessaries (cyclogest 400 mg bd) or progesterone im (gestone 100 mg daily).

Maintenance of intravascular volume

The aim is to replace fluids in the vascular compartment to allow resumption of normal urine output (>30 ml/hour).

To expand intravascular compartment with colloid, give 2 units of iv gelofusine or haemaccel daily and encourage oral fluids. Try to minimize the use of crystalloids as these solutions diffuse directly into the extracellular space.

Diuretics should be avoided as they remove fluid from the vascular compartment only. Monitoring of fluid replacement by CVP measurement and urinary catheterization may be required.

Paracentesis

Drainage of ascites or pleural effusions is symptomatically helpful if these are marked or compromising respiratory or renal function. Paracentesis should only be done under ultrasound control to avoid damage to bowel or ovaries. The ascites may rapidly accumulate and the paracentesis may exacerbate protein loss. This is rarely of clinical significance and should not influence the decision if symptomatic relief is required.

Aboulghar *et al.* (1990) reported on 21 patients with severe OHSS who were admitted to hospital over a three-year period. Ten patients in Group A were treated conservatively. Eleven patients in Group B also underwent transvaginal aspiration of ascitic fluid. Hospital stay was significantly shorter in Group B. There were no adverse haemodynamic effects as a result of the aspiration of large volumes of ascitic fluid. Replacement of the plasma proteins was important because of the high protein content of the ascitic fluid. Repeated aspiration was required in 30% of the patients.

Anticoagulation

Prophylactic subcutaneous heparin and TED stockings are beneficial in severe OHSS. Full anticoagulation is given if there is evidence of thromboembolism.

Transfer to intensive treatment unit (ITU)

The gynaecology team admitting a patient with severe OHSS must liaise closely with the renal and ITU physicians as appropriate.

Transfer to ITU should be considered if:

• Poor urine output persists despite colloid rehydration.
• Poor oxygen saturation.
• Severe ascites/pleural effusions.

Surgical treatment

In general, laparotomy should be avoided in OHSS. The management of bleeding from multiple corpora lutea could be very difficult and only haemostatic measures should be undertaken to preserve the ovaries. Surgery should always be performed by an experienced gynecologist.

Ectopic pregnancy can co-exist with OHSS and present a diagnostic dilemma. Aboulghar *et al.* (1991) surgically treated a case of ectopic pregnancy complicated by severe OHSS. The diagnosis of ectopic pregnancy was delayed because the symptoms were masked by severe OHSS.

Laparoscopy

The first case of successful laparoscopic management of ovarian torsion after OHSS was reported by Hurwitz (1983). Mashiach (1990) has since reported 12 pregnant women who presented with torsion of hyperstimulated ovaries. They suggested that ovarian torsion after hyperstimulation should be considered a special entity, which requires vigilance to achieve early diagnosis and management.

Is there an ideal protocol to prevent ovarian hyperstimulation syndrome?

Theoretically, a protocol that incorporates the following components would result in the safest profile. Pretreatment with oral contraceptives followed by follicular phase gonadotrophins, GnRH-antagonist to prevent LH surge, GnRH-agonist to trigger ovulation and progesterone for luteal phase support (Rizk, 2001).

Ovarian hyperstimulation syndrome information for patients

Ovarian hyperstimulation syndrome is an uncommon complication resulting from the use of fertility injections (gonadotrophins). Despite careful monitoring, it occurs in about two in 100 women receiving this treatment. It can be a serious condition so it is important that you are aware of the symptoms.

Over-stimulation of the ovaries is most likely to occur in young women with polycystic ovaries who have plenty of eggs available. An ultrasound scan before starting treatment can tell whether a woman has polycystic ovaries.

During your treatment cycle you will have further scans to monitor your progress. If it looks as though the ovaries are over-responding to the drugs then this will be discussed with you. If necessary the treatment will be stopped and you will be advised not to have intercourse and to avoid pregnancy in that cycle. (Usually it is possible to start treatment again after a few weeks with a lower dose of drugs.)

Usually the symptoms of ovarian hyperstimulation occur a few days after the egg releasing injection of HCG is given. The symptoms get better by the time the menstrual period comes – but if the treatment is successful and results in pregnancy, the symptoms may worsen and last longer. In ovarian hyperstimulation syndrome, the ovaries swell and leak fluid into the abdomen, which leads to dehydration, with the risk of kidney damage and thrombosis.

The symptoms to watch for are:
• Nausea and vomiting, abdominal discomfort and bloating (this is common), abdominal swelling, thirst, passing only small amounts of concentrated dark urine and breathlessness.

If you experience any of these you should:
• Drink plenty of clear fluids.
• Take paracetamol as a painkiller, if necessary.
• Rest.
• Contact telephone number for office and out of hours.

REFERENCES

Abdalla, H. I., Ah-Moye, M., Brinsden, P., Howe, D. L., Okonofua, F. & Craft, I. (1987). The effect of the dose of human chorionic gonadotropin and the type of gonadotropin stimulation on oocyte recovery rates in an in vitro fertilization program. *Fertil. Steril.* **48**: 958–63.

Aboulghar, M. A., Mansour, R. T., Serour, G. I. & Amin, Y. (1990). Ultrasonically guided vaginal aspiration of ascites in the treatment of ovarian hyperstimulation syndrome. *Fertil. Steril.* **53**: 933–5.

Aboulghar, M. A., Mansour, R. T., Serour, G. I. & Ramsy, A. M. (1991). Severe ovarian hyperstimulation syndrome complicated by ectopic pregnancy. *Acta Obstet. Gynecol. Scand.* **70**: 371–2.

Aboulghar, M. A., Mansour, R. T., Serour, G. I., Elhelw, B. A. & Shaarawy, M. (1998). Elevated levels of angiogenin in serum and ascitic fluid from patients with severe ovarian hyperstimulation syndrome. *Hum. Reprod.* **13**: 2068–71.

Abramov, Y., Schenker, J. G., Lewin, A., Friedler, S., Nisman, B. & Barak, V. (1996). Plasma inflammatory cytokines correlate to the ovarian hyperstimulation syndrome. *Hum. Reprod.* **11**: 1381–6.

Amso, N. N., Ahuga, K. K., Morris, N. & Shaw, R. W. (1990). The management of predicted ovarian hyperstimulation involving gonadotrophin-releasing hormone analogue with elective cryopreservation of all pre-embryos. *Fertil. Steril.* **53**: 1087–90.

Asch, R. H., Li, H. P., Balmaceda, J. P., Weckstein, L. N. & Stone, S. C. (1991). Severe ovarian hyperstimulation syndrome in assisted reproductive technology: definition of high risk groups. *Hum. Reprod.* **6**: 1395–9.

Asch, R. H., Ivery, G., Goldsman, M., Frederick, J. L., Stone, S. C. & Balmaceda, J. P. (1993). The use of intravenous albumin in patients at high risk for ovarian hyperstimulation syndrome. *Hum. Reprod.* **8**: 1015–20.

Balasch, J., Carmona, F., Llach, J., Arroyo, V., Jore, I. & Vanrell, J. A. (1990). Acute prerenal failure and liver dysfunction in a patient with ovarian hyperstimulation syndrome. *Hum. Reprod.* **5**: 348–51.

Balasch, J., Tur, R., Creus, M. *et al.* (1994). Triggering of ovulation by gonadotropin releasing hormone agonist in gonadotropin-stimulated cycles for prevention of ovarian hyperstimulation syndrome and multiple pregnancy. *Gynecol. Endocrinol.* **8**: 7–12.

Balasch, J., Fabregues, F., Tur, R. *et al.* (1995). Further characterization of the luteal phase inadequacy after gonadotrophin-releasing hormone agonist-induced ovulation in gonadotrophin-stimulated cycles. *Hum. Reprod.* **10**: 1377–81.

Belaisch-Allart, J., Belaisch, J., Hazout, A., Testart, J. & Frydman, R. (1998). Selective oocyte retrieval: a new approach to ovarian hyperstimulation. *Fertil. Steril.* **50**: 654–6.

Blankstein, J., Shalev, J., Saadon, T. *et al.* (1987). Ovarian hyperstimulation syndrome prediction by number and size of preovulatory ovarian follicles. *Fertil. Steril.* **47**: 597–602.

Bracero, M. W., Jurema, M. N., Posada, J. G., Whelan, J. G., Garcia, J. E. & Vlahos, N. P. (2001). Triggering ovulation with leuprorelide acetate (LA) instead of human chorionic gonadotropin (hCG) after the use of ganirelix for in vitro fertilization-embryo transfer (IVF-ET) does not compromise cycle outcome and may prevent ovarian hyperstimulation syndrome. *American Society Reproductive Medicine Fifty-Seventh Annual Meeting*, General Program Prize, Abstracts of the scientific oral and poster sessions program supplement, Abstract 0-245, S-93.

Chillik, C. F., Itskovitz, J., Hahn, D. W., Mcguire, J. L., Danforth, D. R. & Hodgen, G. D. (1987). Characterizing pituitary response to a gonadotropin-releasing hormone (GnRH) antagonist in monkeys: tonic follicle-stimulating hormone/luteinizing hormone secretion versus acute GnRH challenge tests before, during, and after treatment. *Fertil. Steril.* **48**: 480–5.

de Jong, D., Macklon, N. S., Mannaerts, B. M., Coelingh Bennink, H. J., Fauser, B. C. (1998). High dose gonadotrophin-releasing hormone antagonist (ganirelix) may prevent ovarian hyperstimulation syndrome caused by ovarian stimulation for in-vitro fertilization. *Hum. Reprod.* **13** (3): 573–5.

Egbase, P., Al-Awadi, S., Al-Sharhan, M. & Grudzinskas, J. G. (1998). Unilateral ovarian diathermy prior to successful in vitro fertilization: a strategy to prevent ovarian hyperstimulation syndrome? *J. Obstet. Gynaecol.* **18**: 171–3.

Emperaire, J. C. & Ruffie, A. (1991). Triggering ovulation with endogenous luteinizing hormone may prevent the ovarian hyperstimulation syndrome. *Hum. Reprod.* **6**: 506.

Felberbaum, R. E., Reissmann, T., Kupker, W., Bauer, O., Hasani, S., Diedrich, C. & Diedrich, K. (1995). Preserved pituitary response under ovarian stimulation with hMG and GnRH antagonists (Cetrorelix) in women with tubal infertility. *Eur. J. Obstet. Gynecol. Reprod. Biol.* **61**: 151–5.

Fukaya, T., Murakakmi, T., Tamura, M., Watanabe, T., Terada, Y. & Yajima, A. (1995). Laser vaporization of the ovarian surface in polycystic ovary disease results in reduced ovarian hyperstimulation and improved pregnancy rates. *Am. J. Obstet. Gynecol.* **173**: 119–25.

Gerris, J., De Vits, A., Joostens, M. *et al.* (1995). Triggering of ovulation in human menopausal gonadotrophin-stimulated cycles: comparison between intravenously administered gonadotrophin-releasing hormone (100 and 500 micrograms), GnRH agonist (buserelin 500 micrograms) and human chorionic gonadotrophin (10 000 IU). *Hum. Reprod.* **10**: 56.

Gomez, R., Simon, C., Remohi, J. & Pellicer, A. (2001). Vascular Endothelial Growth Factor 121 and 164 (VEGF-121 and VEGF-164) Iso-forms increase vascular permeability (VP) in hyperstimulated rats that is prevented by blocking the VEGF receptor-2 (VEGFR-2), *American Society Reproductive Medicine 57th Annual Meeting*, General Program Prize, Abstracts of the scientific oral and poster sessions program supplement, Abstract 0-1, S-1.

Gonen, Y., Balakier, H., Powell, W. & van Royen, E. (1990). Use of gonadotropin-releasing hormone agonist to trigger follicular maturation for in vitro fertilization. *J. Clin. Endocrinol. Metab.* **71**: 918–22.

Graf, M. A., Fischer, R., Naether, O., Bakloh, V., Tafel, J. & Nuckel, M. (1997). Reduced incidence of ovarian hyperstimulation by prophylactic infusion of hydroxyaethyl starch solution in an in-vitro fertilization program. *Hum. Reprod.* **12**: 2599–602.

Hurwitz, A., Milwidsky, A., Yagel, S. & Adoni, A. (1983). Early unwinding of torsion of an ovarian cyst as a result of hyperstimulation syndrome. *Fertil. Steril.* **40**: 393–4.

Imoedemhe, D. A., Chan, R. C., Sigue, A. B., Pacpaco, E. L. & Olazo, A. B. (1991). A new approach to the management of patients at risk of ovarian hyperstimulation in an in vitro fertilization programme. *Hum. Reprod.* **6**: 1088–91.

Itskovitz, J., Boldes, R., Levron, J., Erlik, Y., Kahana, L. & Brandes, J. M. (1991). Induction of pre-ovulatory luteinizing hormone surge and prevention of ovarian hyperstimulation syndrome by gonadotropin-releasing hormone agonist. *Fertil. Steril.* **56**: 213–20.

Itskovitz-Eldor, J., Kol, S. & Mannaerts, B. (2000). Use of a single bolus of GnRH agonist triptorelin to trigger ovulation after GnRH antagonist ganirelix treatment in women undergoing ovarian stimulation for assisted reproduction, with special reference to the prevention of ovarian hyperstimulation syndrome: preliminary report: short communication. *Hum. Reprod.* **15** (9): 1965–8.

Krasnow, J. S., Berga, S. L., Guzick, D. S., Zeleznik, A. J. & Yeo, K. T. (1996). Vascular permeability factor and vascular endothelial growth factor in ovarian hyperstimulation syndrome: a preliminary report. *Fertil. Steril.* **65**: 552–5.

Kulikowski, M., Wolczynski, S., Kuczynski, W., Grochowski, D. & Szamatowicz, M. (1995). Use of GnRH analog for induction of the ovulatory surge of gonadotropins in patients at risk of the ovarian hyperstimulation syndrome. *Gynecol. Endocrinol.* **9**: 97–102.

Lanzone, A., Fulghesu, A. M., Apa, R., Caruso, A. & Mancuso, S. (1989). LH surge induction by GnRH agonist at the time of ovulation. *Gynecol. Endocrinol.* **3**: 213–20.

Lanzone, A., Fulghesu, A. M., Villa, P. *et al.* (1994). Gonadotropin-releasing hormone agonist versus human chorionic gonadotropin as a trigger of ovulation induction in polycystic ovarian disease gonadotropin hyperstimulated cycles. *Fertil. Steril.* **62**: 35–41. (Erratum appears in *Fertil. Steril.* **63**: 684–5.)

Levy, T., Orvieto, R., Homburg, R., Peleg, D., Dekel, A. & Ben Rafael, Z. (1996). Severe ovarian hyperstimulation syndrome despite low oestradiol concentration in a hypogonadotrophic hypogonadal patient. *Hum. Reprod.* **11**: 1177–9.

Lewit, N., Kol, S., Manor, D. *et al.* (1995). The use of GnRH analogues for induction of the pre-ovulatory gonadotropin surge in assisted reproduction and prevention of the ovarian hyperstimulation syndrome. *Gynecol. Endocrinol.* **4** (Suppl.): 13.

Mashiach, S. Bider, D., Moran, O., Goldenberg, M. & Ben-Rafael, Z. (1990). Adnexal torsion of hyperstimulated ovaries in pregnancies after gonadotropin therapy. *Fertil. Steril.* **53**: 76–80.

McClure, N., Healy, D. L., Rogers, P. A., Sullivan, J., Beaton, L., Haning, R. V. Jr., Connolly D. T. & Robertson, D. M. (1994). Vascular endothelial growth factor as capillary permeability agent in ovarian hyperstimulation syndrome. *Lancet* **344**: 235–6.

Morris, R. S. & Paulson, R. J. (1994). Letter to the editor. *Hum. Reprod.* **9**: 753.

Mukherjee, T., Copperman, A. B., Sandler, B., Bustillo, M. & Grunfeld, L. (1995). Severe ovarian hyperstimulation despite prophylactic albumin at the time of oocyte recovery for in vitro fertilization and embryo transfer. *Fertil. Steril.* **64**: 641–2.

Ng, E., Leader, A., Claman, P., Domingo, M. & Spence, J. E. (1995). Intravenous albumin does not prevent the development of severe ovarian hyperstimulation syndrome in an in-vitro fertilization programme. *Hum. Reprod.* **10**: 807–10.

Olivennes, F., Fanchin, R., Bouchard, P., Taieb, J. & Frydman, R. (1996). Triggering of ovulation by a gonadotropin-releasing hormone (GnRH) agonist in patients pretreated with GnRH antagonist. *Fertil. Steril.* **66**: 151–3.

Penarrubia, J., Balasch, J., Fabregues, F. *et al.* (1998). Human chorionic gonadotropin luteal support overcomes luteal phase inadequacy after gonadotropin-releasing hormone agonist-induced ovulation in gonadotropin-stimulated cycles. *Hum. Reprod.* **13**: 3315.

Rabinovici, J., Kushnir, O., Shalev, J., Goldenberg, M. & Blankstein, J. (1987). Rescue of meno-tropin cycles prone to develop ovarian hyperstimulation. *Br. J. Obstet. Gynecol.* **94**: 1098–102.

Revel, A. & Casper, R. F. (2001). The use of LH-RH agonist to induce ovulation. In *Infertility and Reproductive Medicine Clinics of North America*, ed. P. Devroey, vol.12, pp. 105–18. Philadelphia: W. B. Saunders.

Rimington, M. R. Walker, S. M. & Shaw, R. W. (1997). The use of laparoscopic ovarian electro-cautery in preventing cancellation of in-vitro fertilization treatment cycles due to risk of ovarian hyperstimulation syndrome in women with polycystic oavries. *Hum. Reprod.* **12**: 1443–7.

Rizk, B. (1993). Ovarian hyperstimulation syndrome. In *Progress in Obstetrics and Gynecology*, ed. J. Studd, vol. 11. Edinburg: Churchill Livingston.

Rizk, B. (2001). Ovarian hyperstimulation syndrome. *American Society for Reproductive Medicine, 34th Annual Postgraduate Course, Advances and Controversies in Ovulation Induction*, October 2001, pp. 23–46, Orlando, Florida.

Rizk, B. & Smitz, J. (1992). Ovarian hyperstimulation syndrome after superovulation using GnRH agonists for IVF and related procedures. *Hum. Reprod.* **7**: 320–7.

Rizk, B. & Aboulghar, M. A. (1999). Classification, pathophysiology and management of ovarian hyperstimulation syndrome. In *A Textbook of In Vitro Fertilization and Assisted Reproduction*, ed. P. R. Brinsden, 2nd edn, pp. 131–55. Carnforth: Parthenon Publishing.

Romeu, A., Monzo, A., Peiro, T. *et al.* (1997). Endogenous LH surge versus hCG as ovulation trigger after low-dose highly purified FSH in IUI: a comparison of 761 cycles. *J. Assist. Reprod. Genet.* **14**: 518.

Schmidt-Sarosi, C., Kaplan, D. R., Sarosi, P. et al. (1995). Ovulation triggering in clomiphene citrate-stimulated cycles: Human chorionic gonadotrophin versus a gonadotrophin releasing hormone agonist. *J. Assist. Reprod. Genet.* **12**: 167–74.

Scott, R. T., Bailey, S. A., Kost, E. R., Neal, G. S., Hofmann, G. E. & Illions, E. H. (1994). Comparison of leuprorelide acetate and human chorionic gonadotropin for the induction of ovulation in clomiphene citrate-stimulated cycles. *Fertil. Steril.* **61**: 872–9.

Segal, S. & Casper, R. F. (1992). Gonadotropin-releasing hormone agonist versus human chorionic gonadotropin for triggering follicular maturation in in vitro fertilization. *Fertil. Steril.* **57**: 1254–8.

Shalev, E., Geslevich, Y. & Ben-Ami, A. (1994). Induction of pre-ovulatory luteinizing hormone surge by gonadotrophin-releasing hormone agonist for women at risk for developing the ovarian hyperstimulation syndrome. *Hum. Reprod.* **9**: 417–19.

Shalev, E., Geslevich, Y., Matilsky, M. & Ben-Ami, A. (1995a). Gonadotrophin-releasing hor-mone agonist compared with human chorionic gonadotrophin for ovulation induction after clomiphene citrate treatment. *Hum. Reprod.* **10**: 2541–4.

Shalev, E., Geslevich, Y., Matilsky, M. & Ben-Ami, A. (1995b). Induction of pre-ovulatory go-nadotropin surge by gonadotrophin-releasing hormone agonist compared to pre-ovulatory injection of human chorionic gonadotrophins for ovulation induction in intrauterine insem-ination treatment cycles. *Hum. Reprod.* **10**: 2244–7.

Sher, G., Salem, R., Feinman, M., Dodge, S., Zouves, C. & Knutzen, V. (1993). Eliminating the risk of life-endangering complications following overstimulation with menotropin fertility agents: a report on women undergoing in vitro fertilization and embryo transfer. *Obstet. Gynecol.* **81**: 1009–11.

Shoham, Z., Weissman, A., Barash, A., Borenstein, R., Schachter, M. & Insler, V. (1994). Intra-venous albumin for the prevention of severe ovarian hyperstimulation syndrome in an in vitro fertilization program: a prospective, randomized, placebo controlled study. *Fert. Steril.* **62**: 137–42.

Sueldo, C. E., Price, H. M., Bachenberg, K., Steinleitner, A., Gitlin, N. & Swanson, J. (1988). Liver dysfunction in ovarian hyperstimulation syndrome. A case report. *J. Reprod. Med.* **33**: 387–90.

Tozer, A. J., Al-Shawaf, T., Zosmer, A., Hussain, S., Wilson, C., Lower, A. M. & Grudzinskas, J. G. (2001). Does laparoscopic ovarian diathermy affect the outcome of in vitro fertilization-emryo transfer in women with polycystic ovary syndrome? A retrospective study. *Hum. Reprod.* **16**: 91–5.

Tulchinsky, D., Nash, H., Brown, K. *et al.* (1991). A pilot study of the use of gonadotropin-releasing hormone analog for triggering of ovulation. *Fertil. Steril.* **55**: 644.

Urman, B., Pride, S. M. & Yuen, B. H. (1992). Management of overstimulated gonadotrophin cycles with a controlled drift period. *Hum. Reprod.* **7**: 213–17.

Van der Meer, S., Gerris, J., Joostens, M. & Tas, B. (1993). Triggering of ovulation using a gonadotrophin-releasing hormone agonist does not prevent ovarian hyperstimulation syndrome. *Hum. Reprod.* **8**: 1628–31.

Wada, I., Matson, P. L., Troup, S. A., Morroll, D. R., Hunt, L. & Lieberman, B. A. (1993). Does elective cryopreservation of all embryos from women at risk of ovarian hyperstimulation syndrome reduce the incidence of the condition? *Br. J. Obstet. Gynecol.* **100**: 265–9.

9

Early pregnancy complications after assisted reproductive technology

Eric Jauniaux and Natalie Greenwold

Department of Obstetrics and Gynaecology, University College London, London, UK

The availability of prenatal diagnosis has expanded, in particular with great advances in ultrasound imaging enabling investigation of the fetus from three weeks after conception. Because pregnancies resulting from assisted reproductive technology (ART) undergo regular ultrasound examination, often on a weekly basis, they have been an invaluable source of information on normal and abnormal human development in utero. For example, most measurement charts used in early pregnancy units have been constructed from the investigation of ART pregnancies.

Miscarriage is the most common complication of spontaneous and artificial gestations (Table 9.1). In cases of miscarriage the diagnosis of a specific anomaly has important epidemiological value and may help to elucidate unclear mechanisms implicated in some cases of early pregnancy loss (EPL). Because of the perceived need to stimulate excess follicles and transfer more than two embryos to achieve high pregnancy rates, multiple gestation pregnancy (MGP) rates are higher in ART cycles and because perinatal mortality rates are four to six times higher for MGP than singleton, MGP must be considered a serious complication of ART. This chapter presents the different aspects of early investigation and management of pregnancy failure and MGP, including sections on the clinical aspects of miscarriage, the ultrasound diagnosis of EPL and ectopic pregnancy, and the differential diagnosis between monozygotic and dizygotic twinning. The role of multifetal pregnancy reduction (MFPR) in the management of MGP resulting from ART is also discussed.

Clinicopathology and epidemiology of early pregnancy complications: definitions

Early pregnancy loss

This is defined as a miscarriage occurring within the first 12 weeks of gestation. There are four different clinical forms of EPL:

Good Clinical Practice in Assisted Reproduction, ed. P. Serhal & C. Overton.
Published by Cambridge University Press. © Cambridge University Press 2004.

Table 9.1. Frequency of pregnancy loss

Variable	(%)
Total loss of conception	50–70
Total clinical miscarriages	25–30
Before 6 weeks' gestation	18
Between 6 and 9 week's gestation	4
After 9 weeks' gestation	3
EPL in primigravidas	6–10
Risk of EPL after three miscarriages	25–30
Risk of EPL of women aged 40 years	30–40
Ectopic pregnancies per live births	1–2

Note: EPL: early pregnancy loss.

- *Threatened miscarriage*
  According to the World Health Organization (WHO) nomenclature (FIGO News, 1976), threatened miscarriage is defined as painless vaginal bleeding occurring any time between implantation and 24 weeks of gestation. Probably a quarter of all pregnancies are complicated by threatened miscarriage, although many women may be unaware of their pregnancy at the time they present with vaginal bleeding. It is certainly one of the most common indications (together with suspected ectopic pregnancy) for emergency referral of a young woman to a Accident & Emergency (A&E) department. The bleeding may resolve spontaneously in a few days, never to recur. It may also continue, or stop and start over several days or weeks. It is only when abdominal cramps supervene that the process may move in the direction of inevitability, in particular if the cervix opens. It usually happens between six and nine weeks of gestation when the definitive placenta forms.
- *Inevitable miscarriage*
  Inevitable miscarriage can be complete or incomplete depending on whether or not all fetal and placental tissues have been expelled from the uterus. The typical features of incomplete miscarriage are heavy (sometimes intermittent) bleeding with passage of clots and tissue, together with lower abdominal cramps. If these symptoms improve spontaneously, a complete miscarriage is more likely.
- *Missed miscarriage*
  Missed miscarriage is a gestational sac containing a dead embryo/fetus before 20 weeks of gestation without clinical symptoms of expulsion. The diagnosis is usually made by failure to identify fetal heart action on ultrasound. Within this context, the woman often complains of chronic but light vaginal bleeding.

- *Recurrent miscarriage*

  Recurrent miscarriage is defined as three or more consecutive spontaneous miscarriages. The aetiologies of recurrent pregnancy failure are diverse, not well understood and will be discussed later. They may present clinically as any of the previously described forms of EPL.

Gestational trophoblastic disease (GTD)

GTD is a term commonly applied to a spectrum of interrelated diseases originating from the placental trophoblast (Jauniaux, 1999). The main categories of GTD are complete hydatidiform mole, partial hydatidiform mole and choriocarcinoma. Complete or classical hydatidiform moles are described as a generalized swelling of the villous tissue, diffuse trophoblastic hyperplasia and no embryonic or fetal tissue. Partial hydatidiform moles are characterized by focal swelling of the villous tissue, focal trophoblastic hyperplasia and embryonic or fetal tissue. The abnormal villi are scattered within macroscopically normal placental tissue, which tends to retain its shape (Jauniaux, 1998). Both complete and partial hydatidiform moles can transform into choriocarcinoma (Seckl *et al.*, 2000).

Epidemiology

It has been estimated that about 60% of all fertilized ova are lost before the end of the first trimester (Edmonds *et al.*, 1982). Most are lost during the first month after the last menstrual period and are often ignored as conceptions, particularly if they occur around the time of an expected menstrual period. Pregnancy wastage during the first three cycles accounts for 31% of the pregnancies detected (Zinaman, 1996). About 40% of these losses are detected only by urine human chorionic gonadotrophin (HCG) testing.

The rate of pregnancy loss is known to decrease with gestational age. The precise incidence of early pregnancy loss at different stages of gestation has been more clearly defined with the routine use of transvaginal ultrasound. In women with positive urinary pregnancy tests and no antecedent history of vaginal bleeding, pregnancy loss is virtually complete by the end of the embryonic period (70 days after the onset of the last menstrual period). Once a gestational sac has been documented on scan, subsequent loss of viability in the embryonic stage is still 11.5%. If an embryo has developed up to 5 mm, subsequent loss of viability occurs in 7.2% (Goldstein, 1994). Loss rates drop rapidly to 3.3% for embryos measuring 6–10 mm and to 0.5% for embryos >10 mm. The fetal loss rate after 11 weeks is 2–3% (Pandya *et al.*, 1996).

Estimates of the incidence of the various forms of GTD vary mainly because few countries have registers and complete and partial moles have often been treated as a single entity in epidemiological studies. The estimated incidence of complete moles is one per 1000–2000 pregnancies whereas the incidence of partial moles is around one per 700 pregnancies (Jauniaux, 1999). The vast majority of complete and partial moles abort spontaneously during the first trimester of pregnancy and the incidence of molar pregnancies has been estimated to account for 2% of all miscarriages. The incidence of choriocarcinoma varies from one in 10 000 to one in 50 000 pregnancies. Expressed as a percentage of hydatidiform moles it ranges from 3% to 10%.

Etiopathology

The risk of pregnancy loss will increase with maternal age, and a woman aged 40 years carries twice the risk of a woman aged 20 years. Past obstetric history also influences the risk. The pregnancy loss rate among primigravidas is 6–10% whereas after three or more losses the risk increases to 25–30%. The only well established epidemiological fact about EPL is that about 50–60% are associated with a chromosomal defect of the conceptus and that the frequency of abnormal chromosomal complement increases up to 90% when the embryonic demise occurs earlier in gestation (Edwards, 1986).

Autosomal trisomies are the most common chromosomal defect with an incidence of 30–35%, followed by triploidies and monosomies X. Triploidy and tetraploidy are frequent but extremely lethal chromosomal abnormalities and are rarely found in late miscarriages (Simpson & Bombard, 1987). Structural chromosomal rearrangements such as translocation or inversions are present in only 1.5% of sporadic miscarriages but are a significant cause of recurrent miscarriages (Li, 1998).

Complete hydatidiform moles have a diploid chromosomal constitution totally derived from the paternal genome usually resulting from the fertilization of an oocyte by a diploid spermatozoon. The maternal chromosomes may be either inactivated or absent, remaining only inside the mitochondria. Partial moles are usually triploid and of diandric origin, having two sets of chromosomes from paternal origin and one from maternal origin. Most have a 69,XXX or 69,XXY genotype derived from a haploid ovum with either reduplication of the paternal haploid set from a single sperm, or less frequently, from dispermic fertilization (Jauniaux, 1999). Triploidy of digynic origin, due to a double maternal contribution are not associated with placental hydatidiform changes. Maternal age and a previous history of molar pregnancy have consistently been shown to influence the risk of hydatidiform mole, whereas the evidence that the rate of molar pregnancies varies according to dietary habits of some ethnic groups remains controversial.

Other causes of miscarriage include, endocrine diseases, anatomic abnormalities of the female genital tract, infections, immune factors, chemical agents, hereditary disorders, trauma, maternal diseases and psychological factors (Barnea, 1992). Prospective epidemiological surveys indicate that none of these etiologies can quantitatively be shown to cause more than a small percentage of EPL. Etiologies such as exposure to certain toxins were rarely reported but are becoming an important issue in the context of voluntary and passive smoking or of ecological disasters. In the case of recurrent miscarriages, some other causes such as thrombophilia may be relatively more frequently found. Mullerian tract fusion and cervical abnormalities are well accepted causes of second trimester losses, but are not associated with a higher rate of first trimester EPL.

Early pregnancy outcome after ART

Miscarriage after ART

The rate of miscarriage after ART ranges between 10% and 30% depending on the technique used (Lam *et al.*, 1989; Wennerholm *et al.*, 1997; Aytoz *et al.*, 1999; Westergaard *et al.*, 2000), the number of embryos transferred (Balen *et al.*, 1993) and maternal age (Lass *et al.*, 1998; Pantos *et al.*, 1999; Nikolettos *et al.*, 2000). In spontaneous gestations and pregnancies resulting from ART, maternal age is the most important parameter in the evaluation of the risk of pregnancy complications, and in women aged 45 or more the risk of miscarriage is around 75% (Nybo *et al.*, 2000). In infertile women there is an overall fivefold increase in early pregnancy loss from the age of 40 years compared to 31–35 years, independent of the diagnosed cause of infertility, mode of insemination and ovulation induction protocol (Smith & Buyalos, 1996).

Studies have described the outcome of ART pregnancies following prenatal diagnosis but there appear to be no cytogenetic data regarding pregnancy loss before 11 weeks of gestation. The rate of miscarriage in IVF quoted in the literature is widely variable and displays the same increase in incidence with maternal age as in spontaneous miscarriage. Cryopreservation in IVF and intracytoplasmic sperm injection (ICSI) do not appear to alter the rates of miscarriage in relation to 'fresh' procedures but ICSI is associated with a higher incidence of sex-chromosomal de novo aberrations (Tarlatziz & Grimbizis, 1999). However, there are no karyotype results in cases of miscarriage in the studies on the pregnancy outcome after ICSI. Overall, there is a need for more information on the epidemiology of chromosome abnormalities in miscarriage after ART.

Molar pregnancy after ART

Molar pregnancies may be complete (diploid and androgenetic usually arising from fertilization by a haploid sperm which doubles its chromosomes and takes over the ovum) or partial (triploid and predominantly genetically male). Partial moles may, albeit rarely, coexist with a live fetus. The incidence of molar pregnancy after ART is not clear from the literature, with case reports accounting for the majority of articles. Cases of repeated molar pregnancies have been reported in certain individuals. In such cases a strategy for prevention using ICSI and preimplantation genetic diagnosis with fluorescence in situ hybridization (FISH) has been suggested (Reubinoff *et al.*, 1997). Using this strategy, complete moles arising from dispermic fertilization are avoided by the use of ICSI, followed by preimplantation selection against the transfer of 46,XX embryos thus preventing transfer.

Conservative management of a live pregnancy coexisting with a complete mole has been reported (Manase *et al.*, 2000). In this case a complete mole, alongside a live fetus at 13 weeks of gestation was diagnosed after a pregnancy conceived following gamete intrafallopian transfer (GIFT). At 36 weeks of gestation a live male infant was delivered by caesarean section due to elevated serum HCG levels.

Diagnosis of EPL

Maternal serum biochemistry

Maternal serum levels of many proteins and hormones of fetal and placental origin have been tested to predict the outcome of women with vaginal bleeding in early pregnancy. These assays were very popular in the 1970s and 1980s before the advent of high resolution ultrasound. The idea that some forms of EPL may be associated with abnormal serum levels of specific placental protein before the appearance of any clinical symptoms is a matter of debate. In general, the concentration of placental products is reduced in a threatened miscarriage in which the outcome is fetal loss, but normal in cases in which pregnancy proceeds (Salem *et al.*, 1984; Stewart *et al.*, 1995). As a clinically predictive tool, measurement of these compounds is often unnecessary if fetal life can be demonstrated by ultrasound examination (Stabile *et al.*, 1989). In particular, if on high resolution transvaginal ultrasound the gestational sac is inside the uterine cavity but the fetal heart is not evident ultrasonically after five weeks of gestation, then abnormally low levels of any fetoplacental products will not provide additional clinical information.

Progesterone and HCG have both been used extensively in the diagnosis, management and treatment of abnormal early pregnancy. The predictive value of these hormones remains important in the follow-up of extrauterine pregnancies or very early EPL. A logistic model using transvaginal ultrasound features and HCG and progesterone levels has been proposed in the case of early pregnancy of unknown location (Banerjee *et al.*, 1999). The majority of these pregnancies are abnormal and at the initial visit the logistic model will identify those that will resolve without the need for further intervention. Serum progesterone appears to be the single most specific biomarker for distinguishing viable from nonviable pregnancy (Phipps *et al.*, 2000). The measurement of plasma or urine HCG has always been pivotal in the diagnosis and follow-up of GTD.

HCG remains a reliable predictor of successful implantation and pregnancy viability. An ovulation +14 days HCG level <50 iu/l is often predictive of a nonviable outcome, while ovulation +21 days HCG <200 iu/l always indicates a nonviable pregnancy (Sunder & Lenton, 2000). A small proportion of fetuses with a heart action will subsequently spontaneously abort and a single serum free β-HCG measurement taken in early pregnancy has a 88% sensitivity and 83% positive predictive value in the diagnosis of EPL and long-term prognosis of viability (al-Sebai *et al.*, 1996). In this small group of women, the levels of PAPP-A and SP-1 are reduced before fetal death. Low progesterone levels and low β-HCG levels at four to seven weeks of gestation have been shown to have 59% and 68% sensitivity in the prediction of early pregnancy loss (Lower & Yovich, 1992). This suggests that there may be relationships between trophoblast dysfunction and some forms of miscarriage. Furthermore, the pattern of the reduction in the circulating levels of the placental proteins in later miscarriages suggests the function of specific cell types may be impaired in these cases (Johnson *et al.*, 1993).

At an experimental level, an early pregnancy factor (EPF) has been studied in sera of women with unexplained spontaneous miscarriage. It was found that low levels of EPF are associated with a poor prognosis (Shu-Xin & Zhen-Qun, 1993). Inhibin A is mainly produced by the feto-placental unit and inhibin pro-alpha C by the corpus luteum (Lockwood *et al.*, 1998). Low levels herald pregnancy failure despite luteal supplementation with progesterone. Relaxin and progesterone have also been studied in the luteal phase of stimulated cycles by gonadotrophins and it has been found that pregnancies resulting in a miscarriage have low inhibin and progesterone levels. Relaxin induces placental protein 14 (PP14) expression in a receptive endometrium, and measurements of serum PP14 may be of value as a screening test for implantation potential (Sunder & Lenton, 2000). Finally, in the serum of women with recurrent pregnancy loss LH concentration is inappropriately raised in 81%. High LH levels may have adverse effects on the developing oocyte or endometrium either directly or indirectly by causing an elevation in testosterone and oestrogen levels (Watson *et al.*, 1993).

Ultrasound diagnosis of EPL

The presence or absence of an intrauterine gestational sac is the main point of distinction between intrauterine and tubal pregnancy. In 10–20% of ectopic

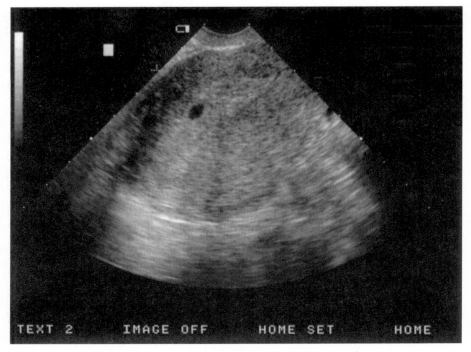

Figure 9.1.   Transvaginal ultrasound image showing a pseudogestational sac – characteristically centrally located endometrial fluid collection surrounded by a single echogenic ring.

pregnancies, a pseudogestational sac is seen (Figure 9.1) as a small, centrally located endometrial fluid collection surrounded by a single echogenic rim of endometrial tissue undergoing decidual reaction (Cadkin & McAlpin, 1984). Distinction between a very early intrauterine sac and pseudogestational sac may be difficult on ultrasound scan. In a true gestational sac, the decidua vera and adjacent decidua capsularis usually form two concentric rings that surround a portion of the gestational sac forming 'the double decidual sac sign' and can be seen during the fifth week. However, this is not always specific in appearance and careful analysis is required before a final diagnosis is made.

The other common diagnostic problem is the distinction between abnormal intrauterine pregnancy and ectopic pregnancy. In cases of incomplete and complete miscarriages the scan will reveal variable amounts of echogenic tissue inside the uterine cavity, which may represent either blood clots or retained placental tissue. This finding often leads to inconclusive diagnosis, reported in up to 21% of cases (Cacciatore et al., 1990).

A strong correlation exists between the occurrence of a miscarriage and the following ultrasound criteria; fetal bradycardia, discrepancy between the diameter of

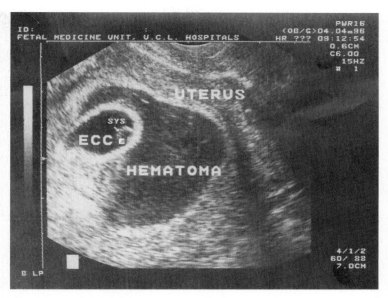

Figure 9.2. Transvaginal ultrasound image – haematoma at five weeks gestation. SYS: secondary yolk sac; ECC: extra embryonic coelom – coelomic cavity; E: embryo.

the gestational sac and the crown–rump length, and discrepancy between menstrual and sonographic age of >one week. The risk of EPL is 6% when none of the above risk factors are present and is as high as 84% when all are present (Falco *et al.*, 1996). The role of combining ultrasound and endocrinology in predicting this type of early pregnancy complication remains controversial. Nevertheless, the evaluation of the size of the gestational sac or the embryo and demonstration of embryonic heart action are important in the management, psychological support and counselling of women with this common pregnancy complication.

Intrauterine haematomas can be subchorionic (between the membranes and the uterine wall) and retro-placental (between the placenta and the myometrium), or both. The incidence of haematomas in the general population of early pregnancies varies greatly between studies, ranging from 4% to 48% (Jauniaux *et al.*, 1996), and their aetiology remains unclear. Even large haematomas in the first trimester (Figure 9.2) are not considered to pose a serious threat to the pregnancy. Much emphasis has been put on the intrauterine haematoma volume and/or the presence of vaginal bleeding but not on the location of the haemorrhage. It is likely that if the bleeding occurs at the level of the definitive placenta (under the cord insertion), it may result in placental separation and subsequent miscarriage. By contrast, a subchorionic haematoma detaching only the membrane opposite to the cord insertion may reach a significant volume before it affects normal pregnancy development (Figure 9.3).

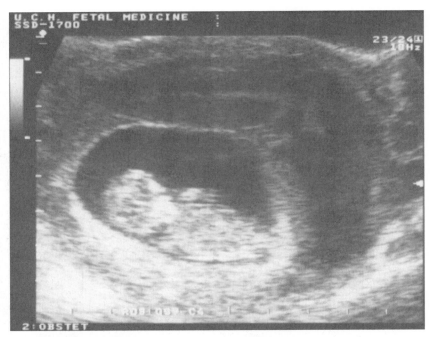

Figure 9.3.   Transvaginal ultrasound image showing a subchorionic haematoma – the haematoma lies
between the membranes and the uterine wall.

The sonographic feature of incomplete miscarriage is thick irregular echoes in
the midline of the uterine cavity. However, this is often not diagnostic of retained
products, as blood clots may look remarkably similar on scan. The finding of a
well-defined regular endometrial line can effectively exclude this diagnosis. The
reliability of ultrasonography in the detection of complete miscarriage is highly
effective in correctly identifying 98% of women with an empty uterus, who do not
need a surgical operation (Rulin *et al.*, 1993; Haines *et al.*, 1994).

About one-third of normal embryos with a crown–rump length <5 mm have
no demonstrable cardiac activity (Levi *et al.*, 1990). Thus the diagnosis of missed
miscarriage should not be made in embryos smaller than this. With the wider
use of transvaginal ultrasound equipment, an increasing number of instances in
which fetal death has been erroneously diagnosed by ultrasound examination have
been reported within the context of medical litigation. The sonographic features
of a missed miscarriage include the presence of a gestational sac, which is often
collapsed, and a dead fetus or no embryonic echoes within a gestational sac large
enough for such structures to be visible (Figure 9.4). Provided that both operator
and equipment are technically adequate, a mean gestational sac diameter >15 mm

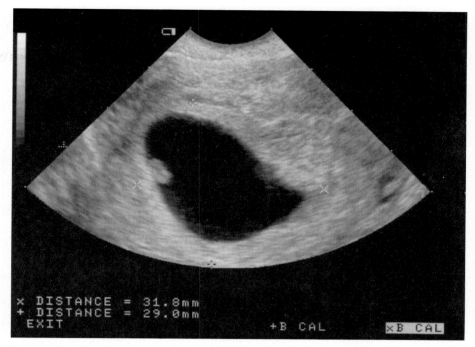

Figure 9.4. Transvaginal ultrasound image showing gestational sac (diameter 31.8 mm × 29 mm, including trophoblast) and fetal pole. The sac is collapsed and irregular in shape.

(using transvaginal probe) or >17 mm (using a transabdominal probe) are necessary before diagnosing this anomaly.

When the gestational sac is at least 25 mm in diameter but no fetal part can be seen, the terms 'blighted ovum' or 'anembryonic pregnancy' have often been used by pathologists and more commonly by ultrasonographers. Recent findings suggest that the most likely explanation for this early pregnancy complication is the early death and resorption of an embryo with persistence of the placental tissue, rather than a pregnancy originally without an embryo. Most pregnancies traditionally classified as anembryonic gestation result from early embryonic demise, the embryo having developed for at least up to 14 days after ovulation, corresponding to the stage of embryonic life when the secondary yolk sac starts to form (Jauniaux *et al.*, 1995).

The vast majority of complete and partial hydatidiform moles abort spontaneously during the first trimester of pregnancy resulting in a total incidence of molar placenta of about 1% of all conceptions (Palmer, 1994). Following uterine evacuation, 10% of patients with a complete mole develop persistent gestational trophoblastic disease. The ultrasound diagnosis of a complete mole is usually

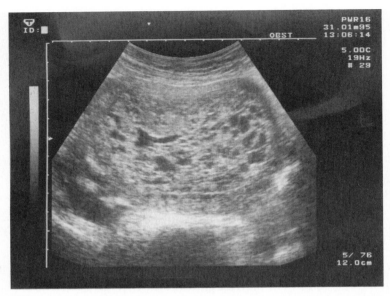

Figure 9.5. Transvaginal ultrasound image showing typical snowstorm appearance of complete mole.

straightforward after nine weeks of amenorrhea (Jauniaux, 1998). Prior to this, the ultrasound demonstration of an abnormal trophoblast may be very difficult and inaccurate. Characteristically, the uterine cavity is filled with hydropic, vesicular placental tissue giving a typical snowstorm appearance on ultrasound (Figure 9.5). The diagnosis of a partial mole is usually more complex both in utero and after delivery. The presence of any form of placental molar changes and a coexistent fetus is often referred to as a partial mole. As demonstrated by our recent study there are at least three different categories of placental lesion to be considered when sono-lucent areas are found within the placenta on ultrasound examination (Jauniaux & Nicolaides, 1997).

Colour Doppler imaging

Comparing the blood flow velocity waveforms and pathological features in missed miscarriages and normal pregnancies, it has been demonstrated that in missed miscarriages, high mean pulsatility index (PI) and premature intervillous flow were associated with abnormal placentation and dislocation of the trophoblastic shell (Jauniaux et al., 1994). The premature entry of maternal blood into the intervillous space at this stage of pregnancy disrupts the placental shell and is probably the mechanical cause of miscarriage. The predictive value of Doppler measurements in early pregnancy is limited. All Doppler studies in the first trimester have failed to show abnormal blood flow indices in the uteroplacental circulation of pregnancies that subsequently ended in miscarriage or missed miscarriage.

Early management of MGP after ART

Ultrasound diagnosis

The use of ultrasound has dramatically improved the antenatal diagnosis and pre-natal outcome of multiple pregnancies and early information is vital for coun-selling patients. The vanishing twin phenomenon is the spontaneous miscarriage or resorption of one twin and occurs in about 20% of twins recognized in the first trimester, although vaginal bleeding is reported in only 20% (Jauniaux *et al.*, 1988). If as in the majority of the cases of first trimester vanishing twins the pregnancy outcome was not otherwise affected, this may be a traumatizing psychological ex-perience for the parents.

The degree of prenatal outcome in twins is primarily related to chorionicity, which is the major factor in determining pregnancy outcome. It is already known that in monochorionic twins, perinatal morbidity and mortality is twice as high as in dichorionic twins. Conjoined twins or shared placenta is the cause for the pathologic events of twin–twin transfer syndrome and twin reversed atrial perfusion syndrome. Furthermore, the death of a monochorionic twin jeopardizes the co-twin, putting it at high risk of sudden death or severe neurological impairment (Machin & Keith, 1999). Therefore, accurate identification of monochorionic twins would enable close monitoring of these very high risk fetuses that would greatly benefit from more intensive surveillance.

It is possible to identify more than one gestational sac as early as five to six weeks of gestation by transabdominal scanning, although more details regarding the fetal pole, beating heart and yolk sac may be visible later. It is very important to visualize the entire uterine cavity for proper identification of its whole content, as well as the entire pelvis to rule out the rare combination of heterotopic pregnancy. Sono-graphic criteria, similar to those used in singleton gestations, should be applied to document the viability and the correct gestational age. However, there are some typical scanning landmarks for twin gestations during the first trimester deserv-ing special consideration, such as placentation, chorionicity and the presence of major typical congenital anomalies (i.e. conjoined twins). Based on first trimester ultrasound parameters, including the growth of the gestational sac, yolk sac, fetal pole and fetal heart rate, it may be possible to predict that the smallest twin or the one with a fetal heart rate of <85 bpm is more likely to become a vanishing twin.

The traditional diagnostic scanning methods of chorionicity include visualiza-tion of two sacs before 10 weeks of gestation, different fetal sexes and two complete

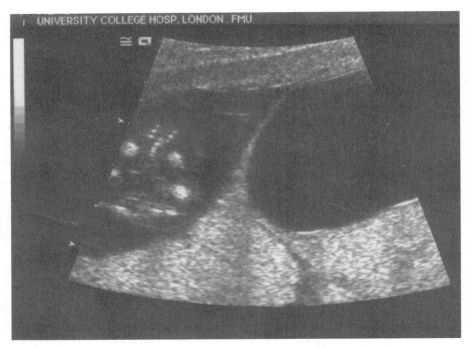

Figure 9.6.   Transvaginal ultrasound image of dichorionic twin pregnancy showing the triangular project at the base of the intertwin membrane, known as the twin peak or lambda sign.

separate placentas. Another important scanning target is intertwin membrane characteristics, such as width and number of layers (<2 mm and four layers are more echogenic typically for dichorionic/diamniotic twins) (D'Alton & Dudley, 1989; Winn *et al.*, 1989). Another sonographic feature of dichorionicity is the extension of placental tissue in a triangular projection between the base of the intertwin membrane known as the twin peak or lambda sign (Figure 9.6) and Epsilon sign in triplet pregnancies (Fineberg, 1992; Sepulveda *et al.*, 1996a). Based on these scanning criteria, 94% sensitivity and 88% specificity was found in determining chorionicity of twin pregnancies between 12 and 40 weeks (Wood *et al.*, 1996). However, a high reliability for determining chorionicity in twin pregnancies was found based on intertwin membrane assessment on transabdominal first trimester scanning (Sepulveda *et al.*, 1996b).

Multifetal pregnancy reduction (MFPR)

ART has resulted in a worrying increase in MGP. MFPR was introduced in the mid-1980s in the management of triplets and higher order MGP but it remains controversial both medically and ethically (Finnerety *et al.*, 2000). Gestational age at delivery and thus perinatal morbidity and mortality is inversely proportional to the number of fetuses. In those small areas of the world where the long-term morbidity of severe prematurity can be prevented or limited by high-tech neonatal care, there is now little difference in the outcome of triplet compared to twin pregnancies (Angel *et al.*, 1999; Leondires *et al.*, 2000). However, even in these areas there are few neonatal centres with a limited number of intensive care cots that can deal with extreme prematurity. Because of high feto-maternal morbidity and mortality and the cost, it is obvious that better use of ART world-wide to avoid MGP is in the best interest of the patients and of society as a whole. In a recent study over a two-year period in one American hospital, the cost estimates for neonatal intensive care unit admission were compared to charges for MFPR and it was found that costs averted in the MFPR population exceeded $28 million (Miller *et al.*, 2000). For couples with long-standing infertility, the decision to reduce a pregnancy is extremely difficult and a limit on embryos transferred to one or two, with three under exceptional clinical conditions has been suggested as the only way forward (Gerris & Van Royen, 2000).

MFPR can be performed transcervically, transvaginally, or transabdominally under ultrasound guidance with the latter two approaches having been favoured. MFPR by the transabdominal route is generally carried out between 10 and 13 weeks of gestation, whereas the transvaginal technique can be used earlier. Transcervical or transvaginal MFPR may be safer very early in gestation and transabdominal safer later in the first trimester (Evans *et al.*, 1994). The experience and preference of the operator are probably the key determinants for an individual patient. The primary advantage of the transvaginal approach is the improved ultrasound visualization, prompting proponents of this technique to suggest that fetal reduction could be accomplished as early as seven to eight weeks. However, the vanishing twin phenomenon may occur as frequently as 20% after a fetal heart rate has been documented and delaying the procedure to after 10 weeks would avoid unnecessary procedures in those cases.

Injection of a concentrated potassium chloride solution into the chest of a fetus is the most commonly used method. The pregnancy loss rate after the procedure is about 8–10% in triplets and quadruplets, and is greater for higher order pregnancies. The largest reported series is a multicentre registry, which includes 1789 completed MFPR cases (Evans *et al.*, 1996). The overall pregnancy loss was 11.7% but varied from a low of 7.6% for triplets to twins and increased with each additional starting number to 22.9% for sextuplets or higher. Pregnancy losses up to 24 weeks were observed in 13.1% of transcervical or transvaginal cases and in 16.2% of transabdominal cases early in the series (Evans *et al.*, 1994) but decreased to 8.8% later in the series.

In addition to total pregnancy loss there are a number of theoretical risks associated with MFPR. In particular, disseminated intravascular coagulation in the mother has been reported in cases of prolonged retention of a spontaneously occurring intrauterine fetal demise. In all series of MFPR, no case of disseminated intravascular coagulation was observed. Other risks associated with invasive procedures such as infection or amniotic fluid leakage are also extremely rare after MFPR. There are no studies evaluating the long-term effects of MFPR on both the surviving fetuses and their parents.

REFERENCES

al-Sebai, M. A., Diver, M. & Hipkin, L. J. (1996). The role of a single free beta-human chorionic gonadotrophia measurement in the diagnosis of early pregnancy failure and the prognosis of fetal viability. *Hum. Reprod.* **11**: 881–8.

Angel, J. L., Kalter, C. S., Morales, W. J., Rasmussen, C. & Caron, L. (1999). Aggressive perinatal care for high-order multiple gestations: does good perinatal outcome justify aggressive assisted reproductive techniques? *Am. J. Obstet. Gynecol.* **181**: 253–9.

Aytoz, A., Van den Abbeel, E., Bonduelle, M. *et al.* (1999). Obstetric outcome of pregnancies after the transfer of cryopreserved and fresh embryos obtained by conventional in-vitro fertilization and intracytoplasmic sperm injection. *Hum. Reprod.* **10**: 2619–24.

Balen, A. H., McDougall, J. & Tan, S. L. (1993). The influence of the number of embryos transferred in 1060 in-vitro fertilization pregnancies on miscarriage rates and pregnancy outcome. *Hum. Reprod.* **8**: 1324–8.

Banerjee, S., Aslam, N., Zosmer, N., Woelfer, B. & Jurkovic, D. (1999). The expectand management of women with early pregnancy of unknown location. *Ultrasound Obstet. Gynecol.* **14**: 231–6.

Barnea, E. (1992). Epidemiology, etiology of early pregnancy disorders. In *The First Twelve Weeks of Gestation*, ed. E. Barnea, J. Hustin & E. Jauniaux, pp. 263–79. Heidelberg: Springer-Verlag.

Cacciatore, B., Stenman, U. H. & Ylstalo, P. (1990). Diagnosis of ectopic pregnancy by vaginal ultrasonography in combination with a discriminatory serum hCG level of 1000 IU/l (IRP). *Br. J. Obstet. Gynaecol.* **97**: 904–8.

Cadkin, A. V. & McAlpin, J. (1984). The decidua-chorionic sac: A reliable sonographic indicator of intrauterine pregnancy prior to detection of a fetal pole. *J. Ultrasound Med.* **3**: 539–48.

D'Alton, M. E. & Dudley, D. K. (1989). The ultrasound prediction of chorionicity in twin gestation. *Am. J. Obstet. Gynecol.* **160**: 557–61.

Edmonds, D. K., Lindsay, K. S., Miller, J. F., Williamson, E. & Wood, P. (1982). Early embryonic mortality in woman. *Fertil. Steril.* **38**: 447–53.

Edwards, R. G. (1986). Causes of early embryonic loss in human pregnancy. *Hum. Reprod.* **1**: 185–98.

Evans, M. I., Dommergues, M., Timor-Tritsch, I. *et al.* (1994). Transabdominal versus transcervical and transvaginal multifetal pregnancy reduction: international collaborative experience of more than one thousand cases. *Am. J. Obstet. Gynecol.* **170**: 902–9.

Evans, M. I., Dommergues, M., Wapner, R. J. *et al.* (1996). International, collaborative experience of 1789 patients having multifetal pregnancy reduction: a plateauing of risks and outcomes. *J. Soc. Gynecol. Investig.* **3**: 23–6.

Falco, P., Milano, V., Pilu, G., David, C., Grisolia, G., Rizzo, N. & Bovicelli, L. (1996). Sonography of pregnancies with first trimester bleeding and a viable embryo: a study of prognostic indicators by logistic regression analysis. *Ultrasound Obstet. Gynecol.* **7**: 165–9.

FIGO News (1976). List of gynaecologic and obstetric terms and definitions. *Int. J. Gynaecol. Obstet.* **14**: 570–6.

Fineberg, J. (1992). The twin peak sign: reliable evidence of dichorionic twinning. *J. Ultrasound Med.* **11**: 571–7.

Finnerty, J. J., Pinkerton, J. V., Moreno, J. & Ferguson, J. E. (2000). Ethical theory and principles: do they have any relevance to problems arising in everyday practice? *Am. J. Obstet. Gynecol.* **183**: 301–6.

Gerris, J. & Van Royen, E. (2000). Avoiding multiple pregnancies in ART: a plea for single embryo transfer. *Hum. Reprod.* **15**: 1884–8.

Goldstein, S. R. (1994). Embryonic death in early pregnancy: A new look at the first trimester. *Obstet. Gynecol.* **84**: 294–7.

Haines, C. J., Chung, T. & Leung, D. Y. (1994). Transvaginal sonography and the conservative management of spontaneous abortion. *Gynecol. Obstet. Invest.* **37**: 14–17.

Jauniaux, E., Elkhazen, N., Leroy, F., Wilkin, P., Rodesch, F. & Hustin, J. (1988). Clinical and morphologic aspects of the vanishing twin phenomenon. *Obstet. Gynecol.* **72**: 577–81.

Jauniaux, E., Zaidi, J., Jurkovic, D., Campbell, S. & Hustin, J. (1994). Comparison of color Doppler features and pathologic findings in complicated early pregnancy. *Hum. Reprod.* **9**: 2432–7.

Jauniaux, E., Gulbis, B., Jurkovic, D., Gavriil, P. & Campbell, S. (1995). The origin of alpha-fetoprotein in first trimester anembryonic pregnancies. *Am. J. Obstet. Gynecol.* **173**: 1749–53.

Jauniaux, E., Gavriil, P. & Nicolaides, K. H. (1996). Ultrasonographic assessment of early pregnancy complications. In *Ultrasound and Early Pregnancy*, ed. D. Jurkovic & E. Jauniaux, pp. 53–64. Carnforth: Parthenon.

Jauniaux, E. & Nicolaides, K. H. (1997). Early ultrasound diagnosis and follow-up of molar pregnancies. *Ultrasound Obstet. Gynecol.* **9**: 17–21.

Jauniaux, E. (1998). Ultrasound diagnosis and follow-up of gestational trophoblastic disease. *Ultrasound Obstet. Gynecol.* **11**: 367–77.

Jauniaux, E. (1999). Partial moles: From postnatal to prenatal diagnosis. *Placenta* **20**: 379–88.

Johnson, M. R., Riddle, A. F., Sharma, V., Collins, W. P., Nicolaides, K. H. & Grudzinskas, J. G. (1993). Placental and ovarian hormones in anembryonic pregnancy. *Hum. Reprod.* **8**: 112–15.

Lam, S. Y., Baker, H. W., Evans, J. H. & Pepperell, R. J. (1989). Factors affecting fetal loss in induction of ovulation with gonadotropins: increased abortion rates related to hormonal profiles in conceptual cycles. *Am. J. Obstet. Gynecol.* **160**: 621–8.

Lass, A., Croucher, C., Duffy, S., Dawson, K. *et al.* (1998). One thousand initiated cycles of in vitro fertilization in women > or = 40 years of age. *Fertil. Steril.* **70**: 1030–4.

Levi, C. S., Lyons, E. A., Zheng, X. H., Lindsay, D. J. & Holt, S. C. (1990). Endovaginal US: demostration of cardiac activity in embryos of less than 5.0 mm in crown-rump length. *Radiology* **176**: 71–4.

Leondires, M. P., Ernst, S. D., Miller, B. T. & Scott, R. T. (2000). Triplets: outcomes of expectant management versus multifetal reduction for 127 pregnancies. *Am. J. Obstet. Gynecol.* **183**: 454–9.

Li, T. C. (1998). Recurrent miscarriage: principles of management. *Hum. Reprod.* **13**: 478–82.

Lockwood, G. M., Ledger, W. L., Barlow, D. H., Groome, N. P. & Muttukrishna, S. (1998). Identification of the source of inhibins at the time of conception provides a diagnostic role for them in very early pregnancy. *Am. J. Reprod. Immunol.* **40**: 303–8.

Lower, A. M. & Yovich, J. L. (1992). The value of serum levels of oestradiol, progesterone and beta-human chorionic gonadotrophin in the prediction of early pregnancy loss. *Hum. Reprod.* **7**: 711–17.

Machin, G. A. & Keith, L. G. (1999). *An Atlas of Multiple Pregnancy: Biology and Pathology.* New York: Parthenon.

Manase, K., Henmi, H. & Yamanata, I. (2000). Complete hydatidiform mole coexisting with a live fetus after gamete intrafallopian transfer. A case report. *J. Reprod. Med.* **45**: 227–30.

Miller, V. L., Ransom, S. B., Shalhoub, A., Sokol, R. J. & Evans, M. I. (2000). Multifetal pregnancy reduction: perinatal and fiscal outcomes. *Am. J. Obstet. Gynecol.* **182**: 1575–80.

Nikolettos, N., Kupker, W., Al-Hasani, S., Demirel, L. C., Schopper, B., Sturm, C. & Diedrich, K. (2000). ICSI outcome in patients of 40 years age and over: a retrospective analysis. *Eur. J. Obstet. Gynecol. Reprod. Biol.* **91**: 177–82.

Nybo, A. A. M., Wohlfahrt, J., Christens, P., Olsen, J. & Melbye, M. (2000). Maternal age and fetal loss: populations based register linkage study. *BMJ* **320**: 1708–12.

Palmer, J. R. (1994). Advances in the epidemiology of gestational trophoblastic disease. *J. Reprod. Med.* **39**: 155–62.

Pandya, P., Snijders, R. J. M., Psara, N., Hibert, L. & Nicolaides, K. H. (1996). The prevalence of non-viable pregnancy at 10–13 weeks of gestation. *Ultrasound Obstet. Gynaecol.* **7**: 170–3.

Pantos, K., Athanasiou, V., Stefanidis, K. *et al.* (1999). Influence of advanced age on the blastocyst development rate and pregnancy rate in assisted reproductive technology. *Fertil. Steril.* **71**: 1144–6.

Phipps, M. G., Hogan, J. W., Peipert, J. F., Lambert-Messerlian, G. M., Canick, J. A. & Seifer, D. B. (2000). Progesterone, inhibin, and HCG multiple marker strategy to differentiate viable from nonviable pregnancies. *Obstet. Gynecol.* **95**: 227–31.

Reubinoff, B. S., Lewin, A., Verner, M., Safran, A., Schenker, J. G. & Abeliovich, D. (1997). Intracytoplasmic sperm injection combined with preimplantation genetic diagnosis for the prevention of recurrent gestational trophoblastic disease. *Hum. Reprod.* **12**: 805–8.

Rulin, M. C., Bornstein, S. G. & Campbell, J. D. (1993). The reliability of ultrasonography in the management of spontaneous abortion, clinically thought to be complete: a prospective study. *Am. J. Obstet. Gynecol.* **168**: 12–15.

Salem, H. T., Ghaneimah, S. A., Shaaban, M. M. & Chard, T. (1984). Prognostic value of biochemical tests in the assessment of fetal outcome in threatened abortion. *Br. J. Obst. Gynaecol.* **81**: 382–5.

Seckl, M. J., Fisher, R. A., Salerno, G., Rees, H., Paradinas, F. J., Foskett, M. & Newlands, E. S. (2000). Choriocarcinoma and partial hydatidiform moles. *Lancet* **356**: 36–9.

Sepulveda, W., Sebire, N. J., Odibo, A., Psarra, A. & Nicolaides, K. H. (1996a). Prenatal determination of chorionicity in triplet pregnancy by ultrasonographic examination of the Ipsilon zone. *Obstet. Gynecol.* **88**: 855–8.

Sepulveda, W., Sebire, N. J., Hughes, A., Odibo, D. & Nicolaides, K. H. (1996b). The lambda sign at 10–14 weeks of gestation as a predictor of chorionicity in twin pregnancies. *Ultrasound Obstet. Gynecol.* **7**: 421–3.

Shu-Xin, H. & Zhen-Qun, Z. A. (1993). Study of early pregnancy factor activity in the sera of patients with unexplained spontaneous abortion. *Am. J. Reprod. Immunol.* **29**: 77–81.

Simpson, J. L. & Bombard, A. T. (1987). Chromosomal abnormalities in spontaneous abortion: Frequency, pathology and genetic counselling. In *Spontaneous Abortion*, ed. K. Edmonds & M. J. Bennett, pp. 51–76. London: Blackwell.

Smith, K. E. & Buyalos, R. P. (1996). The profound impact of patient age on pregnancy outcome after early detection of fetal cardiac activity. *Fertil. Steril.* **65**: 35–40.

Stabile, I., Campbell, S. & Gruzinskas, G. (1989). Ultrasound and circulating placental protein measurements in complications of early pregnancy. *Br. J. Obstet. Gynaecol.* **96**: 1182–91.

Stewart, B. K., Nazar-Stewart, V. & Toivola, B. (1995). Biochemical discrimination of pathologic pregnancy from early, normal intrauterine gestation in symptomatic patients. *Am. J. Clin. Pathol.* **103**: 386–90.

Sunder, S. & Lenton, E. A. (2000). Endocrinology of the peri-implantation period. *Baillières Best Pract. Res. Clin. Obstet. Gynaecol.* **14**: 789–800.

Tarlatzis, B. C. & Grimbizis, G. (1999). Pregnancy and child outcome after assisted reproduction techniques. In *ART in the Year 2000. Hum. Reprod.* **14** (1): 231–42.

Watson, H., Kiddy, D. S., Hamilton Fairley, D., Scanlon, M. J., Barnard, C., Collins, W. P., Bonney, R. C. & Franks, S. (1993). Hypersecretion of luteinizing hormone and ovarian steroids in women with recurrent early miscarriage. *Hum. Reprod.* **8**: 829–33.

Wennerholm, U. B., Hamberger, L., Nilsson, L. *et al.* (1997). Obstetrics and perinatal outcome of children conceived from cryopreserved embryos. *Hum. Reprod.* **12**: 1819–25.

Westergaard, H. B., Johansen, A. M., Erb, K. & Andersen, A. N. (2000). Danish National IVF Registry 1994 and 1995. Treatment, pregnancy outcome and complications during pregnancy. *Acta. Obstet. Gynecol. Scand.* **79**: 384–9.

Winn, H. N., Gabrielli, S., Reece, E. A., Roberts, J. A., Salafia, C. & Hobbins, J. C. (1989). Ultrasonographic criteria for the prenatal diagnosis of placental chorionicity in twin gestations. *Am. J. Obstet. Gynecol.* **161**: 1540–2.

Wood, S. L., Onge, R. S. T., Connors, G. & Elliot, P. D. (1996). Evaluation of the twin peak or lambda sign in determining chorionicity in multiple pregnancy. *Obstet. Gynecol.* **88**: 6–9.

Zinaman, M. J., Clegg, E. D., Brown, C. C., O'Connor, J. & Selevan, S. G. (1996). Estimates of human fertility and pregnancy loss. *Fertil. Steril.* **65**: 503–9.

10

Oocyte donation

Paul Serhal

Assisted Conception Unit, UCLH, London, UK

To women traditionally considered irreversibly sterile due to ovarian failure, oocyte donation and exogenous steroid replacement to create an endometrial milieu receptive to embryonic implantation offers the prospect of achieving a successful pregnancy. Irrespective of the age of the oocyte recipient, it is possible to achieve a high fertility potential with a low miscarriage rate, reflecting the improved biological performance of oocytes obtained from young donors. It is now feasible to dissociate the stages of embryonic development and endometrial maturation in oocyte recipients. Hence, oocyte donation can provide insights into as yet unresolved questions, such as the duration of the 'implantation window' in humans. In human reproduction, oocyte donation undoubtedly complements basic IVF in elucidating the biological interactions between the conceptus, endometrium and steroid environment.

In 1983, Trounson *et al.* reported the first successful transfer of an in vitro fertilized donated oocyte embryo to a menstrually cyclic recipient using luteinizing hormone (LH) synchronization between the donor and the recipient to time the transfer. In 1984, Lutjen *et al.* reported the first successful pregnancy in a primary ovarian failure patient, following a sequential steroid replacement regimen and transfer of in vitro fertilized donated oocyte embryos. In 1983, Buster *et al.* reported the successful transfer of an in vivo fertilized donated ovum. In 1986, Serhal and Craft introduced the notion that women older than 40 years who have already entered the menopause might extend their reproductive potential through oocyte donation. Oocyte donation is a well-established technique and a large proportion of IVF units now run oocyte donation programs.

Good Clinical Practice in Assisted Reproduction, ed. P. Serhal & C. Overton.
Published by Cambridge University Press. © Cambridge University Press 2004.

Indications for oocyte donation

Women requiring oocyte donation comprise two main groups:

(1) Women with primary or secondary ovarian failure:
  • gonodal dysgenesis (Turner's syndrome, XY karyotype, major deletions on one X chromosome);
  • premature ovarian failure;
  • surgically ablated ovaries;
  • previous chemotherapy and/or radiotherapy;
  • menopause.

(2) Women with normal menstrual cycles:
  • IVF failure (poor response to ovarian stimulation, repetitive poor oocyte harvest, recurrent or persistent ovarian cysts, failed IVF due to oocyte abnormality).
  • women older than 45 years;
  • women with familial genetic disorders difficult to diagnose by early prenatal or preimplantation genetic diagnosis.

Donors

There will always be an imbalance between supply of and demand for donated oocytes due to ethical considerations, concerns about potential health risks to the donor, and the relatively invasive techniques involved in ovarian stimulation and oocyte collection. Ideally, the oocyte donor should be aged <35 years, be free of major medical or psychiatric illnesses and have no history of familial genetic disorders.

Screening the donor

As stipulated in the screening guidelines (Aird *et al.*, 2000) in addition to psychological counselling, medical screening of oocyte donors includes cytomegalovirus (CMV), hepatitis B and C, cystic fibrosis, blood group, full blood count, karyotyping, VDRL, HbsAg and HIV status. In addition, women of ethnic origin groups must be screened for haemoglobin electrophoresis, sickle cell and Tay–Sachs disease.

Donor recruitment

In the United Kingdom, the Human Fertilisation and Embryology Authority (HFEA) stipulates that oocyte donors may be paid no more that £15 for each donation in addition to reasonable expenses. Reasonable expenses are defined in the

HFEAs Code of Practice and are intended to reimburse the donor for out of pocket expenses, not as an incentive to donate. Payment of oocyte donors is permitted in the United States.

Women who donate oocytes comprise three main groups:

(1) Anonymous donor – this may be an individual simply with an altruistic motivation to help a childless couple or a patient who has agreed to donate oocytes in combination with undergoing laparoscopic sterilization. Anonymously advertising for a donor is permitted under the HFEA guidelines.

(2) Donor known to the recipient – the acceptability of a sibling sister oocyte donor is high amongst oocyte recipient women (Sauer *et al.*, 1988). Oocyte donation by other women known to the recipient is possible.

(3) IVF patient donating excess oocytes (egg sharing).

Steroid replacement for non-menstrually cyclic recipients

Adequate and sustained steroid hormone secretion by the corpus luteum of the ovulatory cycle is required for establishing and maintaining pregnancy in humans for the first seven to nine weeks, following which the placenta assumes these functions (Csapo *et al.*, 1972). Endogenous ovarian steroid production is deficient in women with primary or secondary ovarian failure and exogenous oestrogen and progesterone replacement therapy is needed to stimulate endometrial receptivity to embryonic implantation. In primates, little is known about hormonal requirements for implantation although it is thought that only progesterone is required, with oestradiol playing a facilitatory role (Hearn, 1980).

Oestrogen replacement

The first step in preparing the endometrium for embryo implantation is priming with a natural oestrogen. 17-β oestradiol (E2) is the predominant oestrogen in ovulating women and is the most potent oestrogen at the receptor site (Wiegerinck *et al.*, 1983). It has been used less frequently for general therapeutic purposes than nonphysiological agents because it is rapidly metabolized in the gastrointestinal tract and liver. One method to improve absorption has been micronization (Fincher, 1968), a process involving reduction in particle size to increase the absorptive area.

The E2 concentration achieved via the oral route is sufficient to prime the endometrium in spite of rapid metabolism through the enterohepatic circulation. If necessary, oestradiol valerate may be given sublingually to bypass the enterohepatic circulation. Using the same dosages sublingually, higher plasma concentrations of E2 are achieved than via the oral route (Serhal & Craft, 1989). As with the oral route, there is an increase in the oestrone (E1):E2 ratio. The vaginal route (using E2-impregnated vaginal rings) has also been used to bypass the enterohepatic circulation and higher and steadier E2 concentrations can be achieved without an accompanying increase in E1 to nonphysiological levels (Fincher, 1968). Transdermal E2 patches have been successfully used in priming the endometrium in oocyte recipients (Rosenwaks, 1987), the advantages being that the plasma E2 and E1 concentrations remain within the physiological range during treatment and peak concentrations and variable availability are avoided. Nevertheless, oral administration of micronized E2 valerate (Progynova, Schering) remains the most commonly used route for cycle replacement in oocyte recipients.

Since the endometrium is an effective bioassay of oestrogen supplementation, during the treatment cycle the recipient is monitored with ultrasound scans to assess endometrial response in terms of thickness and receptivity. The ultrasonographic texture of the endometrium is of great prognostic value for implantation. Relatively unanimous in the current literature is that the endometrium is unreceptive when it is hyperechoic compared with myometrium, and a much higher pregnancy rate is reported in association with a 'triple' layered appearance of the uterus (Zaidi *et al.*, 1995). Cervical mucus production can also be assessed during the treatment cycle.

Usually, the endometrium is primed with oestrogen for approximately two weeks before starting progesterone supplementation, but pregnancies have been achieved in recipients who have been treated with E2 valerate for as little as one week and as much as five to six weeks (Navot *et al.*, 1989). Therefore, it can be concluded that either short or prolonged priming of the endometrium with E2 can result in adequate secretory changes following progesterone supplementation. This is of practical importance in terms of synchronization, as it allows greater flexibility in cycle management when the donor and the recipient are out of phase.

Progesterone replacement

Embryonic implantation is dependent upon adequate secretory changes induced by progesterone, in an endometrium suitably primed with oestrogen, and 'natural' progesterone is used for this purpose. The 19-norsteroids are testosterone derivatives with residual androgenic effects, as shown by androgen receptor studies (Bergink, 1984), and must not be used in replacement cycles. Progesterone can be administered orally or vaginally in the micronized form (Uterogestan capsules, Besins Iscovesco), vaginal suppositories (Cyclogest, Hoechst) or intramuscularly in ethyl oleate (Gestone, Pains and Barnes).

Replacement protocols

Different replacement regimens can be used in preparing the endometrium of donor oocyte recipients and the suitability of any given regimen depends on the histological

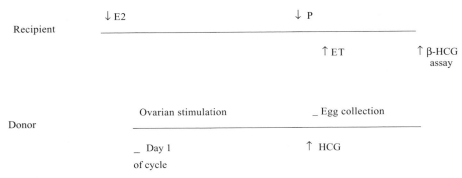

Figure 10.1. Simplified method of hormonal regimen for preparing the endometrium of donor oocyte recipients. E2: 17-beta oestradiol; P: progesterone; ET: embryo transfer; HCG: human chorionic gonadotrophin.

assessment of the endometrium in a pretreatment cycle. Lutjen *et al.* (1986) recommends a steroid replacement regimen administered on a sequential and incremental basis to mimic the steroid profile occurring throughout the natural menstrual cycle. Briefly, every morning up to 2 mg of E2 valerate is administered in single daily doses. On cycle days 10–13 the maximum dose of E2 valerate 6 mg per day is given as three equal doses morning, noon and evening. On the evening of cycle day 15 progesterone is commenced with a single 25 mg vaginal suppository, continuing on cycle day 16 with a 25 mg suppository morning and evening, and on cycle days 17–26 with 50 mg suppository morning and evening.

Although such an approach may result in circulating steroid levels similar to those occurring in a natural cycle, this may not be essential for implantation to occur. Therefore, Serhal & Craft (1987a) developed a simplified method of preparing the recipient by using a simple hormonal regimen of fixed dosages of E2 valerate 2 mg orally tds and progesterone 100 mg intramusculatly daily (Gestone) or 100 mg vaginally tds (uterogestan) or 400 mg vaginally tds (cyclogest) daily (Serhal & Craft 1987a) (Figure 10.1). Progesterone administration is commenced one day before oocyte collection from the donor.

Oocyte donation in menstrually cyclic recipients

Cycle control in women with normal menstrual cycles who require oocyte donation is much more complex than in non-menstrually cyclic recipients because of the normal pituitary ovarian cyclicity. Four methods may be used for cycle control in menstrually cyclic recipients:

- LH synchronization – the donor LH surge must be within 24–48 hours of that of the expected LH surge of the recipient (Trounson *et al.*, 1983) and this method requires taking repeated blood or urine samples from potential donors and

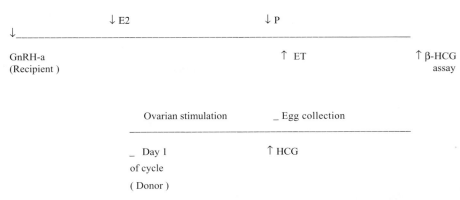

Figure 10.2. Down-regulation of the pituitary gland followed by the administration of oestrogen at the onset of the donor treatment cycle to prime the recipient endometrium. GnRHa: gonadotrophin releasing hormone agonist; E2: 17-beta oestradiol; ET: embryo transfer P: progesterone; HCG: human chorionic gonadotrophin.

the recipient for LH determination to synchronize LH peaks. Several potential donors need to be recruited for the benefit of an individual recipient and in a clinical setting this is impractical.

• Combined oral contraceptive pill – starting in the mid-luteal phase to allow synchronization of the LH peaks between donor and recipient. Bustillo *et al.* (1986) suggests the use of oral contraceptive preparations starting on the seventh day after the recipient LH peak to prolong the luteal phase, thus allowing synchronization of the LH peaks. Although LH synchronization allows transfer of the conceptus into a well-defined milieu, this approach is time-consuming and unnecessarily complex.

• Cryopreservation – cryopreservation and transfer of frozen–thawed embryos can circumvent the problem of synchronicity between donor and recipient (Devroey *et al.*, 1986). The inconvenience of this method in menstrually cyclic recipients is that the LH surge has to be monitored to time the embryo transfer.

• Down-regulation with LH–RHa – the administration of effective cycle control can be achieved in menstrually cyclic recipients by using an LH–RHa preparation to down-regulate the pituitary gland, followed by the administration of oestrogen at the onset of the donor treatment cycle to prime the recipient endometrium (Serhal & Craft, 1989) (Figure 10.2). For the purpose of down-regulation, a short-acting LH–RHa (Buserelin Suprefact, Hoechst) nasal spray 100 µg six-hourly is administered, or a Depo LH–RHa (Goserelin acetate) pellet 3.6 mg (Zoladex ICI) is injected subcutaneously in the abdominal wall. Down-regulation is started either during the first few days of the recipient menstruation or in the recipient mid-luteal phase. On average, menstrually cyclic recipients are suppressed for one to two weeks before starting oestrogen treatment.

The advantages of down-regulation of menstrually cyclic recipients with LH–RHa are:

- LH synchronization between donor and recipient is no longer required.
- Patient management is easier (fewer hospital visits are required of the recipient prior to the transfer procedure).
- The simplicity of this method enhances patient compliance.
- The ability to down-regulate the recipient and the donor allows greater flexibility in planning the transfer procedure.

Controlled preparation of the endometrium can also be achieved with exogenous E2 without prior ovarian suppression with a GnRHa in menstrually cyclic recipients using the E2 sublingually (Serhal, 1990) or transdermally (De Ziegler *et al.*, 1991) in order to bypass the enterohepatic circulation. Oral E2 therapy may not always be effective in suppressing ovulation in some women, especially the younger menstrually cyclic woman (Serhal, 1990).

Implantation window

For successful embryo transfer in animals, the donor and the recipient should be synchronous in oestrus or be asynchronous within a limited interval. In the bovine model, asynchrony of two days or more in the luteal phase results in poor pregnancy rates (Newcomb & Rowson, 1975). In mice, synchrony between donor and recipient must be within six hours for implantation to occur (Beatty, 1951). In sheep, a 75% pregnancy rate was reported in the recipients when synchronization was precise, and a high pregnancy rate was obtained when the asynchrony was up to two days. However, when there was asynchrony of three or more days, only 8% of ewes conceived (Rowson & Moor, 1966). In humans, the duration of the receptive phase, the 'implantation window', is still under investigation. In human IVF, embryos between 2 and 8 cells are usually transferred 48 to 72 hours after egg collection. Therefore, studies on implantation and endometrial–embryo interaction have been limited. In oocyte donation, it is now possible to dissociate the stages of embryonic development and endometrial maturation and at the same time avoid any possible effect of multiple follicular development on the endometrium.

To optimize the success of IVF treatment in oocyte recipients, treatment has been synchronized to perform the embryo transfer procedure on cycle day 18–19 (Table 10.1). Lutjen *et al.* (1985) performed embryo transfers on cycle day 17 and the recipient was started on progesterone on the day before oocyte collection from the donor. In the case of eight oocyte recipients Navot *et al.* (1986) performed embryo transfer on days 16–21. Two pregnancies were established by transfer on days 18 and 19, suggesting that transfer should be performed around this time to achieve embryonic implantation. Similarly, Rosenwaks (1987) performed 32 transfers on

Table 10.1. IVF pregnancy rates in relation to the day of embryo transfer

	No. of embryo transfers	Days of transfer	No. of pregnancies	No. of viable pregnancies
Salat-Baroux *et al.* (1988)	12	14	4	4
Lutjen *et al.* (1985)	15	17–18	4	4
Navot *et al.* (1986)	8	16–21	2	2
Rosenwaks (1987)	21	17–19	8	6
Rosenwaks (1987)	11	20–24	0	0
Edwards (1988)	1	24	1	0
Schulte & Serhal (1996)	1	21	1	1

different days of the luteal phase. Eight of the 21 transfers performed on days 17–19 of the cycle resulted in pregnancy, while none of the patients who had transfers on days 20 or later became pregnant.

Pregnancies have been reported with early as well as late transfers. Salat-Baroux *et al.* (1988) performed frozen–thawed embryo transfers as early as cycle day 14 (on the second day of progesterone supplementation) and achieved four successful transfers in 21 replacement cycles (31%). On the other hand, Formigli *et al.* (1987) reported that a blastula might implant when placed in a cycle day 22 endometrium. Similarly, Edwards (1988) performed an embryo transfer on day 10 of the luteal phase (seven days after the usual time of replacement). The patient conceived and a gestational sac was documented on ultrasound scan, but a miscarriage occurred at six weeks of gestation. Schulte & Serhal (1996) reported a successful transfer of a donated oocyte embryo on cycle day 21, resulting in a viable twin pregnancy carried to term.

Based on these clinical data, it is reasonable to assume that although the receptive phase is probably at its peak around cycle days 17–19, it may be possible to transfer embryos to an endometrium that is out of phase. Oocyte recipients can provide a unique model to investigate the implantation window in humans and to determine whether precise embryo–endometrial synchrony is essential for implantation to occur. Similarly, another biological approach involves transferring cryopreserved–thawed embryos in a natural cycle.

The successful implantation and maintenance of pregnancy in the uterus of older women is an interesting observation. Gosden (1985) has reviewed the effect of ageing in mammals (including humans) and believes that the vasculature of the ageing uterus becomes increasingly deficient in patients aged >40 years. In the opinion of the author implantation in older women depends mainly on the quality of the embryo and the receptivity of the endometrium, which in oocyte recipients is under the direct influence of exogenous hormones.

Procedures

Different techniques can be used in treatment with donated oocytes:

- IVF (Trounson *et al.*, 1983; Feichtinger & Kremeter, 1985; Lutjen *et al.*, 1985; Serhal & Craft, 1987) and gamete intrafallopian transfer (GIFT) (Ash, 1986; Serhal & Craft, 1987) have been commonly used approaches. Nonsurgical transfer of an in vivo fertilized ovum removed by uterine lavage from a fertile donor who has been inseminated with the recipient husband's sperm has also been performed (Buster *et al.*, 1983). This procedure involves certain risks to the donor, such as semen exposure and retained or ectopic pregnancy.

- Pronuclei stage tubal transfer (PROST) has also been used in oocyte recipients (Yovich *et al.*, 1987). The donated oocytes are fertilized in vitro and the pronuclear oocytes transferred to the fallopian tubes of the recipient. The advantage of PROST versus GIFT in oocyte donation is that fertilization of the donated oocytes is documented prior to tubal transfer and the recipient procedure is performed on the day after the donor has been discharged. Hence, anonymity is more easily preserved.

- Transfer of cryopreserved–thawed embryos to oocyte recipients has the advantage of preserving anonymity and obviating the need for synchronization between donor and recipient, and offers the benefit of quarantine.

Steroid maintenance of pregnancy

In natural conception, from nidation to two weeks later (three to five weeks menstrual age), the serum E2 levels are slightly higher than those normally occurring during the luteal phase of the cycle. The duration of the corpus luteum activity is limited. After the fifth week the continuous rise of E2 and oestrone is due to the production by the trophoblast (Tulchinsky & Hobel, 1973; Ryan, 1980) and thereafter the corpus luteum contributes little to the production of E2. As for progesterone secretion, there is also a reduction in the serum levels of 17α-hydroxyprogesterone after the fifth week of gestation. The level of 17α-hydroxyprogesterone reflects the activity of the corpus luteum only, as the placenta lacks the enzyme 17α-hydroxylase and is unable to produce this substance. The rise of progesterone after nine weeks indicates that the trophoblast has taken over the steroid maintenance of pregnancy. This is called the luteoplacental shift (Yoshimi *et al.*, 1969; Tulchinsky & Hobel, 1973). In oocyte recipients, the phase during which exogenous steroid supplementation is an absolute necessity is relatively short and with progressive trophoblastic proliferation exogenous steroids assume a supplemental role.

A beta HCG assessment is usually performed 13–14 days after embryo transfer procedure. If the result is negative, the patient is asked to discontinue her medication and menstruation will usually occur within three to four days. If it is positive, it is assumed that embryo implantation has occurred and the steroid requirement of early pregnancy must be met by maintaining exogenous replacement therapy until the time of the luteoplacental shift. When the Australian replacement regimen is used, the dose of E2 is increased from 2 mg to 8–9 mg per day. In our simplified regimen, a fixed dose of E2 valerate (2 mg tds) and progesterone (400 mg vaginally twice a day or 100 mg intramuscularly daily) is used from the start of the replacement and the same dose is maintained to meet the demand of early pregnancy.

The optimal concentrations of E2 and progesterone needed for implantation and maintenance of pregnancy are still unknown. Lutjen et al. (1985) aimed to keep the plasma levels of these steroids within the range of a normal pregnancy and maintained E2 at 100–500 pmol/l and progesterone within 100–200 nmol/l.

The precise timing of withdrawal of replacement steroids for the maintenance of successful pregnancy is difficult to ascertain at this stage. Based on studies of spontaneous abortion and associated fall in steroid levels in luteo-ectomized women with and without replacement treatment, Csapo et al. (1973) showed that the shift from ovarian steroid maintenance of pregnancy to the placenta took place at around 50–60 day's gestation. Progesterone replacement after luteo-ectomy during the first 50 days of gestation maintained plasma progesterone and E2 levels over a seven-day observation and prevented cervical dilatation and abortion from occurring. E2 alone failed to prevent abortion after luteo-ectomy.

Pregnancies achieved following oocyte donation are ideal cases for studying the critical period of placental take-over and self-sufficiency. In general, when a fixed steroid dose is used it is easier to assess the endogenous E2 and progesterone production by the placenta. Lutjen et al. (1985) monitored the plasma levels of E2 and progesterone on a weekly basis and the medication was withdrawn when a rise in endogenous steroids from the placenta was noted. An early increase in steroid production enabling gradual withdrawal of exogenous steroids from days 57 to 65 of pregnancy in two patients respectively was reported. Exogenous replacement was discontinued on day 80. Earlier patients required greater dosages for replacement and steroids were discontinued in the second trimester (Lutjen et al., 1984). Salat-Baroux (1988) and Devroey et al. (1986) noted that the E2 levels increased quickly from the fifth week of pregnancy, even with the same dose of E2 supplementation indicating that the luteoplacental shift may occur earlier than the tenth week. On the other hand, Navot et al. (1986) observed a rise in E2 during the eleventh week and began gradual withdrawal of E2 around that time. Progesterone started to rise during the twelfth week of pregnancy. For practical purposes, exogenous steroid replacement can be safely discontinued around 14 weeks of gestation without the need of monitoring of endogenous steroid levels.

If bleeding occurs during the first trimester of pregnancy, the dose of E2 and progesterone is increased. This is done on the assumption that the bleeding may be due to suboptimal steroid supplementation.

Pregnancy outcome

Serhal and Craft reported a high incidence of multiple pregnancy in oocytes recipients (Serhal, 1990) and an increased risk of pre-eclampsia (Serhal & Craft, 1987b), a finding subsequently confirmed (Pados *et al.*, 1994; Yaron *et al.*, 1995).

Multiple pregnancies are associated with a higher incidence of obstetric and perinatal complications, the adverse effects of which are exacerbated in older recipients. Caution needs to be exercised regarding the number of embryos transferred in oocyte recipients.

It should be borne in mind that the risk of aneuploidy of any resulting pregnancy reflects the age of the donor and not the age of the recipient. Prenatal diagnosis carries the risk of miscarriage and should be carefully considered in these precious pregnancies.

As average life expectancy and quality of life increase, pregnancy from oocyte donation to post-menopausal women becomes more possible. The increased risk of obstetric complications (Sauer *et al.*, 1993) is an important consideration as is the welfare of the child in respect of maternal age (see Chapter 19).

REFERENCES

Aird, I., Barrat, C., Murdoch, A. & the BFS Committee (2000). BFS recommendations for good practice on the screening of egg and embryo donors. *Hum. Fertil.* **3**(3): 162–5.

Ash, R. H. (1986). Pregnancy following gamete intrafallopian tube transfer in premature ovarian failure. *Hum. Reprod.* **1**(Suppl. 2): 17–18.

Beatty, R. A. (1951). Transplantation of mouse eggs. *Nature* **168**: 2995.

Bergink, E. W. (1984). Binding of contraceptive progesterone to receptor proteins in human myometrium and MCF-7 cells. *Br. J. Family Planning* **10**: 33.

Buster, J. E., Bustillo, M., Thorneycroft, I. H. *et al.* (1983). Non-surgical transfer of in vivo fertilised donated ova to five infertile women: report of two pregnancies. *Lancet.* **i**: 816–18.

Bustillo, M., Cohen, S. W., Thornycroft, I. H., & Buster, J. E. (1986). Use of combination oral contraceptives to synchronise recipient-donor LH peaks for ovum transfer. *42nd Annual Meeting of the American Fertility Society*, p. 54 (Abstr. 152).

Csapo, A. I., Pulkkinen, M. O., Ruttner, B., Sauvage, J. P. & Wiest, W. G. (1972). The significance of the human corpus luteum in pregnancy maintenance. I. Preliminary studies. *Am. J. Obstet. Gynecol.* **112**(8): 1061–7.

Csapo, A. I., Pulkkinen, M. O. & Wiest, W. G. (1973). Effects of luteectomy and progesterone replacement therapy in early pregnant patients. *Am. J. Obstet. Gynecol.* **115**(6): 759–65.

De Ziegler, D., Cornel, C., Bergeron, C., Hazout, A., Bouchard, P. & Frydman, R. (1991). Controlled preparation of the endometrium with exogenous estradiol and progesterone in women having functioning ovaries. *Fertil. Steril.*, **56**(5): 851–5.

Devroey, P., Braeckmans, P., Camus, M. *et al.* (1986). Pregnancies after replacement of fresh and frozen-thawed embryos in a donation program. In *Future Aspects in Human In Vitro Fertilisation*, ed. W. Feichtinger & P. Kremeter, p. 133. Berlin: Springer-Verlag.

Edwards, R. G. (1988). Human uterine endocrinology and the implantation window. *Ann. NY Acad. Sci.* **541**: 445–54.

Feichtinger, W. & Kremeter, P. (1985). Pregnancy after total ovariectomy achieved by ovum donation. *Lancet* **2**: 722–3.

Fincher, J. H. (1968). Particle size of drugs and its relationship to absorption and activity. *J. Pharm. Sci.* **57**: 1825–35.

Formigli, L., Formigli, G. & Roccio C. (1987). Donation of fertilized uterine ova to infertile women. *Fertil. Steril.* **47**(1): 162–5.

Gosden, R. G. (1985). Maternal age: a major factor affecting the prospects and outcome of pregnancy. *Ann. NY Acad. Sci.* **442**: 45–7.

Hearn, J. P. (1980). Primate models for early human pregnancy. In *Animal Models in Human Reproduction*, ed. M. Serio & L. Martini, pp. 319–32. New York: Raven Press.

Lutjen, P., Trounson, A., Leeton, J., Findlay, J., Wood, C. & Renou, P. (1984). The establishment and maintenance of pregnancy using in vitro fertilization and embryo donation in a patient with primary ovarian failure. *Nature* **307**: 174–5.

Lutjen, P. J., Findlay, J. K., Trounson, A. O., Leeton, J. F. & Chan, L. K. (1986). Effect on plasma gonadotropins of cyclic steroid replacement in women with premature ovarian failure. *J. Clin. Endocrinol. Metab.* **62**(2): 419–23.

Lutjen, P. J., Leeton, J. F. & Findlay, J. K. (1985). Oocyte and embryo donation in IVF programmes. *Clin. Obstet. Gynaecol.* **12**(4): 799–813.

Navot, D., Anderson, T. L., Droesch, K., Scott, R. T., Kreiner, D. & Rosenwaks, Z. (1989). Hormonal manipulation of endometrial maturation. *J. Clin. Endocrinol. Metab.* **68**(4): 801–7.

Navot, D., Laufer, N., Kopolovic, J. *et al.* (1986). Artificially induced endometrial cycles and establishment of pregnancies in the absence of ovaries. *N. Engl. J. Med.* **314**(13): 806–11.

Newcomb, R. & Rowson, L. E. (1975). Conception rate after uterine transfer of cow eggs, in relation to synchronization of oestrus and age of eggs. *J. Reprod. Fertil.* **43**(3): 539–41.

Pados, G., Camus, M., Van Steirteghem, A., Bonduelle, M. & Devroey, P. (1994). The evolution and outcome of pregnancies from oocyte donation. *Hum. Reprod.* **9**(3): 538–542.

Rosenwaks, Z. (1987). Donor eggs: their application in modern reproductive technologies. *Fertil. Steril.* **47**(6): 895–909.

Rowson, L. E. & Moor, R. M. (1966). Embryo transfer in the sheep: the significance of synchronizing oestrus in the donor and recipient animal. *J. Reprod. Fertil.* **11**(2): 207–12.

Ryan, K. J. (1980). In *Maternal–fetal Endocrinology*, ed. D. Tulchinsky & K. J. Ryan, pp. 3–16. Philadelphia: Saunders.

Salat-Baroux, J., Cornet, D. & Alvarez, S. (1988). Pregnancies after replacement of frozen-thawed embryos in a donation program. *Fertil. Steril.* **49**(5): 817–21.

Sauer, M. V., Rodi, I. A., Scrooc, M., Bustillo, M. & Buster, J. E. (1988). Survey of attitudes regarding the use of siblings for gamete donation. *Fertil. Steril.* **49**(4): 721–2.

Sauer, M. V., Paulson, R. J. & Lobo, R. A. (1993). Pregnancy after age 50: application of oocyte donation to women after natural menopause. *Lancet* **341**: 321–3.

Schulte, A. & Serhal, P. (1996). Twin pregnancy following embryo transfer on day 7 of the luteal phase in an oocyte donation programme. *Hum. Reprod.* **11**(4): 893–4.

Serhal, P. (1990). Oocyte donation and surrogacy. *Br. Med. Bull.* **46**(3): 796–812.

Serhal, P. & Craft, I. (1987a). Ovum donation – a simplified approach. *Fertil. Steril.* **48**(2): 265–9.

Serhal, P. & Craft, I. (1987b). Immune basis for pre-eclampsia evidence from oocyte recipients. *Lancet* **2**: 744.

Serhal, P. & Craft, I. (1989). Oocyte donation in 61 patients. *Lancet* **i**: 1185–7.

Trounson, A., Leeton, J., Besanko, M., Wood, C. & Conti, A. (1983). Pregnancy established in an infertile patient after transfer of a donated embryo fertilised in vitro. *BMJ* **286**: 835–7.

Tulchinsky, D. & Hobel, C. J. (1973). Plasma human chorionic gonadotropin, estrone, estradiol, estriol, progesterone, and 17 alpha-hydroxyprogesterone in human pregnancy. 3. Early normal pregnancy. *Am. J. Obstet. Gynecol.* **117**(7): 884–93.

Wiegerinck, M. A., Poortman, J., Donker, T. H. & Thijssen, J. H. (1983). In vivo uptake and subcellular distribution of tritium-labeled estrogens in human endometrium, myometrium, and vagina. *J. Clin. Endocrinol. Metab.* **56**(1): 76–80.

Yaron, Y., Amit, A., Brenner, S. M., Peyser, R., David, M. P. & Lessing, J. B. (1995). In vitro fertilization and oocyte donation in women 15 years of age and older. *Fertil. Steril.* **63**(1): 71.

Yoshimi, T., Strott, C. A., Marshall, J. R & Lipsett, M. B. (1969). Corpus luteum function in early pregnancy. *J. Clin. Endocrinol. Metab.* **29**(2): 225–30.

Yovich, J. L., Blackledge, D. G., Richardson, P. A. *et al.* (1987). PROST for ovum donation. *Lancet* **1**: 1209–10.

Zaidi, J., Campbell, S., Pittrof, R., & Tan, S. L. (1995). Endometrial thickness, morphology, vascular penetration and velocimetry in predicting implantation in an in vitro fertilization program. *Ultrasound Obstet. Gynaecol.* **6**(3): 191–8.

11

Surrogacy

Peter R. Brinsden

Bourn Hall Clinic, Cambridge, UK

In the United Kingdom (UK) and the United States (US) surrogacy is an accepted treatment option for certain specific causes of childlessness, but most countries do not allow it (Jones & Cohen, 2001). Until IVF produced an alternative, 'natural surrogacy' was the only treatment option available to women with congenital absence of a uterus or women who had lost their uterus to surgery. In vitro fertilization surrogacy is required by relatively few couples and accounts for approximately 1% of IVF treatment cycles at Bourn Hall (Brinsden *et al.*, 2000) and only 0.1% of assisted reproductive treatment cycles in the UK (Human Fertilisation and Embryology Authority, 2000).

Definition of terms

Considerable confusion exists over the terms used in connection with surrogacy. 'Natural surrogacy', sometimes known as 'partial surrogacy', refers to an arrangement in which a female surrogate, sometimes known as the 'surrogate mother', agrees to be inseminated with the sperm of the male partner of the couple wanting a child, sometimes known as the 'commissioning couple', and this is often done without medical supervision. The resulting child is genetically the child of the female surrogate and of the male partner of the couple wanting the child, but genetically unrelated to the female partner of the couple wanting the child. 'IVF-surrogacy', sometimes known as 'gestational surrogacy' or 'full surrogacy', refers to an arrangement where the couple wanting a child provide both sets of gametes and, following fertilization *in vitro*, their embryos are transferred to the female surrogate. The resulting child is genetically the child of the couple wanting the child and genetically unrelated to the female surrogate. In this chapter the terms 'IVF-surrogacy' and 'natural surrogacy' will be used. The couple wanting a child

Good Clinical Practice in Assisted Reproduction, ed. P. Serhal & C. Overton.
Published by Cambridge University Press. © Cambridge University Press 2004.

Table 11.1. Indications for treatment by IVF-surrogacy

- Following hysterectomy
- Congenital absence of the uterus
- Repeated failure of IVF treatment
- Recurrent miscarriage
- Severe medical conditions incompatible with pregnancy

Source: Adapted from: Brinsden *et al.*, 2000, with permission.

and requesting treatment by IVF-surrogacy will be referred to as the 'genetic couple' and the female surrogate will be referred to as the 'surrogate host'.

Indications for treatment by IVF-surrogacy

The major indications for treatment by IVF-surrogacy (Table 11.1) are congenital absence of the uterus and previous hysterectomy for haemorrhage or malignancies. Other indications include recurrent miscarriage, repeated failure of IVF treatment, and medical conditions such as severe heart or kidney disease rendering a woman unfit for pregnancy but fit enough to care for a child when it is born.

Assessment for treatment

The genetic couple

Usually, couples seeking IVF-surrogacy are referred by their consultant gynaecologist with a clear indication for treatment following full investigation and referral with inappropriate indications like social reasons are rare.

In the first instance, the genetic couple are seen in consultation so that a full history can be taken and a full examination carried out. The indications for treatment are reviewed with the couple and details of that treatment should be supported with written information. It must be explained to couples that, by law in the UK, they must find their own surrogate host as clinics providing treatment are not permitted to make these arrangements, and that commercial arrangements for surrogacy are not permitted. In the US, commercial surrogacy is allowed and agencies, often run by legal advisors, can make surrogacy arrangements.

Evidence of normal ovarian function of the genetic mother may be assessed by:

- Symptoms of monthly cycling, such as breast and emotional changes.
- Estimations of serum follicle stimulating hormone (FSH), luteinizing hormone (LH) and oestradiol and, if cyclical symptoms are present, serum progesterone in the estimated luteal phase.

- Serial pelvic ultrasound scans for evidence of follicular development.
- A well-kept basal temperature chart (BTC).

The male partner of the genetic couple should receive counselling and should be informed that by Law in the UK (Surrogacy Arrangements Act, 1985), his semen must be frozen for six months prior to use, just as if he were acting as a sperm donor. His HIV status is checked before freezing and checked again prior to use at the end of the six months 'quarantine'. An alternative to freezing the semen for six months is to create embryos by IVF and freeze the embryos for the six months 'quarantine' before checking HIV status and transferring to the surrogate host. In the UK this is standard practice but is not mandatory for surrogacy programs in other countries.

The surrogate host

A surrogate host may be a relative of the genetic couple or a close friend. In the UK the surrogate host may be previously unknown to the genetic couple and introduced through an agency such as childlessness overcome through surrogacy (COTS) or in the US through commercial agencies. A surrogate host should be fit, less than 38 years of age, should have had at least one child, and preferably have completed her own family. It is preferable that a surrogate host is in a stable relationship and that her partner is made fully aware of the implications of what she is undertaking. In the work-up to treatment, reliable contraception of the surrogate host must be emphasized. A surrogate host on the contraceptive pill may continue the pill right up to the start of treatment. In-depth counselling should be arranged for the surrogate host, her partner and her family as appropriate. Surrogate hosts being introduced through an agency may already have received counselling from that agency or from contact with other surrogate hosts within support organizations.

The surrogate host must undergo the following preliminary tests:
- Physical examination.
- Cervical smear.
- Blood group.
- Hepatitis B (HBV), hepatitis C (HBC) and HIV testing. The male partner of the surrogate host is also tested once.

Counselling

Counselling and appropriate legal advice is essential to all parties of a surrogacy arrangement. The role of counselling is to guide all parties contemplating treatment to consider all aspects of the arrangement and the factors that will influence their future lives. Counselling should not only involve imparting comprehensive information about surrogacy, but should enable all involved to be confident and comfortable with their decision. Counselling should enable trust between all the parties involved, so that no one party will feel they are being taken advantage of or that the legal and ethical rules and regulations to which they are subject are being exploited. In its 1990 report, the British Medical Association stated that, when advising couples about surrogacy, 'the aggregate of foreseeable hazards should not be so great as to place unacceptable burdens on any of the parties – including the future child' (British Medical Association, 1990).

At Bourn Hall Clinic, Cambridgeshire, counselling usually takes place in the home of the genetic couple, with whom the hoped-for child will be raised. All parties to the arrangement, including the genetic couple, the surrogate host and her partner, and any children of the surrogate host who are old enough to take part, are seen together and separately as appropriate. The counsellor reviews all aspects of treatment by IVF-surrogacy including an assessment of the compatibility of all parties and the motivation of the surrogate host.

The surrogacy arrangement is presented anonymously to the clinic's Ethics Committee where it is reviewed and an opinion given as to the suitability of the arrangement, and any potential problems highlighted. The Ethics Committee will either recommend that treatment proceed as arranged, recommend further investigation and counselling followed by review, or recommend that the arrangement not proceed. Arrangements for treatment to commence are only made upon approval by the Ethics Committee.

Management of the genetic mother

Usually, the genetic mother will undergo an IVF cycle with a standard follicular stimulation regimen and oocyte collection. At Bourn Hall Clinic this involves:

- Standard 'down-regulation' with a LH/RH analogue started in the estimated mid-luteal phase, combined with follicular stimulation using recombinant-FSH in a dose of 150 to 300 iu daily depending on the woman's age, previous serum FSH levels and any experience of previous stimulation cycles.
- Standard follicular monitoring by estimations of serum oestradiol and follicle size by pelvic ultrasound.
- Administration of HCG 10 000 iu when two or more follicles have developed to 18 or more millimetres in diameter.
- Standard vaginal ultrasound oocyte collection procedure, either under sedation or general anaesthesia. Occasionally trans-abdominal oocyte collection may be necessary if the ovaries are situated outside the pelvis.
- Standard laboratory procedures for in vitro fertilization of the oocytes with the prepared semen sample.

- Transfer of a maximum of two embryos to the surrogate host.
- Cryopreservation of any supernumerary embryos for future use.

Management of the surrogate host

After the process of examination, counselling and Ethics Committee approval, the surrogate host is reviewed and her treatment cycle arranged. If it has been agreed that the cycles of the female of the genetic couple and the surrogate host are to be synchronized, this can be achieved if both parties are given the LH/RH analogue. At Bourn Hall Clinic the host surrogate is placed on the LH/RH analogue, starting in the mid-luteal phase of the cycle prior to the transfer cycle. Menstruation usually occurs about 7–10 days after the start of the analogue and oral oestradiol valerate tablets are started in a standardized regimen (Marcus & Brinsden, 1999). The surrogate host's cycle is monitored by pelvic ultrasound scan and the 'quality' of the endometrium assessed two to four days prior to planned embryo transfer. The standard embryo transfer technique is used (Brinsden, 1999) and a maximum of two embryos transferred to the uterus of the surrogate host. The LH/RH analogue is discontinued two days prior to embryo transfer and oral oestradiol valerate in the standard regimen (Marcus & Brinsden, 1999) is continued with progesterone by vaginal suppository or intramuscularly.

Some clinics prefer to transfer the embryos in a 'natural cycle' without LH/RH analogue or oestradiol support. In a natural cycle replacement, the monitoring of the surrogate host takes place daily from about day 8 of the natural cycle until an LH surge is detected. The embryos are transferred 48 hours after the LH surge. Luteal support is not usually necessary. At Bourn Hall, natural cycles are used only if the surrogate host expresses a strong preference for this treatment. However, it is often necessary to cancel these cycles because of poor response or inappropriate synchronization.

Results of treatment

To date, relatively few reports of large series of IVF-surrogacy treatments have been published. In our own series of 49 genetic couples treated, we reported live birth rates of 37% per genetic couple and 34% per host surrogate with a mean of two embryos transferred (Brinsden *et al.*, 2000; Table 11.2).

Utian and his colleagues (1985) were the first group to report a successful IVF-surrogacy pregnancy and reported a series of 59 women treated at their unit who achieved an 18% pregnancy rate (Utian *et al.*, 1989). Goldfarb *et al.* (2000) reviewed 180 IVF-surrogacy treatment cycles from between 1984 and 1999 on a total of 112 couples and the live birth rate per treatment cycle was 15.8%.

Table 11.2. Summary of results of treatment by IVF Surrogacy at Bourn Hall Clinic 1990 – 1998

• *Treatment of genetic couples*		
Number of patients started treatment	49	
Mean age at start (years)	32.9	Range = 22–40
Total stimulated cycles	80	Range = 1–5
• *Treatment of host surrogates*		
Number of hosts started treatment	53	
Number of cycles to embryo transfer	87	Mean transfers/host = 1.6
• *Final outcomes*		
Delivered/ongoing pregnancies/host transfer cycle	18/87	21%
Clinical pregnancies/surrogate host	31/53	58.5%
Delivered/ongoing pregnancies/surrogate host	18/53	34%
Clinical pregnancies/genetic couple	31/49	63%
Delivered/ongoing pregnancies/genetic couple	18/49	37%

Source: (Adapted from: Brinsden *et al.*, 2000, with permission.)

Batzofin *et al.* (1999) reported another series from the US, giving an ongoing or delivered pregnancy rate of 36% (172 out of 484 surrogate hosts), with a mean of 5 ± 1.3 embryos transferred. Also from the US, Corson *et al.* (1998) have reported a clinical pregnancy rate of 58% per genetic couple and 33.2% per embryo transfer in surrogate hosts when the genetic female was aged <40 years.

Meniru & Craft (1997) reported the only other series from the UK. In a series of 22 women with previous hysterectomy, a pregnancy rate of 37.5% per surrogate host and 27.3% per cycle of treatment begun was achieved.

Although some of the series cited above have reported live birth rates, very little effort has been made to monitor the live birth rate resulting from IVF-surrogacy. Parkinson *et al.* (1999) compared the perinatal outcome of pregnancies from IVF-surrogacy to those of pregnancies from standard IVF. The main finding was that pregnancy-induced hypertension and bleeding in the third trimester of pregnancy was five times more frequent in the surrogate host. Similarly, very few long-term studies have been done on the women who have acted as surrogate hosts or their surrogacy babies, but there is little to suggest any long-term harm or regret among them (Fisher & Gillman, 1991; Blyth, 1994; Van den Akker, 1999).

Complications of treatment

The major complications arising out of treatment by IVF-surrogacy have involved legal issues, the custody of the resulting child being the main example. The majority of these have occurred in the US and have arisen from natural surrogacy arrangements. The major ethical and practical problems that cause concern are that:

- the surrogate host might wish to keep the child once it is born. All practitioners and counsellors providing treatment are concerned about this but, with proper counselling and legal advice, it is unlikely to occur;
- if a child were born and found to be abnormal, he or she might be rejected by both sets of 'parents'. Detailed counselling about this possibility should occur before treatment starts;
- in the UK, the surrogate host can receive 'reasonable expenses', whereas in the US full commercial arrangements with the surrogate host are legal;
- the long-term psychological and emotional well-being of children born as a result of surrogacy, and of the surrogate hosts, has not been adequately followed to date. This issue is being addressed and it is hoped that information on this important issue will soon become available;
- some genetic couple females respond poorly to follicular stimulation, particularly if post-hysterectomy, and this possibility should be included in the counselling process. Often it is possible to improve follicular response in subsequent cycles;
- genetic couple females with Rokitansky–Kuster–Hauser (RKH) syndrome have reasonably expressed concern that they might produce children similarly affected with congenital absence of the uterus. Petrozza *et al.* (1997) attempted to address this question and have published reassuring data showing no increased incidence of congenital absence of the uterus and vagina in the offspring of women with RKH syndrome.

Regulation of surrogacy

IVF-surrogacy has been practised in the UK and US for more than 13 years and has now become an accepted treatment in these countries. Worldwide there are a few other countries where IVF-surrogacy is permitted, but as yet there is no published data on their experience. In Europe, the majority of countries do not allow IVF-surrogacy, with Belgium and The Netherlands the exceptions.

Religious issues

The attitude of major religions to surrogacy is summarized in Table 11.3.

Conclusion

Treatment by IVF-surrogacy is straightforward, involving the resources and skills that already exist in centres practising IVF (Figure 11.1). What makes the treatment

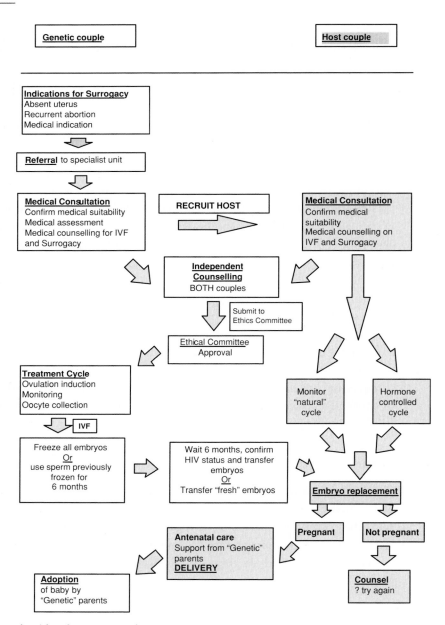

Figure 11.1. Algorithm for treatment by IVF surrogacy.

special is the care that must be exercised in ensuring that the arrangements are appropriate and that the genetic couple and their surrogate host are entirely compatible with each other and fully informed of all aspects of the treatment, including potential complications. Those who have treated reasonable numbers of women by

Table 11.3. Religious attitudes to surrogacy

- *Christian view*
  Not acceptable – Catholic or Anglican
  'Contrary to unity of marriage and dignity of the creation of
  the person . . .'
- *Jewish view*
  Not forbidden
  'The child belongs to the father who gave the sperm'
- *Islamic view*
  Not acceptable
  'Pregnancy should be the fruit of a legitimate marriage'
  'If a host did deliver, the child would be hers'
- Buddhist view
  Not prohibited, but generally against, because of family ties and
  legal and moral reasons

Source: Adapted from: Brinsden *et al.*, 2000, with permission.

IVF-surrogacy in the past 10 or more years, have shown it is a successful treatment option and relatively free of complications, especially when compared with natural surrogacy arrangements. Couples requesting treatment require careful assessment and in-depth counselling, and should be provided with support throughout their treatment and for as long as they need it afterwards. Ideally, all IVF-surrogacy treatment should be provided by a few of the larger assisted conception centres that have experience in managing these cases. Surrogacy arrangements should not be undertaken lightly or without the full support of an experienced team of fertility specialists, counsellors and an independent ethics committee. IVF-surrogacy remains controversial (British Medical Association, 1996; Department of Health, 1997) but, where it is practised within accredited or licensed clinics with full counselling facilities and the support of an independent ethics committee, the treatment is effective in helping a small group of women with their unique reproductive problems.

REFERENCES

Batzofin, J., Nelson, J., Wilcox, J., Potter, D., Rogoff, R., Norbryhn, G., Hatkoff, C. & Feinman, M. (1999). Gestational surrogacy: is it time to include it as part of ART? *American Society for Reproductive Medicine Programme Supplement*: P-017 (Abst).

Blyth, E. (1994). Interviews with surrogate mothers in Britain. *J. Reprod. & Infertil. Psychol.* **12**: 189–98.

Brinsden, P. R. (1999). Oocyte recovery and embryo transfer techniques for *in vitro* fertilization. In *A Textbook of In Vitro Fertilization and Assisted Reproduction*, 2nd edn., ed. P. R. Brinsden, pp. 171–84. Carnforth: Parthenon Publishers.

Brinsden, P. R., Appleton, T. C., Murray, E., Hussein, M., Akagbosu, F. & Marcus, S. F. (2000). Treatment by in vitro fertilisation with surrogacy: experience of one British centre. *BMJ* **320**: 924–8.

British Medical Association. (1990). *Surrogacy: Ethical Considerations. Report of the Working Party on Human Infertility Services.* (London: BMA Publications).

British Medical Association (1996). *Changing Conceptions of Motherhood. The Practice of Surrogacy in Britain.* London: BMA Publications.

Corson, S. L., Kelly, M., Braverman, A. & English, M. E. (1998). Gestational carrier pregnancy. *Fertil. Steril.* **69**: 670–4.

Department of Health (1997). *Surrogacy. Review for the UK Health Ministers of Current Arrangements for Payments and Regulation. Consultation Document.* London: Department of Health.

Fisher, S. & Gillman, I. (1991). Surrogate Motherhood: Attachment, Attitudes and Social Support. *Psychiatry* **54**: 13–20.

Goldfarb, J., Austin, C., Peskin, B., Lisbona, H., Desai, N. & Loret De Mola, J. R. (2000). Fifteen years experience with an in vitro fertilisation surrogate gestational pregnancy programme. *Hum. Reprod.* **15**: 1075–8.

Human Fertilisation and Embryology Authority (2000). *Ninth Annual Report 2000.* London: Human Fertilisation and Embryology Authority.

Jones, H. W. & Cohen, J. (2001). IFFS Surveillance 01. ASRM report on worldwide IVF surrogacy. *Fertil. Steril.* **76** (Suppl. 2): S26.

Marcus, S. F. & Brinsden, P. R. (1999). Oocyte donation. In *A Textbook of In Vitro Fertilization and Assisted Reproduction*, 2nd edn., ed. P. R. Brinsden, pp. 343–54. Carnforth: Parthenon Publishers.

Meniru, G. I. & Craft, I. L. (1997). Experience with gestational surrogacy as a treatment for sterility resulting from hysterectomy. *Hum. Reprod.* **12**: 51–4.

Parkinson, J., Tran, C. & Tan, T. (1999). Perinatal outcome after in-vitro fertilisation – surrogacy (IVF-surrogacy) *Hum. Reprod.* **14**: 671–6.

Petrozza, J. C., Gray, M. R., Davies, A. J. & Reindollar, R. H. (1997). Congenital absence of the uterus and vagina is not commonly transmitted as a dominant genetic trait: Outcomes of surrogate pregnancies. *Fertil. Steril.* **67**: 387–9.

Utian, W. F., Goldfarb, J. M., Kiwi, R. *et al.* (1989). Preliminary experience with in vitro fertilization-surrogate gestational pregnancy. *Fertil. Steril.* **52**: 633–8.

Utian, W. H., Sheean, L. A., Goldfarb, J. M. & Kiwi, R. (1985). Successful pregnancy after in vitro fertilisation and embryo transfer from an infertile woman to a surrogate. *N. Engl. J. Med.* **313**: 1351–2.

Van den Akker, O. B. A. (1999). Organisational selection and assessment of women entering a surrogacy agreement in the UK. *Hum. Reprod.* **14**(1): 262–6.

12

Clinical aspects of preimplantation genetic diagnosis

Joyce C. Harper and Joy D. A. Delhanty

Department of Obstetrics and Gynaecology, University College London, London, UK

Introduction

Preimplantation genetic diagnosis (PGD) is a procedure developed to help couples who are at risk of transmitting an inherited disease to have a healthy family. Apart from PGD, the main option for these couples is prenatal diagnosis (amniocentesis or chorionic villous sampling) between 10 and 16 weeks' gestation to determine if the fetus is affected. If prenatal diagnosis shows an affected fetus, the couple must then decide whether to continue with the pregnancy or undergo a termination. Other options are natural conception with the associated risk of having an affected child, gamete donation or to remain childless.

Couples referred for PGD are known to be at genetic risk due to an affected family member or the birth of an affected child and may:

- have a previous history of prenatal diagnosis and termination of an affected pregnancy;
- have moral or religious objections to termination of pregnancy;
- have a previous history of recurrent spontaneous miscarriages due to chromosomal abnormalities;
- be infertile and carrying a genetic abnormality (which may or may not be causing their infertility).

PGD involves three stages: IVF, embryo biopsy and single cell diagnosis. Although many PGD couples are fertile, routine IVF procedures are required so that embryos are generated outside the body for biopsy and PGD and unaffected embryos can be subsequently transferred to the woman. It is possible to remove cells from the embryo at three stages (Table 12.1), but the most common method is cleavage stage biopsy. Polymerase chain reaction (PCR) or fluorescent in situ hybridization (FISH) are used for single cell diagnosis (Table 12.2).

Good Clinical Practice in Assisted Reproduction, ed. P. Serhal & C. Overton.
Published by Cambridge University Press. © Cambridge University Press 2004.

Table 12.1. Methods of embryo biopsy

- Polar body biopsy; removal of the first and second polar body either sequentially or simultaneously. Only used by a few centres
- Cleavage stage biopsy; removal of 1–2 blastomeres from the 6–8 cell embryo. Used by the majority of PGD centres
- Blastocyst biopsy; removal of some of the trophectoderm cells from the blastocyst. To date has not been clinically applied

Note: PGD: preimplantation genetic diagnosis.

Table 12.2. Methods of diagnosis

PCR – analyse mutation in a gene:
- single gene defects (dominant and recessive)
- sexing for X-linked disease, or specific diagnosis of X-linked disease
- triplet repeat disorders

FISH – analyse presence or absence of a chromosome or part of a chromosome:
- sexing for X-linked disease
- chromosomal abnormalities, e.g. translocations
- aneuploidy screening (to help increase pregnancy rates for IVF patients)

Note: PCR: polymerase chain reaction; FISH: fluorescent in situ hybridization.

PCR is used for the diagnosis of single gene defects such as cystic fibrosis, screening of specific diagnosis of X-linked diseases and the triplet repeats disorders such as myotonic dystrophy (reviewed in Wells & Sherlock, 1998). FISH is used for the analysis of chromosomes. This can be for sexing by using probes for the X and Y chromosomes and for PGD of chromosome abnormalities, such as translocations, by using probes for the chromosomes involved in the specific translocation (reviewed in Harper & Delhanty, 2000). PGD has been used in an effort to improve pregnancy rates for older women undergoing IVF, by using probes for the chromosomes commonly involved in aneuploidy (Munné *et al.*, 1999).

Single cell FISH and PCR are both technically challenging techniques. PCR can be problematic due to contamination and a phenomenon known as 'allele dropout' (ADO) (Table 12.3). One of the main contaminants can be sperm embedded in the zona pellucida that may be dislodged during the embryo biopsy procedure. Therefore, the intracytoplasmic sperm injection (ICSI) technique is used to inject a single sperm into the oocyte, so that sperm do not become embedded in the zona pellucida. FISH PGD can be contaminated by cumulus cells that surround the embryo, and PGD for chromosomal abnormalities is complicated by the presence of chromosomal mosaicism in human preimplantation embryos. Usually, after

Table 12.3. Possible causes of misdiagnosis in preimplantation genetic diagnosis

PCR – important for dominant disorders or when only one mutation analysed in heterozygotes:
    contamination (sperm, cumulus cells, cells in atmosphere, DNA)
    allele dropout (ADO)
    mosaicism

FISH – important for the analysis of chromosome abnormalities:
    mosaicism
    hybridization failure

Note: PCR: polymerase chain reaction; FISH: fluorescent in situ hybridization.

transfer following PGD, any remaining embryos are used to confirm the original diagnosis.

Clinical aspects of PGD

When couples are referred for PGD, usually they have already had genetic counselling. At University College London Centre for PGD they are given a preliminary consultation to describe in detail the IVF and PGD procedures (Appendix 12.1). If the couple wishes to proceed with PGD, the next stage is diagnosis workup. Besides embryo sexing for X-linked disease, all other PGDs involve a test specific to that couple, and so the workup may take several months or longer. In the UK, all PGDs need to be approved by the Human Fertilisation and Embryology Authority (HFEA), which licenses all IVF and PGD procedures, and application must be made before any treatment is commenced.

When the diagnosis workup is complete, couples require a full IVF and PGD consultation, including gynaecological and fertility tests routine to IVF procedures (such as sperm count, hormone tests, examination of the uterus, trial embryo transfer) (Appendix 12.2). For PGD patients, especially those carrying fragile X syndrome, a test of ovarian reserve is recommended (at UCL we use the GnRH-agonist ovarian stimulation test – G-test). PGD is identical to regular IVF except that ovarian stimulation aims to maximize the number of eggs retrieved. For PGD to be successful, at least nine oocyte cumulus complexes are required (Vandervorst *et al.*, 1998), to improve the chances of good quality, unaffected embryos for replacement. In some cycles, all embryos will be affected and no embryos will be available for replacement (ESHRE PGD Consortium, 1999, 2000). In PGD the diagnosis is made from one or two cells. Due to the problems of single cell diagnosis and mosaicism, it is recommended that pregnant women undergo prenatal diagnosis but only 50% of patients opt for this (ESHRE PGD Consortium, 1999, 2000).

Table 12.4. Aims of the ESHRE Preimplantation Genetic Diagnosis (PGD) Consortium

- To survey the availability of PGD for different conditions facilitating cross referral of patients
- To collect prospectively and retrospectively data on accuracy, reliability and effectiveness of PGD
- To initiate follow-up studies of pregnancies and children born
- To produce guidelines and recommended PGD protocols to promote best practice
- To formulate a consensus on the use of PGD

The European Society of Human Reproduction and Embryology (ESHRE) PGD Consortium was set up in 1997 and its aims are shown in Table 12.4. Two data collections have been reported (ESHRE PGD Consortium, 1999, 2000), the second including cycles from centres in Australia, Belgium, Denmark, France, Greece, Italy, South Korea, Spain, Israel, The Netherlands, Sweden, United Kingdom, and the United States. Although some of the patients are fertile, over the two years the pregnancy rate is low (17% and 19% per oocyte retrieval), probably because of the reduction in the number of embryos considered suitable for transfer (ESHRE PGD Consortium, 2000). The different types of diseases diagnosed by PGD have remained small, due to the technical nature of the diagnosis. A follow-up of all PGD pregnancies submitted to the consortium is in progress. Besides the PGD Consortium data, which does not account for all PGD cycles, it is estimated that worldwide approximately 200 babies have been born following PGD.

Embryo biopsy

Theoretically there are three stages at which cells can be removed from human embryos for PGD: polar bodies from the oocyte/zygote; one to two blastomeres from cleavage stage embryos; and 10 or so trophectoderm cells from the blastocyst (Table 12.1). However, the majority of PGD centres use cleavage stage biopsy (ESHRE PGD Consortium 1999, 2000).

Removal of the first polar body was first performed with the view that it would be a method of preconceptional diagnosis (Verlinsky et al., 1990), since the first polar body is a waste product of oocyte meiosis. However, it was soon realized that for an accurate diagnosis the first and second polar body are required, and the second polar body is not produced until fertilization occurs. Since the first polar body degenerates quite rapidly, the first and second polar body should ideally be removed sequentially (Strom et al., 1997) rather than simultaneously (Verlinsky et al., 1996).

The method of polar body biopsy involves making a hole in the zona pellucida that surrounds the oocyte and zygote, by using a laser, a bevelled pipette, or by mechanical ripping of the zona (partial zona dissection). The polar body or bodies can then be aspirated and used for the diagnosis. Polar body diagnosis has been used for the analysis of age-related aneuploidy (Munné *et al.*, 1999; Verlinsky *et al.*, 1996), translocations (Munné *et al.*, 1998) and single gene defects (Verlinsky *et al.*, 1997). The advantages of this procedure are that it may be ethically more acceptable in some countries where embryo manipulation is prohibited, e.g. Malta and Germany, and the polar bodies probably are not required for embryo development. However, it is limited as it can only examine maternal chromosomes and the oocytes/zygotes may be subjected to two manipulations.

Cleavage stage biopsy is the most commonly used procedure to remove embryonic material. In the ESHRE PGD Consortium data (2000), from 759 cycles with PGD, 755 used cleavage stage biopsy (only three used polar body biopsy and one polar body biopsy and cleavage stage biopsy). Cleavage stage biopsy was the original method reported in the first cases of PGD (Handyside *et al.*, 1990), and the method used today is almost unchanged (Van de Velde *et al.*, 2000). Embryos at the 6–8 cell stage are immobilized and a small hole drilled in the zona pelludica. This is most commonly achieved using acid Tyrodes solution, but the use of a compact diode 1.48 micron noncontact laser is becoming more common (ESHRE PGD Consortium, 1999, 2000). Partial zona dissection, in a technique similar to that used for polar body biopsy, has been reported for cleavage stage zona breaching. Once a hole has been made in the zona, the usual method for removal of the blastomeres is aspiration ((ESHRE PGD Consortium, 1999, 2000). One problem originally encountered was blastomere lysis as at the 8-cell stage, human embryos start to undergo compaction where the blastomeres increase their intercellular connections. Therefore, removal of one blastomere may be difficult if it is attached to other blastomeres. However, the use of Ca^{2+}/Mg^{2+}-free biopsy medium (which breaks the cellular contacts in a reversible way as they are Ca^{2+} dependent) has increased the efficiency of the embryo biopsy procedure (Dumoulin *et al.*, 1998). From the ESHRE PGD Consortium data (2000), 96% of embryo biopsies were successfully carried out.

The advantages of cleavage stage biopsy (Figure 12.1) are that the procedure is relatively easy to perform and the blastomeres aspirated can be selected (often the presence of an interphase nucleus can be seen before biopsy). However, the limitations are that there are only one or two cells for the analysis and chromosomal mosaicism is observed at this stage, which may result in the biopsied blastomere not being representative of the rest of the embryo. There has been much discussion in the PGD community on whether one or two blastomeres should be taken for the diagnosis (Van de Velde *et al.*, 2000), as a number of misdiagnoses have been reported (reviewed in Harper & Delhanty, 2000). Therefore, taking two blastomeres will increase the chance of a successful diagnosis, especially in the case of chromosomal analysis. However, taking two blastomeres may lower the implantation rate when compared to taking one. This issue is yet to be resolved.

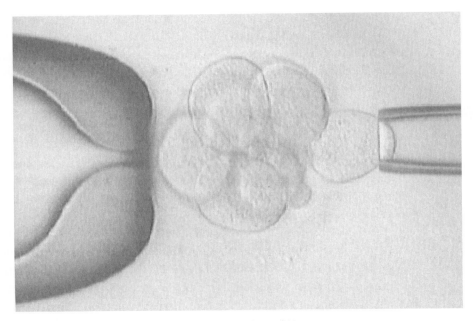

Figure 12.1. Cleavage stage embryo biopsy. (Courtesy Alpesh Doshi.)

Blastocyst biopsy has not been applied clinically to PGD, mainly because only 50% of human embryos reach the blastocyst stage in vitro. For PGD to be successful it is important to start the procedure with a high number of embryos (Vandervorst *et al.*, 1998) to ensure that some good quality, unaffected embryos are available for transfer. Therefore, reducing the original number of embryos with blastocyst culture would affect the success of the procedure.

The method of blastocyst biopsy involves zona drilling, either with acid Tyrodes or a laser, and then culturing the embryo until some of the trophectoderm cells herniate through the zona. These can then be removed and used for the diagnosis (Veiga *et al.*, 1997). The advantages of the procedure are that there would be 10–20 cells for the diagnosis. The limitations are that few embryos will be available, the time available for the diagnosis would be very short as embryos start to implant at this stage and so would need to be returned to the uterus, and the trophectoderm may differ in chromosomal constitution to the inner cell mass (which goes on to make the embryo proper) (Evsikov & Verlinsky, 1998; Ruangvutilert *et al.*, 2000).

Diagnosis of single gene disorders

Table 12.5 lists those single gene disorders for which successful PGD protocols have been reported. In principle, PGD can be developed for any condition caused by

Table 12.5. Reported polymerase chain reaction diagnoses for single gene disorders

Recessive disorders
Cystic fibrosis (various mutations)
Tay–Sachs disease
β-thalassaemia
Sickle cell anaemia
Rh blood typing
Spinal muscular atrophy
Adrenogenital syndrome
Congenital adrenal hyperplasia
Plakophilin-1 (PKP1)
Medium chain acyl CoA dehydrogenase deficiency

Dominant disorders
Marfan syndrome
Familial adenomatous polyposis coli
Charcot–Marie–Tooth disease (type 1A)
osteogenesis imperfecta
Crouzon syndrome
Neurofibromatosis type 2
Li–Fraumeni syndrome

Triplet repeat disorders
Myotonic dystrophy
Huntington's disease
Fragile X syndrome

Specific diagnosis of X-linked disease
Lesch–Nyhan syndrome
Duchenne muscular dystrophy
Charcot–Marie–Tooth disease
Retinitis pigmentosum
Ornithine transcarbamylase deficiency

a single gene mutation providing the molecular basis of the disease is understood (Wells & Sherlock, 1998). This enables specific DNA primers to be designed to allow amplification of the region of interest in the gene via the PCR. When starting from a single genome a large number of PCR cycles is needed to obtain sufficient product for analysis and this can exaggerate problems such as contamination encountered with routine PCR analysis. A strict regime is necessary to prevent contamination as far as possible.

Cellular contamination is likely to come from extra sperm or from maternal cumulus cells and the latter must be carefully removed prior to biopsy. The use of

Table 12.6. Mutation detection methods applied to preimplantation genetic diagnosis for single gene disorders

Heteroduplex formation
Restriction enzyme digestion
Single strand conformation polymorphism
Denaturing gradient gel electrophoresis
Fluorescent polymerase chain reaction
Use of lined markers, with or without above techniques

ICSI prevents sperm contamination but the most frequent source of contamination is from the products of previous PCR reactions that become airborne in the laboratory. This requires the provision of containment facilities for the handling of single cells. One of the most significant problems related to analysis of DNA from a single cell is ADO. This occurs when the gene sequence present on one chromosome fails to amplify or does so with reduced efficiency so that it is underrepresented in the final PCR product. This may lead to misdiagnosis of a heterozygous cell as homozygous. This is particularly important for dominant disorders but is equally so in the case of compound heterozygotes when the analysis system used is designed only to detect one of the mutations. The testing of two independent cells will minimize the risk of misdiagnosis due to ADO.

Once the DNA from a single blastomere has been amplified to a level where analysis is possible a wide variety of mutation detection approaches are available for PGD. These include restriction enzyme digestion of amplified DNA, heteroduplex formation, single strand conformation polymorphism (SSCP) and denaturing gradient gel electrophoresis (DGGE) (Wells & Sherlock, 1998). Table 12.6 lists the methods that have been applied clinically in PGD cycles.

Currently, the use of fluorescent PCR technology is having a wide impact on the PGD of single gene disorders. Since the sensitivity of fluorescent PCR product detection is over a thousand times greater than for conventional methods of analysis, a great reduction in the number of amplification cycles needed for single cell analysis is possible. The increased sensitivity also reduces the risk of ADO, as an underrepresented product from one of the alleles may still be detected.

When the exact disease causing mutation is unknown, PGD may still be possible by the use of linked markers, preferably a combination of two, either within or closely flanking the gene. This is one method of tackling PGD for the group of diseases caused by large expansions in the number of trinucleotide repeats within or close to a gene, for example fragile X syndrome or myotonic dystrophy. These mutations pose particular problems for PGD partly because the developmental timing of the expansions is not fully understood but also because the large number of repeat sequences present in affected embryos is not detectable by PCR at the single cell level. It is becoming increasingly common to devise protocols for PGD that include the detection of a linked or unlinked polymorphic marker in addition to analysis of the mutation site (Harper & Wells, 1999). This allows not only detection of contaminating DNA but also its possible source.

Chromosome detection by FISH

FISH is a molecular cytogenetic technique in which DNA probes are labelled directly or indirectly with fluorochromes and hybridized in situ to metaphase or interphase nuclei. A major advantage is that FISH can be used to determine the number of copies of a particular chromosome or region of a chromosome when it is difficult or impossible to obtain good quality metaphase preparations. This situation applies in the case of blastomeres from cleavage stage human embryos. There are a number of different FISH probes that can be used in interphase nuclei, including repeat probes, locus specific probes and sub-telomeric probes (Figure 12.2).

Sexing for X-linked disease

Sexing the embryo to avoid X-linked disease is one of the major indications for PGD. There are over 400 X-linked diseases and for the majority no specific diagnosis is available. Options for these families are limited to refraining from reproduction or

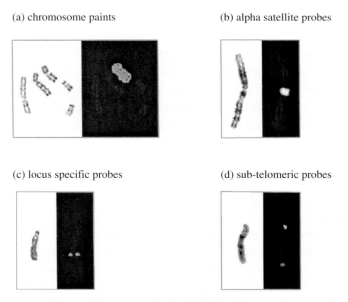

(a) chromosome paints   (b) alpha satellite probes

(c) locus specific probes   (d) sub-telomeric probes

Figure 12.2. Types of FISH (fluorescent in situ hybridization) probes. (With permission from Harper, Delhanty & Handyside, 2001.)

agreeing to pregnancy termination for all male fetuses, despite the fact that only half would be expected to be affected.

Although the first clinical application of PGD was the diagnosis of sex by PCR amplification of a repeat sequence from the long arm of the Y chromosome in embryonic DNA (Handyside *et al.*, 1990), the use of FISH is now generally preferred for this purpose (Staessen *et al.*, 1999; Delhanty *et al.*, 1997) because of the low risk of contamination. The presence of an amplified band by PCR indicates only that an X or Y chromosome is present and gives no information about copy number. Hence, a 45,X karyotype (Turner syndrome) cannot be distinguished from the normal 46,XX, and 47,XXY (Klinefelter syndrome) cannot be distinguished from a normal 46,XY male. Most important is the fact that since 45,X embryos will have the maternal X in 80% of cases they will be at almost as high a risk of the X-linked disease as the male embryos. Directly labelled X and Y probes together with an autosomal probe to provide additional information on chromosomal status is now routinely applied for embryo sexing in PGD in many centres worldwide (ESHRE PGD Consortium, 1999, 2000).

Detecting chromosome abnormalites

There are two groups of patients for whom the diagnosis of chromosomal abnormalities in the preimplantation embryo has been developed. The first group includes those with an exceptionally high risk due to specific parental chromosome rearrangements or gonadal mosaicism. Although these couples are not usually infertile, many will have experienced repeated miscarriages.

The second group is older women undergoing IVF treatment who are at a generally increased risk of an abnormal conception due to the age-related aneuploidy factor (preimplantation genetic screening – PGS). The detection of patient-specific chromosomal imbalance differs from general aneuploidy screening as combinations of locus-specific probes are required and need to be developed for individual cases. At present PGD for chromosome abnormalities relies on FISH analysis of biopsied first polar body chromosomes and/or interphase blastomere nuclei biopsied from cleavage-stage embryos.

Chromosomal mosacism

One unforeseen outcome of the application of FISH for sexing the cleavage stage embryo was the discovery of the true extent of chromosomal abnormality at this point in human development (Delhanty *et al.*, 1993). Further work led to the classification of chromosomes in cleavage embryos into four types: normal, uniformly abnormal, mosaic or chaotic (Table 12.7) (Harper *et al.*, 1995; Delhanty *et al.*, 1997). The mosaics were mainly diploid with a minority of cells aneuploid,

Table 12.7. Chromosome constitution of human preimplantation embryos

Normal: all chromosomes normal
Abnormal: all chromosomes abnormal
Mosaic: two cell lines present, e.g. diploid/tetraploid, diploid/aneuploid
Chaotic: all nuclei have randomly different chromosomes

haploid or tetraploid whereas the chaotics had chromosome complements varying randomly from cell to cell within one embryo. Typically, when testing two pairs of chromosomes, 30% of apparently normally developing cleavage stage embryos were mosaic, with a small percentage classed as chaotic. The investigation of larger numbers of nontransferred embryos in a group of PGD patients showed that the frequency of this highly abnormal type (chaotics) was strongly patient dependent (Delhanty *et al.*, 1997).

These findings have important implications for the diagnosis of embryo sex. So far, there have been no reports of an XX nucleus in a normally developing embryo that is male and there has been no case of misdiagnosis of sex in PGD when using the FISH technique. However, XO cells are seen in male embryos (Harper *et al.*, 1995), so embryos should only be considered for transfer when two X signals are seen in the absence of a Y signal and an embryo with an XO nucleus should never be transferred.

PGD for couples carrying balanced chromosome rearrangements

This high-risk group includes couples where one partner is a carrier of a chromosomal rearrangement that predisposes to the production of chromosomally unbalanced gametes. The most common types are Robertsonian and reciprocal translocation. Those presenting for PGD are a select group at the extreme end of the normal range, who have suffered recurrent spontaneous or induced abortions as a result of a series of abnormal conceptions.

Other chromosomal rearrangements that predispose the carrier to produce abnormal gametes are pericentric inversions, insertions and ring chromosomes, the latter two are rare. A particular group of couples requiring assisted conception and at high risk of a chromosomally abnormal conception are those requiring ICSI because of a sperm problem. Oligospermic males have an approximate 4% risk of carrying a chromosome rearrangement and should be routinely karyotyped. Once an abnormality is detected, these couples can be offered PGD to counteract the elevated risk of chromosome imbalance at conception.

To date, of the results from the PGD cycles carried out by different groups for specific chromosome rearrangements described here, almost all show very high levels of chromosome abnormalities resulting from abnormal meiotic segregation and post-zygotic mosaicism (Conn *et al.*, 1998, 1999; Munné *et al.*, 1998; Iwarrson *et al.*, 2000), and this is reflected in the poor pregnancy rate for this particular patient group. For this reason, counselling of prospective couples needs to emphasize that although the advantage of PGD is that many embryos can be screened simultaneously, where the majority are abnormal the chance of a normal pregnancy will still be low.

Robertsonian translocations

Analysis of metaphase stage first polar bodies can be carried out to infer the karyotype of oocytes from female Robertsonian translocation carriers using commercially available probes for the two chromosomes involved. This approach has resulted in the birth of babies with normal or balanced chromosomes (Munné *et al.*, 1998).

Detection of the acrocentric chromosomes, 13, 14, 15, 21 and 22, in interphase nuclei poses difficulties since centromere probes cannot be used. Now that commercial locus-specific probes are available for these chromosomes, they can be used for the detection of chromosome imbalance in blastomere nuclei resulting from maternal or paternal Robertsonian translocations, which is relatively straightforward for PGD. However, the chance of pregnancy may still be low (Conn *et al.*, 1998). The evidence is that two factors may be acting to reduce fertility in these couples, the aneuploid segregation of the parental Robertsonian translocation and post-zygotic errors in an exceptionally high proportion of embryos.

Reciprocal translocations

Balanced reciprocal translocations are by far the most frequently encountered chromosome rearrangement found in couples requesting PGD. As breakpoints can occur theoretically at any point on any chromosome, each translocation case represents a unique event with its own risk of chromosome imbalance at conception. Polar body analysis can be used for maternal reciprocal translocation carriers in a similar way to that used for Robertsonian translocations, by inferring the karyotype of the oocyte.

Maternal or paternal reciprocal translocations can be detected in the preimplantation embryo, using 'flanking' probes. It can be demonstrated with the aid of meiotic diagrams that the use of three probes is sufficient to detect all segregations. This involves the use of two probes flanking the breakpoint on one translocation chromosome and a third probe specific for the other chromosome, located in any position (Conn *et al.*, 1999). This approach does not allow embryos with normal or balanced chromosomes to be distinguished, but since the choice of morphologically normal embryos is usually limited in practice this would not be important.

Gonadal mosaicism

The presence of a second aneuploid cell line in a phenotypically normal individual creates a high risk situation. In women aged <35 years, repeated conceptions with trisomy for the same chromosome are likely to be caused by mosaicism for a cell line with the same trisomy that extends to the gonads. This mosaicism may not be detectable in somatic tissues such as lymphocytes that are used for standard karyotyping. PGD can be used in these cases to screen embryos for the specific trisomy (Conn et al., 1999).

Screening for age-related aneuploidy

It can be estimated that the overall risk of aneuploidy and triploidy at conception is about 12% for all maternal ages, but for women aged >40 years this is generally increased to >50%. This is the logic behind attempting to screen for age-related aneuploidy in older IVF patients in an attempt to improve the implantation rate and decrease the miscarriage rate.

To date over half of all PGD cycles carried out world-wide have been performed for this general screening for age-related aneuploidy. Originally probes were used to detect chromosomes X, Y, 18, 13 and 21, which together account for 95% of all postnatal chromosome abnormalities. More recent reports describe the use of probes for nine chromosomes (13, 15, 16, 17, 18, 21, 22, X and Y) in a two-stage FISH procedure (Bahce et al., 2000). Implantation rates and those of ongoing pregnancies have been improved, and the frequency of spontaneous abortions reduced (Munné et al., 1999). The debate on the benefit of screening all IVF embryos from older women is ongoing.

The disadvantages are that PGD is labour intensive and expensive and necessarily reduces the number of embryos available for transfer, which may be very low in older patients. For this reason, this screening may be of more benefit to those aged 35–40 years, which still has an increased risk of aneuploidy but is likely to produce more embryos for analysis than the >40-year age group.

The future

PGD has been marred by a number of misdiagnoses. In the light of our current knowledge, including ADO and chromosome mosaicism, it is hardly surprising that these errors have occurred. Therefore, for the future of PGD we have to ensure that diseases can be diagnosed using more efficient techniques to eliminate misdiagnosis. This can be achieved by basic DNA fingerprinting using STR markers, to ensure that the DNA analysed is embryonic and techniques such as multiplex PCR, which can be used to maximize the information obtained from a single cell.

The development of PGD for couples at risk of chromosome abnormalities has been slow, as for many of these patients appropriate FISH probes are not currently available. However, techniques such as comparative genomic hybridization (CGH) (Wells *et al.*, 1999) and interphase conversion (Willadsen *et al.*, 1999) are two methods that allow all of the chromosomes from an interphase nucleus to be examined.

In CGH, control and test DNA are labelled in different colours (red and green) and co-hybridized onto a control metaphase spread. Analysis of the ratio of red to green can detect whether the test DNA has extra or missing chromosomes or segments of chromosomes. This technique has been applied to analyse every cell from a series of spare, good quality IVF embryos (Wells & Delhanty 2000). This gave a complete picture of the chromosome status of these embryos and proved the existence of human IVF embryos with no aneuploid cells (25%). Sixty per cent were mosaic, with two examples of the chaotic type.

CGH has now been applied clinically (Wilton *et al.*, 2001). Avoiding the transfer of those embryos with lethal abnormalities could lead to an improvement in the implantation rate per embryo transferred and reduce the risk of multiple pregnancies.

Appendix 12.1: PGD patient checklist for preliminary consultation

Name:

Date:

Disorder:

Feasibility:

Bloods taken:

Buccal cells:

Discussed during consultation:

History – any children/miscarriages/terminations

Age female:

Explain:

   IVF

   Embryo biopsy

   Diagnosis

   all embs affected

   only testing their disorder

   IVF/PGD pregnancy rates

   Options – PGD, prenatal, gamete donation

Genetic counselling (had already – yes/no)

Information leaflets (given)

Next step

1. Funding – shall we apply?
2. Wait to hear from patients – ring or email
3. If start work up will incur a charge

Comments:

Appendix 12.2: PGD patient checklist for full consultation

Name:

Date:

Disorder:

Feasibility:

Bloods taken:

Buccal cells:

Discussed during consultation:

History:

Age female:

IVF/G test/HyCoSy

Embryo biopsy

No embryos available for biopsy

Diagnosis

No embryos available for transfer

All embryos affected

Day 3/4 transfer

Only testing for specific chromosomes/disorder

Need result from 2 cells

Mosaicism and misdiagnosis

Spare embryos research/confirmation of diagnosis

IVF/PGD pregnancy rates

Clinical pregnancies from this type of diagnosis

Unprotected sex

Prenatal diagnosis

Follow-up of children

Genetic counselling

Funding status

Information leaflets

Next step

Comments:

REFERENCES

Bahce, M., Escudero, T., Sandalinas, M., Morrison, L., Legaton, M. & Munne, S. (2000). Improvements of preimplantation diagnosis of aneuploidy by using microwave hybridisation, cell recycling and monocolour labelling of probes. *Mol. Hum. Reprod.* **6**: 845–54.

Conn, C. M., Harper, J. C., Winston, R. M. & Delhanty, J. D. (1998). Infertile couples with Robertsonian translocations: preimplantation genetic analysis of embryos reveals chaotic cleavage divisions. *Hum. Genet.* **102**: 117–23.

Conn, C. M., Cozzi, J., Harper, J. C., Winston, R. M. & Delhanty, J. D. (1999). Preimplantation genetic diagnosis for couples at high risk of Down syndrome pregnancy owing to parental translocation or mosaicism. *J. Med. Genet.* **36**: 45–50.

Delhanty, J., Griffin, D., Handyside, A. H. *et al.* (1993). Detection of aneuploidy and chromosomal mosaicism in human embryos during preimplantation sex determination by fluorescent in situ hybridisation (FISH). *Hum. Mol. Genet.* **2**: 1183–5.

Delhanty, J. D. A., Harper, J. C., Ao, A., Handyside, A. H. & Winston, R. M. L. (1997). Multicolour FISH detects frequent chromosomal mosaicism and chaotic division in normal preimplantation embryos from fertile patients. *Hum. Genet.* **99**: 755–60.

Dumoulin, J. C., Bras, M., Coonen, E., Dreesen, J., Geraedts, J. P. & Evers, J. L. (1998). Effect of Ca^{2+}/Mg^{2+}-free medium on the biopsy procedure for preimplantation genetic diagnosis and further development of human embryos. *Hum. Reprod.* **13**: 2880–3.

ESHRE PGD Consortium Steering Committee (1999). ESHRE Preimplantation Genetic Diagnosis (PGD) Consortium. Preliminary assessment of data from January 1997 to September 1998. *Hum. Reprod.* **14**: 3138–48.

ESHRE PGD Consortium Steering Committee (2000). ESHRE Preimplantation Genetic Diagnosis (PGD) Consortium: data collection II (May 2000). *Hum. Reprod.* **15**: 2673–83.

Evsikov, S. & Verlinsky, Y. (1998). Mosaicism in the inner cell mass of human blastocysts. *Hum. Reprod.* **13**: 3151–5.

Handyside, A. H., Kontogianni, E. H., Hardy, K. & Winston, R. M. (1990). Pregnancies from biopsied human preimplantation embryos sexed by Y-specific DNA amplification. *Nature* **344**: 768–70.

Harper, J. C. & Delhanty, J. D. A. (2000). Preimplantation genetic diagnosis. *Curr. Opin. Obstet. Gynaecol.* **12**: 67–72.

Harper, J. C. & Wells, D. (1999). Recent advances and future developments in PGD. *Prenat. Diagn.* **19**: 1193–9.

Harper, J. C., Coonen, E., Handyside, A. H., Winston, R. M. L., Hopman, A. H. N. & Delhanty, J. D. A. (1995). Mosaicism of autosomes and sex chromosomes in morphologically normal monospermic preimplantation human embryos. *Prenat. Diagn.* **15**: 41–9.

Harper, J. C., Delhanty, J. D. A. & Handyside, A. H. (2001). *PGD*. Chichester: Wiley & Sons.

Iwarsson, E., Malmgren, H., Inzunza, J. *et al.* (2000). Highly abnormal cleavage divisions in preimplantation embryos from translocation carriers. *Prenat. Diagn.* **20**: 1038–47.

Munné, S., Scott, R., Sable, D. & Cohen, J. (1998). First pregnancies after preconception diagnosis of translocations of maternal origin. *Fertil. Steril.* **69**: 675–81.

Munné, S., Magli, C., Cohen, J. *et al.* (1999). Positive outcome after preimplantation diagnosis of aneuploidy in human embryos. *Hum. Reprod.* **14**: 2191–9.

Ruangvutilert, P., Delhanty, J. D. A., Serhal, P., Rodeck, C. & Harper, J. C. (2000). FISH analysis on day 5 post insemination of human arrested and blastocyst stage embryos. *Prenat. Diagn.* **20**: 552–60.

Staessen, C., Van Assche, E., Joris, H. *et al.* (1999). Clinical experience of sex determination by fluorescent in-situ hybridization for preimplantation genetic diagnosis. *Mol. Hum. Reprod.* **5**: 382–9.

Strom, C., Rechitsky, S., Cieslak, J. *et al.* (1997). Preimplantation diagnosis of single gene disorders by two-step oocyte genetic analysis. *J. Assist. Reprod. Genet.* **14**: 469.

Vandervorst, M., Liebaers, I., Sermon, K. *et al.* (1998). Successful preimplantation genetic diagnosis is related to the number of available cumulus-oocyte complexes. *Hum. Reprod.* **13**: 3169–76.

Van de Velde, H., De Vos, A., Sermon, K. *et al.* (2000). Embryo implantation after biopsy of one or two cells from cleavage-stage embryos with a view to preimplantation genetic diagnosis. *Prenat. Diagn.* **20**: 1030–7.

Veiga, A., Sandalinas, M., Benkhalifa, M. *et al.* (1997). Laser blastocyst biopsy for preimplantation genetic diagnosis in the human. *Zygote* **5**: 351–4.

Verlinsky, Y., Ginsberg, N., Lifchez, A., Valle, J., Moise, J. & Strom, C. M. (1990). Analysis of the first polar body: preconception genetic diagnosis. *Hum. Reprod.* **5**: 826–9.

Verlinsky, Y., Cieslak, J., Ivakhnenko, V. *et al.* (1996). Birth of healthy children after preimplantation diagnosis of common aneuploidies by polar body fluorescent in situ hybridization analysis. *Fertil. Steril.* **66**: 126–9.

Verlinsky, Y., Rechitsky, S., Cieslak, J. *et al.* (1997). Preimplantation diagnosis of single gene disorders by two-step oocyte genetic analysis using first and second polar body. *Biochem. Mol. Med.* **62**: 182–7.

Wells, D. & Sherlock, J. K. (1998). Strategies for preimplantation genetic diagnosis of single gene disorders by DNA amplification. *Prenat. Diagn.* **18**: 1389–401.

Wells, D., Sherlock, J. K., Handyside, A. H. & Delhanty, J. D. A. (1999). Detailed chromosomal and molecular genetic analysis of single cells by whole genome amplification and comparative genomic hybridisation (CGH). Nucleic Acids *Res.* **27**: 1214–18.

Wells, D. & Delhanty, J. D. A. (2000). Comprehensive chromosome analysis of human preimplantation embryos using WGA & single cell CGH. *Mol. Hum. Reprod.* **6**: 1055–62.

Willadsen, S., Levron, J., Munne, S. *et al.* (1999). Rapid visualization of metaphase chromosomes in single human blastomeres after fusion with in-vitro matured bovine eggs. *Hum. Reprod.* **14**: 470–5.

Wilton, L., Williamson, R., McBain, J., Edgar, D. & Vouliare, L. (2001). Birth of a healthy infant after preimplantation confirmation of euploidy by CGH. *N. Engl. J. Med.* **345**: 1537–41.

13

Controversial issues in assisted reproduction

Caroline Overton[1] and Colin Davis[2]

[1]St. Michael's Hospital and the Bristol Royal Infirmary, Bristol, UK
[2]Fertility Unit, St Bart's and the London Hospitals, London, UK

Fibroids: remove, leave or embolize?

Fibroids are a frequent finding in women with infertility (Figure 13.1). Many clinicians who have performed myomectomy on infertile women have reported that the treatment is effective and increases the pregnancy rate. However, no randomized controlled trials have been performed to establish the causal relationship. In a review of the literature, Vercellini *et al.* (1992) concluded that fibroids do not cause infertility in the vast majority of cases.

Effective management of the woman with fibroids who wishes to conceive cannot yet be determined by an evidence-based approach using randomized controlled trials. However, it is clear that subfertility resulting from fibroids is not absolute and many women will conceive without intervention. It is sensible to ensure that other causes of infertility have been looked for and if present, treated appropriately in the absence of other causes of infertility. The couple is advised to try for at least two years to conceive naturally, unless the woman is aged 34 years or more, when more rapid intervention becomes advisable, given the negative impact of increasing female age on the likelihood of pregnancy, both naturally and after IVF and embryo transfer (IVF-ET).

Many women with fibroids have favourable obstetric outcomes but it is well accepted that the presence of myomas increases the risk of pregnancy related problems. Pregnant women with fibroids have an increased chance of developing pain, red degeneration, bleeding, premature labour, fetal malpresentation, need for operative delivery, retained placenta and postpartum haemorrhage. In a combined series of 1284 women with fibroids, 13% of pregnancies were complicated by premature labour (Rice *et al.*, 1989).

Fibroids are classified according to site (Figure 13.2).

Good Clinical Practice in Assisted Reproduction, ed. P. Serhal & C. Overton.
Published by Cambridge University Press. © Cambridge University Press 2004.

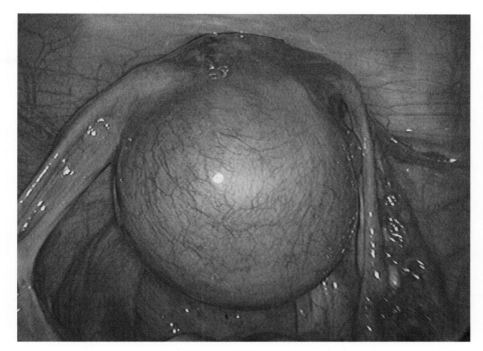

Figure 13.1. Laparoscopic image of a subserosal fibroid.

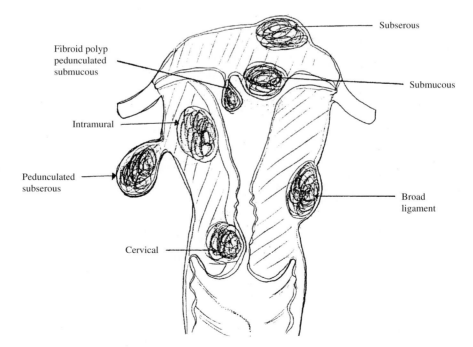

Figure 13.2. Common types of uterine fibroids.

Table 13.1. Effect of fibroids on the outcome of assisted reproductive treatment

Group	Mean fibroid diameter (cm)	Pregnancy rate (%)	Percentage implantation rate	Percentage miscarriage rate
Control		98/318 (31)	15.8	15
Subserosal	2.4 ± 5	14/41 (34)	15.7	14
Intramural	2.4 ± 7	9/55 (16)	6.4	
Submucosal	4.5 ± 2.6	1/10 (10)	4.3	33

Note: From: Elder-Geva *et al.* (1998).

Common types of uterine fibroids

A study by Eldar-Geva *et al.* (1998) demonstrated that the effect of uterine fibroids on fertility is related more to location than to size or number; assisted reproduction technology (ART) success was reduced in women with intramural or submucosal fibroids (Table 13.1).

Eighty-eight fertile women with uterine fibroids completed 106 ART cycles (IVF, intracytoplasmic sperm injection (ICSI) or gamete intrafallopian transfer (GIFT)). Mean age was 35 years (range 25–42) and mean number of previous ART cycles was 2.1. An age-matched control group of 249 women without fibroids or other uterine anomalies completed 318 ART cycles during the same time period. In the fibroid group, 38% had only subserosal fibroids, 52% had intramural fibroids with or without subserosal fibroids and without cavity distortion, and 10% had submucosal fibroids with or without other fibroids with cavity distortion (Table 13.1).

Both fibroid size and location appear to be important variables influencing fertility potential and pregnancy outcome. It is essential to perform a thorough evaluation before deciding whether expectant management or surgical intervention is the most prudent course of action. Ultrasound is helpful in confirming that the mass is of uterine and not adnexal origin and will enable the uterine and fibroid dimensions to be measured. Magnetic resonance imaging (MRI) is less available, more time consuming and expensive, but superior to ultrasound in its ability to measure small fibroids, localize fibroids within the uterus, assess whether fibroids may impinge on the endometrial cavity, differentiate adenomyosis from fibroids and identify the ovaries in cases of large fibroids.

Assessment of the uterine cavity and tubal lumen and ostia is essential before deciding a management plan. A hysterosalpingogram (HSG) is recommended for all patients with fibroids and a history of recurrent pregnancy loss, and poor obstetric history without obvious cause for infertility. The HSG should be done with an antero-posterior view; occasionally a lateral view may help to evaluate whether the fibroid impinges on the uterine cavity. A normal HSG is reliable and hysteroscopy is not necessary to further evaluate the cavity. Abnormalities in the HSG may be followed by diagnostic and possibly operative hysteroscopy. A laparoscopy may help to evaluate the impact of the fibroid on tubo-ovarian relationships.

Most asymptomatic women with subserosal fibroids or smaller intramural or submucosal fibroids can be followed expectantly, with a repeat examination in six months recommended to determine if there is significant uterine growth. If the uterine size is stable, it is reasonable to re-examine every six months, unless a change in menstrual pattern or an increase in symptoms related to an enlarging uterine mass are experienced. In the event of conception, close follow-up is recommended during the pregnancy.

Medical treatment

Gonadotrophin releasing hormone agonists (GnRH-agonist) will cause both uterine and fibroid shrinkage and a reduction or elimination of menstrual flow. After three months of treatment, the mean reduction in uterine volume is 40–50%. Treatment beyond three months rarely results in significant additional shrinkage. Although treatment may cause significant reduction in uterine and myoma size and related symptoms, re-growth of the fibroid after cessation of treatment is usually rapid, with return to pre-treatment size in three to four months. Ovulation may be delayed for one to three months after the cessation of treatment. Therefore, the window of opportunity is narrow and treatment sub-optimal.

Uterine artery embolization

Uterine artery embolization offers an alternative method of treatment that allows conservation of the uterus. Early reports are encouraging but there are no long-term data available. While the safety and efficacy of the technique is being established, we believe that it should be recommended only to women with symptomatic fibroids who might otherwise be advised surgical treatment. Infertile women present particular problems and need to recognize that complications of the procedure may lead to hysterectomy.

Accurate pre-treatment diagnosis is essential. MRI is superior to ultrasound in diagnosing fibroids and more likely to recognize adenomyosis, itself a relative contra-indication to embolization. The value of uterine artery embolization in adenomyosis is unproven but uterine artery embolization may be indicated when fibroids and adenomyosis co-exist. The procedure will be undertaken without a tissue diagnosis and other abnormalities should be excluded. There has been at least one case of failure to respond to uterine artery embolization of an apparent fibroid, which proved to be a sarcoma.

Submucous and interstitial fibroids respond well to embolization and shrink by an average of 60% in six months and 70% in 12 months, and of these patients some will have totally eliminated their fibroids. Information on the rate of occurrence of fibroids after the procedure is not yet available.

MRI guided thermo-ablation of uterine fibroids

Under local anaesthesia and sedation, an 18-gauge needle can deliver heat to a fibroid with localized ablation of a fibroid. Anterior fibroids are most easily accessible. Forty-nine women had a total of 69 ablations and completed 12 months follow-up. There were four re-admissions; one for fluid collection within the fibroid, one for urinary tract infection (cystoscopy was negative) and two minor skin burns at the entry site. The technique was modified and this has not recurred. Four women had surgery, either hysterectomy or myomectomy. There were no peritoneal adhesions, and no extra-uterine or endometrial thermal damage. Menstrual blood loss reduced by 27–45% after one cycle and 58% of the women would recommend the treatment to a friend (Law & Regan, 2000).

High intensity focused ultrasound

In the future, high intensity focused ultrasound may provide a minimally invasive treatment for fibroids. Multiple small area high intensity pulses avoid cavitation and damage to the skin. Women lie face down on a specially designed table. MRI accurately corresponds to the area of damage on histology. Posterior fibroids can also be treated if access avoids the endometrial cavity.

Myomectomy

Myomectomy may be performed endoscopically or at laparotomy (Figure 13.3). Hysteroscopic myomectomy may be considered for women with submucous fibroids less than 3 cm. Pre-treatment with danazol, GnRHa or progestin is not essential but renders the endometrium atrophic and facilitates hysteroscopic visualization and resection. Resection of multiple submucous myomas during a single hysteroscopic surgical procedure may increase the likelihood of developing intrauterine synechiae.

Laparoscopic excision of small subserous or intramural fibroids is possible, but these rarely cause reproductive problems. In a comparison of laparoscopic and abdominal myomectomy (Seracchioli *et al.*, 2000) there was no difference in pregnancy rates (55.9% after laparotomy, 53.6% after laparoscopy), miscarriage rate (12.1% versus 20%), pre-term delivery (7.4% versus 5%) and the use of caesarean section (77.8% versus 65%). Blood loss was higher after laparotomy and three women required a blood transfusion compared to none after laparoscopy. No case of uterine rupture during pregnancy or labour was seen.

Post-myomectomy adhesions may have an adverse effect on fertility. To decrease adhesion formation:

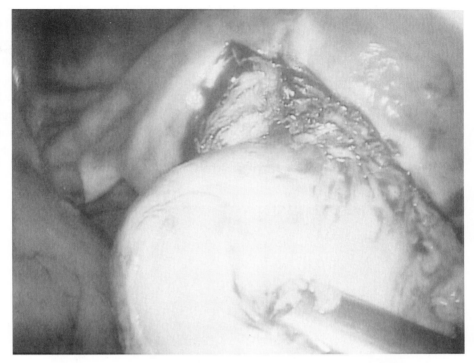

Figure 13.3. Laparoscopic myomectomy. (Courtesy of Dr Ertan Saridogan MRCOG, University College London Hospitals.)

- Anterior uterine incisions are preferable to those on the posterior wall.
- Remove as many fibroids as possible through a single incision.
- Ensure meticulous haemostasis.
- Vertical incisions may be less likely to damage the cornual region than are transverse incisions.
- Use of a vasoconstrictive agent (i.e. vasopressin) or temporary occlusion of the uterine and ovarian vessels may decrease intraoperative blood loss.
- Consider a 'cell saver' autotransfusion device when excessive blood loss is anticipated.

Preoperative use of GnRHa for two to three months decreases the intra-operative blood loss by decreasing myoma size and vascularity. Some surgeons have experienced greater difficulty in fibroid enucleation following GnRH-agonist treatment because of softening and degeneration of some tumours, and thus the difficulty of establishing surgical planes.

Rupture of the gravid uterus following myomectomy is a rare event, a trial of labour may be considered following most myomectomies. Elective Caesarean section is a reasonable option when the uterine cavity has been entered or when extensive myometrial dissection has occurred.

Uterine anomalies

These are seen in 3–5% of the general population, but their frequency increases between 5% and 25% in women with recurrent miscarriages, late miscarriage and pre-term deliveries (Figures 13.4 and 13.5). Uterine septum is the most common congenital abnormality of the female reproductive tract with an incidence of 2–3% in the general population. Its presence is associated with poor reproductive performance, including high incidence of first and second trimester miscarriage, pre-term delivery (often as a result of premature rupture of the membranes) as well as increased abnormal presentations and increased Caesarean section rates.

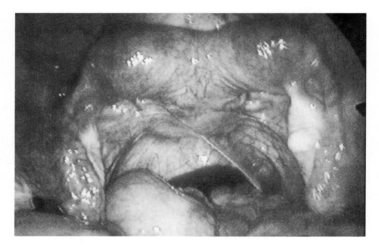

Figure 13.4. Laparoscopic image of uterus didelphus.

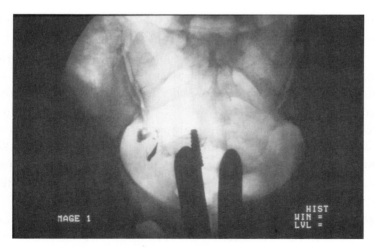

Figure 13.5. Hysterosalpingogram of a unicornuate uterus.

On the other hand, the influence of a septate uterus on a woman's fertility remains a controversial issue.

Several mechanisms have been proposed to explain the adverse effect of a septate uterus on the course of pregnancy. The diminished size of the uterine cavity and cervical incompetence have been suggested as aetiological factors. However, according to the most widely accepted theory, the septum is thought to consist of fibro-elastic tissue with inadequate vascularization and altered relationships between myometrial and endometrial vessels, thus exerting a negative effect on fetal placentation.

Marcus *et al.* (1996) observed increased miscarriage rates and pre-term delivery rates in women with a bicornuate and septate uterus presenting with primary infertility and treated with IVF, without previous correction of the congenital abnormality (Figure 13.5).

The main and absolute indication for the treatment of a woman with a septate uterus is a reproductive history of recurrent abortions or fetal loss. However, a group of patients with septate uteri may present with primary or secondary infertility and this will only be discovered on infertility work-up. In this group hysteroscopic metroplasty is applied mainly as a prophylactic measure to prevent spontaneous abortions and complications during pregnancy and labour. Women with secondary infertility usually have a history of spontaneous miscarriages and hysteroscopic metroplasty is applied as a treatment for their poor reproductive performance. In women with primary infertility, hysteroscopic resection of a septum resulted in a 25% miscarriage rate and 62.5% term delivery rate (Grimbizis *et al.*, 1998). Eight of 11 women conceived after assisted conception treatment and one miscarriage was seen shortly after amniocentesis. These results compare favourably with the poor reproductive performance of the women with secondary infertility. They achieved 45 pregnancies before septum resection; 40 of these (88.9%) ended in spontaneous miscarriage, one was ectopic (2.2%) and only four ended in term deliveries (8.9%).

The septate uterus can be effectively treated by operative hysteroscopy. The incision of the septum can be carried out using scissors, resectoscope or laser, with no obvious advantage from any of these techniques. An accurate diagnosis requires laparoscopy and hysteroscopy for the precise classification of uterine malformations (Appendix 13.1). Hysteroscopic septum resection is accompanied by a significant improvement in reproductive performance. There is no adverse effect in the achievement of pregnancy in women with a history of recurrent miscarriage. Septate uterus does not seem to be an infertility factor, although it may contribute to the delayed spontaneous conception of women with secondary infertility. Women with septate uterus and infertility should be treated mainly for the improvement of their reproductive performance and not for the enhancement of their fertility potential, especially those treated with assisted reproductive techniques.

Hydrosalpinx

Salpingectomy seems to improve the embryo transfer implantation rate in women undergoing IVF in cases of severe tubal pathology. However, many questions are unclear, especially how to determine which women would benefit from salpingectomy. The general consensus is that salpingectomy would benefit conception rates if the hydrosalpinx is visible on ultrasound scan. The evaluation of the severity of the tubal pathology is the crux of the question. Indiscriminate salpingectomy is certainly not the answer.

The presence of one or more hydrosalpinx has been shown to reduce both spontaneous and assisted conception (Figure 13.6). The proposed reasons include: a detrimental effect on mechanical flow within the tubal mucosa, damage to the tubal mucosa, reduction in sperm motility, an embryotoxic effect and reduction in endometrial receptivity. In a larger percentage of cases the only realistic chance of pregnancy is IVF. However, it is essential that the nature of the hydrosalpinx is carefully identified by laparoscopy and salpingoscopy (Figure 13.6). Detailed inspection of the tubal intima allows for classification of the tubal mucosa and grading of the hydrosalpinx (Appendix 13.2). The presence of tubal intimal adhesions and/or absence of mucosal folds is associated with a markedly reduced fecundity.

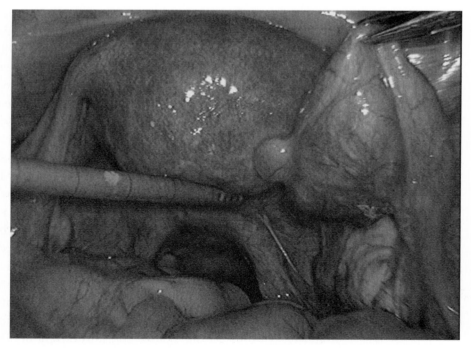

Figure 13.6. Laparoscopic image of hydrosalpinx.

Current debate centres on the issue of salpingectomy for hydrosalpinx. Studies have demonstrated that hydrosalpinx decreases the chance of pregnancy by approximately one half compared to a tubal factor without hydrosalpinx (Camus *et al.*, 1999). In addition, the presence of hydrosalpinx during IVF had adverse effects on pregnancy, implantation, live delivery and early pregnancy loss. This meta-analysis did not address whether or not pregnancy rates were improved by salpingectomy prior to IVF.

In a retrospective review of 348 IVF cycles, including 40 women with hydrosalpinx who had surgical treatment prior to IVF and 45 who did not, Freeman *et al.* (1998) noted that hydrosalpinx was associated with a significantly lower clinical pregnancy rate. The pregnancy loss rate was significantly higher in women with hydrosalpinx, resulting in a significantly lower live birth rate in these patients. Surgical treatment resulted in a decrease in pregnancy loss rate and an increase in live birth rate, comparable to that in the control groups. However, even after surgery the implantation rate and the number of embryos available for transfer did not increase, suggesting that embryo development was permanently impaired. This effect of hydrosalpinx on implantation and early pregnancy loss has also been demonstrated in women undergoing donor oocyte cycles (Cohen *et al.*, 1999).

A prospective randomized study by Strandell *et al.* (1999) examined whether salpingectomy would benefit women with hydrosalpinx. He reported the experience of 204 women available for intention to treat analysis and 192 that actually proceeded to IVF. Clinical pregnancy rates were 36.6% in the women who underwent salpingectomy before IVF and 24% in those who did not. The difference was not significant ($P = 0.67$) but a significant difference was noted in the delivery rates, 28.6% versus 16.3% respectively ($P = 0.045$). A subgroup analysis revealed significant improvement in implantation rates, clinical pregnancy rates and delivery rates in women who had visible hydrosalpinx on ultrasound and underwent salpingectomy prior to IVF.

Options other than salpingectomy such as aspiration of the tubal fluid was unsuccessful as fluid re-accumulated within two days of the procedure. Proximal tubal catheterization has been suggested as an alternative but there are no published series addressing the efficacy and risk, such as infection. Another option is aspiration of the hydrosalpinx at the time of egg retrieval (Van Voorhis *et al.*, 1998). Figure 13.7 gives a schematic representation for the management of hydrosalpinx.

Endometriosis

The primary indication for medical treatment of endometriosis is to relieve pain. However, medical treatment is commonly used to try to reduce the progression of endometriosis and preserve fertility. No medical treatment has ever been shown

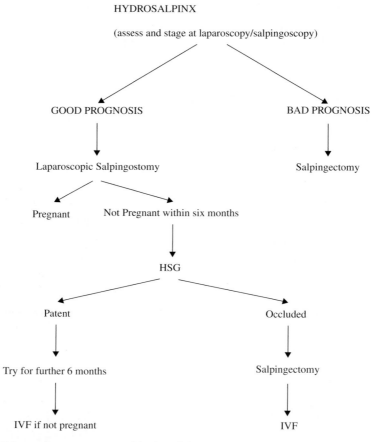

Figure 13.7. Schematic management of hydrosalpinx.

to improve fertility and none is licensed for the treatment of infertility associated with endometriosis.

The American Society of Reproductive Medicine revised classification of endometriosis correlates with the chance of spontaneous conception (Appendix 13.3). The more severe the disease, the smaller the chance of spontaneous conception. The aim of surgical treatment is to destroy or excise endometriotic nodules and divide peritubal or periovarian adhesions (Figures 13.8 and 13.9). Cystectomy rather than drainage of ovarian endometriomata should be considered (Figure 13.10). Drainage alone results in rapid recurrence. Cystectomy may enhance spontaneous pregnancy rates and improve access if IVF is considered. Laparoscopic surgery has increasingly been used to excise large endometrioma.

Surgical ablation of minimal to mild endometriosis improves fertility in infertile women. Marcoux and the Canadian Collaborative study (Marceux *et al.*, 1997) analysed the efficacy of resection or ablation of 341 women with minimal to mild

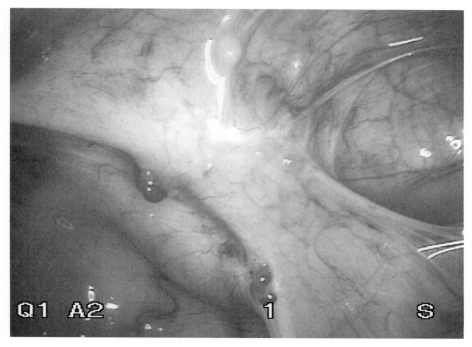

Figure 13.8. Laparoscopic image of blebs of endometriosis over the uterosacral ligament.

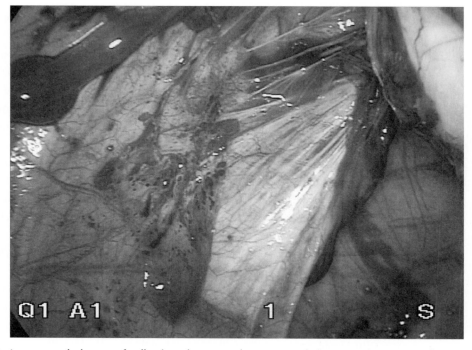

Figure 13.9. Laparoscopic image of adhesions between the ovary and the ovary fossa secondary to endometriosis.

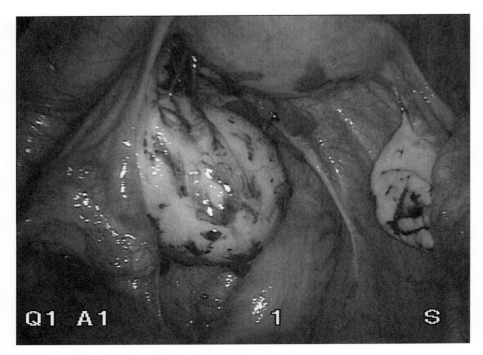

Figure 13.10. Laparoscopic image of ovarian endometriosis.

endometriosis who were undergoing diagnosic laparoscopy. Women were randomly assigned to undergo resection or ablation of visible endometriosis or diagnostic laparoscopy only and were then followed for 36 months. Of the 172 women who had resection or ablation, 50 became pregnant compared to 29 of the 169 women in the diagnostic laparoscopy group (31% versus 18%, $P = 0.006$). The study was well designed, but there was criticism that it was not blind because some women were told that they had had treatment before they went home. Only blue or black lesions were included and the inclusion of adhesiolysis could have introduced bias. However, it seems reasonable to adopt a conservative approach for a year following surgical ablation of endometriosis.

When the presenting symptom is pain, surgery is the treatment of choice in women with stages III and IV disease, and this may also improve fertility (Appendix 13.3). IVF should be considered in these women, either as an alternative to surgery or following unsuccessful surgery. Drawbacks of surgery include postoperative adhesion formation and incomplete removal of the disease.

Assisted reproduction appears to have an overall benefit for all stages of treatment. The treatment of choice will depend on the severity of endometriosis, the woman's age, duration of infertility, past reproductive performance and the presence of other infertility factors such as tubal blockage or male factor infertility.

Endometriosis and ovulation induction

Ovulation induction with clomiphene citrate or gonadotrophins is effective, but is only suitable for young women with healthy fallopian tubes, oligo- or amenorrhoea, minimal or mild endometriosis and no male factor.

Endometriosis and intrauterine insemination

Intrauterine insemination (IUI) of washed and prepared partner/donor sperm is only suitable for young women with healthy fallopian tubes, regular ovulation, minimal or mild endometriosis and no severe male factor.

In subfertile women with minimal to mild endometriosis, ovarian stimulation with IUI is more effective than either expectant management or IUI alone (Tummon *et al.*, 1997). A live birth rate of 10–15% per cycle can be expected (Subspecialty Group in Reproductive Medicine, 2000). IUI is less expensive and less invasive than IVF or GIFT and should be considered initially in suitable patients. About 80% of pregnancies occur in four to six cycles of treatment. If after three or four unsuccessful treatment cycles, then IVF or GIFT should be considered. IUI treatment cycles may be abandoned or converted to IVF or GIFT if excessive follicular development occurs.

GIFT is suitable for women: with patent and healthy fallopian tubes whose endometriosis is not severe; who have failed to conceive by IUI; who are older; with prolonged infertility; and for couples with multiple factor infertility. In women with endometriosis, many studies have demonstrated an acceptable pregnancy and live birth rate following GIFT.

Endometriosis and *in vitro* fertilization

IVF and embryo transfer is an established and successful treatment for endometriosis-related infertility. IVF is suitable for women with damaged or blocked tubes, moderate or severe endometriosis, minimal to mild endometriosis with an infertile male partner, and women who have failed to conceive by IUI.

The use of a GnRH-agonist results in high pregnancy and live birth rates, mainly due to a reduction in cycle cancellation rates because of poor follicular response or premature LH (luteinizing hormone) surge. Other advantages include significantly more supernumerary embryos available for cryopreservation and the ability to programme oocyte collection for convenience. There are several GnRH-agonist protocols available for ovarian stimulation and each has advantages and disadvantages.

Many studies have shown that in women with endometriosis, IVF after prolonged GnRH-agonist treatment results in higher pregnancy rates. Nakamura *et al.* (1992) analysed the outcome of IVF treatment in women with various stages of endometriosis using two different regimens of GnRH-agonist. In the ultra-long protocol ($n = 21$) the agonist was administered for at least 60 days prior to ovarian stimulation. In the long protocol ($n = 11$), the agonist was administered from the mid-luteal phase of the cycle preceding IVF treatment and exogenous gonadotrophin was commenced between the third and seventh day of menstruation after pituitary suppression. The clinical pregnancy rate per embryo transfer was superior in the ultra-long protocol (67% versus 27%). Marcus & Edwards (1994) analysed the outcome of IVF treatment in 84 women with severe endometriosis. The women were assigned to different GnRH-agonist protocols. The long protocol involved administering the agonist in the mid-luteal phase of the cycle preceding IVF treatment, and the ultra-long protocol required the agonist to be given for two to seven months before gonadotrophin was commenced. Pregnancy rates were significantly higher in the group of women who received the ultra-long GnRH-agonist protocol compared with the long protocol (42.8% versus 12.7%, $P < 0.001$).

Many studies have reported the poor outcome of IVF and embryo transfer in women with stages III and IV endometriosis compared to women with stages I and II endometriosis (Azem *et al.*, 1999; Appendix 13.3). However, IVF with prolonged down-regulation using long-acting GnRH-agonist after surgical debulking results in good pregnancy rates comparable to those achieved with other causes of infertility. The presence of small endometriomata does not reduce the success of IVF treatment (Tinkanen & Kujansuu *et al.*, 2000). However, there is an increased risk of developing a pelvic infection following transvaginal oocyte collection (Younis *et al.*, 1997).

Clinical management of ovarian cysts

Most ovarian cysts in women of reproductive age are physiological (functional) and for many years have been treated with oral contraceptives to obtain resolution of the cysts. It has been suggested that expectant management has the same effectiveness as hormonal treatment. In a prospective study, 53 women with ovarian cysts in the first five days of a cycle after ovulation induction were randomized to expectant management (Group A) or to receive oral contraception (Group B) for one cycle. If the cyst persisted, the woman was followed for another cycle without treatment. Of the 50 women who completed the trial, complete resolution of the cysts was observed in 19/25 (76%) and 18/25 (72%) in groups A and B respectively. All the persistent cysts disappeared after a second cycle without treatment. Expectant management is as effective as oral contraceptives for the resolution of functional ovarian cysts induced by ovarian stimulation.

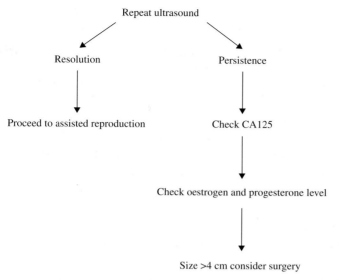

Figure 13.11. Schematic management of an asymptomatic ovarian cyst.

Management of an asymptomatic ovarian cyst

Simple ovarian cysts

Most simple ovarian cysts in women of reproductive age are functional and will resolve spontaneously. If the cyst persists it may be aspirated transvaginally and fluid sent for cytology. If it recurs, formal cystectomy is required.

Endometrioma

The ultrasound scan may suggest an endometrioma with the typical ground glass appearance. If >4 cm, laparoscopy and laparoscopic ovarian cystectomy and ablation or excision of endometriosis may improve spontaneous conception rates.

Small cysts (2–4 cm) can be managed expectantly but it should be remembered that this is without a tissue diagnosis and the possibility of malignancy should be considered, particularly in the older woman. Cysts of 4 cm or more generally require surgery.

Figure 13.11 gives a schematic representation for the management of an asymptomatic ovarian cyst.

Reduced ovarian reserve

Elevated follicle stimulating hormone (FSH)

The ability of the ovaries to respond to gonadotrophins with adequate follicular development leading to ovulation, fertilization and implantation has been referred to as 'ovarian reserve'. Although ovarian reserve declines with age, it is a biological and not just a chronological function. Diminished ovarian reserve may be seen in young women who have had extensive ovarian surgery, radiation or chemotherapy or nonautoimmune premature ovarian failure.

Experience from IVF program indicate that ovarian responsivity decreases as FSH levels increase. This decline is marked by increased numbers of cancelled cycles and decreased pregnancy rates. Once a woman is found to have an elevated basal FSH her response is diminished, even in cycles in which the basal FSH is normal.

However, there are practical difficulties with using basal FSH levels as the determinant of biological age and ovarian responsiveness. There is cycle-to-cycle variation in gonadotrophin levels and a marked variation in what is considered the normal range in different FSH assays. FSH standards reported by one laboratory may not be clinically valid when applied to women whose FSH levels were measured using a different assay. There may be a significant rise in group mean FSH levels while most still remain within the normal range.

An elevated oestradiol level measured early in the menstrual cycle may reflect early follicular recruitment, masking what could be a high FSH level. Early recruitment could lead to a shortened follicular phase and indicates a poor prognosis for the pregnancy. Both age and basal FSH make independent contributions when predicting response to gonadotrophin stimulation. When women with the same basal FSH level are compared, pregnancy rates are lower in the older women.

IVF success rates are proportional to the number of eggs that are retrieved, fertilized and transferred. Age related low responders with a blunted oestradiol rise and poor follicular development have poor pregnancy rates. Increasing the dose of gonadotrophin stimulation in women with elevated cycle day 2–3 FSH levels or poor response to previous stimulation, does not appear to be effective in increasing the pregnancy rate, even if initiated on the first or second day of the cycle.

Although older women produce fewer oocytes when hyperstimulated, the fertilization rate is similar to younger women. The lower implantation rate is primarily due to deficiencies in the embryo. Having fewer fertilized eggs provides fewer opportunities to select embryos with the most favourable morphological appearance for transfer. In addition, abnormal oocytes may produce cleaving embryos that appear normal, but have a decreased chance of implantation.

Although GnRH-agonists generally improve outcome in IVF and GIFT cycles they may also lead to over-suppression of women with diminished ovarian reserve and increase HMG (human menopausal gonadotrophin) requirements with little improvement in ovarian function. Reducing the dose of adjunctive GnRH-agonist or using a follicular 'flare' technique is one option.

It has been recommended that more oocytes should be replaced in older women to increase the pregnancy rate because the risk of multiple gestation is lower than in younger women. The latest published data from IVF program in the UK (Human Fertilisation and Embryology Authority, 1999) reported that 21% of all stimulation cycles were in women aged 38 years or over. In this group, over 5000 retrievals yielded a 12% delivery rate per retrieval without male factor and 10% when a male factor was present. Cancellations were significantly higher in older women and the miscarriage rate was higher.

The older woman's relatively poor response to hyperstimulation, decreased rate of embryo transfer, decreased rate of embryo implantation, higher incidence of clinical and sub-clinical miscarriage and elevated risk of chromosomal abnormalities, present a challenge that has not successfully been overcome by current infertility therapies. Current opinion suggests that most infertility treatments will have exhausted their usefulness after six months of therapy and that very few successful pregnancies will be achieved by medical treatment in women over the age of 43 years. For women between the ages of 40 and 44 years the live birth rate from IVF is 9%, while only one woman over 45 years conceived with IVF using her own oocytes.

While it may be scientifically difficult, psychologically devastating and even legally questionable to assess an upper age limit beyond which treatment should be withheld, the financial and emotional needs of the woman may be better served by helping her make choices, such as adoption or use of donor oocytes, that are more likely to lead to the actual creation of a family or toward a final resolution of her infertility. The National Fertility Association (ISSUE), a non-profit making infertility organization, has a 24-hour, help line for confidential counselling.[1]

Oocyte donation has become a viable option for those women whose fertility is age related. Oocytes collected from superovulated donors are fertilized with sperm from the recipient's partner. The resulting embryos are then transferred to the recipient who has been treated with oestrogen and progestagen to produce an endometrial environment suitable for implantation. This technique has proved to be successful in recipients aged in their 40s and 50s.

The poor responder

The recruitment of a sufficient number of follicles during ovarian stimulation is crucial for the success of assisted conception techniques. A good ovarian response yields a large number of oocytes and a wider choice of embryos for transfer. Failure of the ovaries to respond is usually age related, but may also be unexpectedly found in young women. Screening tests of ovarian reserve have been developed to predict the response to gonadotrophins and tailor treatment to the individual. For tests of ovarian reserve see Chapter 1.

Conventionally, gonadotrophin dosage is decided on the basis of age and baseline FSH measurement. If the response is poor, the cycle may be converted to intrauterine insemination if the tubes are patent. In the case of severe male factor infertility or blocked tubes, then the cycle will have to be abandoned.

Although GnRH-agonists generally improve outcome in IVF and GIFT cycles, they may also lead to over-suppression of women with diminished ovarian reserve and increase HMG requirements with little improvement in ovarian function. The treatment options all aim to reduce or omit the GnRH-agonist dose.

The treatment options are increased gonadotrophin dose and:
- flare-up microdose GnRH-agonist (Scott & Navot, 1994);
- use of the GnRH-agonist in the luteal phase only;
- combination of clomiphene citrate and gonadotrophins with or without GnRH-antagonist (Tanbo *et al.*, 1990).

Women undergoing gonadotrophin stimulation without the use of analogues will require daily urine dipstick and blood tests for premature LH surge.

Thin endometrium

In recipients of donated oocytes, live birth rates are influenced by endometrial thickness with significantly reduced rates in women with endometrial thickness <7 mm. However, pregnancy is still possible.

Additional hormone replacement for three to four months may improve endometrial receptivity for egg recipients. In women having IVF, using their own eggs, there is no treatment available to improve endometrial thickness. Hysteroscopy should be undertaken in order to exclude intrauterine pathology such as adhesions. Aspirin 75 mg can be given empirically to improve endometrial receptivity.

Assisted reproductive techniques: how many gametes to transfer

IVF is associated with a high risk of multiple births, which is a direct consequence of the number of embryos transferred. For every 100 pregnancies after IVF treatment, 27 had more than one fetus (Human Fertilisation and Embryology Authority, 2000). For all donor insemination treatments, this figure was almost seven pregnancies per 100. In comparison, the spontaneous conception rate for multiple pregnancies is fewer than one per 100.

Multiple pregnancies have a greater risk of miscarriage, death and re-absorption of one fetus (vanishing twin syndrome) and higher rate of complications from haemorrhage or hypertensive disorders. Most multiple pregnancies are delivered before full-term and about one-third of twins will be delivered pre-term, i.e. before 37 weeks. The average length of pregnancy is 37 weeks for twins, 34 weeks for triplets and 32 weeks for quadruplets. The birthweight of twins and triplets is generally lower than that of singletons, who have an average weight of 3.5 kg. The average birthweight of a twin infant is 2.5 kg and of a triplet 1.8 kg (Bryan, 1992).

Any pre-term infant is more likely to die than one born at full-term, so that twins and triplets are at much greater risk than singletons. In 1993, the Office for National Statistics recorded that triplets were about six times (twins three times) more likely to be stillborn and 12 times (twins five times) more likely to die than singleton infants in the first year of their life (Office for National Statistics, 1996). In 1993, the perinatal mortality rate of twins was 36.7 (per 1000 live and stillbirths) and 72.6 for triplets, compared with 8.1 for singletons (Office for National Statistics, 1996).

Infants born prematurely are also more likely to have complications which can lead to long-term problems in lung, heart and brain function. One study showed that triplet pregnancies produced an infant with cerebral palsy 47 times more often than a singleton pregnancy. The rate of cerebral palsy for twins was 7.4 per 1000 births and for triplets 26.7 compared with 1.6 for singletons (Petterson *et al.*, 1993). Also, multiple pregnancy imposes additional financial, emotional and logistic burdens on families and health-service providers.

Together these are the arguments for prevention of multiple pregnancy. UK National guidelines recommend fertility clinics to replace a maximum of two embryos in IVF. Three embryos may be transferred in exceptional circumstances. The practice at UCL is to transfer three embryos in poor responders and women ≥ 40 years of age. There is growing recognition that pregnancy rates are influenced by the number of embryos available rather than by the number transferred. Spare embryos can be cryopreserved for transfer in subsequent cycles. Pregnancy rates with cryopreserved embryos are half that with fresh embryos, but any such pregnancy is in addition. Therefore, the birth rate after two-embryo transfer with transfer of surplus cryopreserved embryos in a later cycle should exceed that after three-embryo transfer. Research should be aimed at improving culture conditions and embryo selection, so that fewer but better quality embryos can be transferred with single embryo transfer the ultimate goal.

The factors associated with an increased risk of multiple births were studied using the database established by the Human Fertilisation and Embryology Authority in the UK and 44 236 cycles in 25 240 women were analysed. The chances of a live birth among women undergoing IVF are related to the number of eggs fertilized and thus

Table 13.2. Factors affecting the results of in vitro fertilization (from Templeton & Morris, 1998)

Variable	Odds of a birth (95% CI)	P value	Odds of multiple birth (95% CI)	P value
Maternal factors				
Age (per additional year)	0.9 (0.9–1.0)	<0.001	0.97 (0.95–0.99)	0.013
Tubal infertility (versus no tubal infertility)	0.7 (0.7–0.8)	<0.001	0.8 (0.7–0.9)	<0.001
Previous number of IVF attempts (versus none)				
1–3	0.8 (0.8–0.9)	<0.001	1.0 (0.9–1.1)	0.85
4 or more	0.6 (0.5–0.7)	<0.001	0.6 (0.4–0.8)	<0.001
Infertility duration (per additional year)	0.98 (0.98–0.99)	<0.001	0.98 (0.97–0.99)	0.02
Previous live birth (versus none)				
Not IVF	1.1 (1.0–1.2)	<0.001	Not included in model	
IVF	1.6 (1.4–1.8)	<0.001	Not included in model	
Number of eggs fertilized and embryos transferred				
2 eggs, 2 embryos	0.5 (0.4–0.5)	<0.001	0.5 (0.4–0.7)	<0.001
3 or 4 eggs, 2 embryos	0.6 (0.5–0.7)	<0.001	0.7 (0.6–0.9)	0.008
3 or 4 eggs, 3 embryos	0.7 (0.7–0.8)	<0.001	1.3 (1.1–1.4)	0.008
>4 eggs, 2 embryos	1.01 (0.9–1.1)	–	1.0 (0.9–1.1)	–
>4 eggs, 3 embryos	1.0 (0.9–1.1)	0.78	1.6 (1.5–1.8)	<0.001

the number of embryos available for transfer. When more than four embryos are fertilized and available, transfer of only two embryos will not reduce the woman's chance of becoming pregnant, but it will reduce her chance of multiple pregnancy. This was true for women of all ages, including those aged around 40 years.

Older age, tubal infertility, longer duration of infertility and a higher number of previous attempts at IVF were all associated with a significantly decreased chance of a birth and of multiple births. Previous live birth was associated with an increased chance of a birth but not multiple births.

The higher the number of eggs fertilized, the higher the likelihood of a live birth. When more than four eggs were fertilized, there was no increase in the birth rate for women receiving three-embryo transfer compared to those receiving two, but there was a considerable increase in the rate of multiple births with three-embryo transfer (odds ratio 1.6; 95% confidence intervals 1.5 to 1.8; Table 13.2).

Assisted reproductive technology (ART) is increasingly concerned with making choices from seemingly unlimited options. As a part of the decision-making for each individual, the physical, psychological and financial costs should be weighed against the probability of success. Prognostic models can help to objectively predict the chance of a live birth, although in practice it is impossible to predict accurately the individual chance of a live birth for an individual couple. The development of a better model may be possible by increasing the predictive value by including other promising predictive factors such as basal FSH, cycle day 3 oestradiol or inhibin, rather than age alone (Smeenk *et al.*, 2000).

The ideal ART technique would result in a high probability of singleton pregnancy. Blastocyst transfer has been suggested as a means of facilitating higher pregnancy rates when the number of embryos is limited. The implantation rate of 35.8% achieved when day two embryos at the four-cell stage are transferred suggests that it may not be necessary to culture embryos to the blastocyst stage to obtain acceptable implantation rates. A delay from 48 to 72 hours after oocyte retrieval improved the clinical outcome with an implantation rate of 45.5% when six- to eight-cell embryos were transferred on the third day.

Difficult embryo transfer

If there is difficulty negotiating the cervical canal in previous cycles or dummy embryo transfer mechanical cervical dilatation can be carried out before gonadotrophin stimulation. Alternatively transmyometrial embryo transfer or fallopian tube laparoscopic transfer is an option. See Chapter 7

Lifestyle factors

Smoking reduces fertility (Bolumar *et al.*, 1996) and couples should be advised to give up smoking before assisted conception or to reduce smoking to fewer than 10 cigarettes per day. Moderate alcohol and caffeine intake does not appear to affect fecundability (Bolumar *et al.*, 1997a, b).

In itself, obesity does not appear to be a factor for lowering fertility (Bolumar *et al.*, 2000). However, obesity-induced hormone disorders could contribute to the development of ovulation dysfunction and obesity also affects the hypothalamo-pituitary axis. Weight loss is the best treatment. Drugs such as clomiphene or gonadotrophins can be used in overweight patients. It is important to check that blood glucose is normal before attempting pregnancy and to exclude specific metabolic causes of obesity.

Pregnancy in obese women should be managed as a high risk. The incidence of gestational diabetes and hypertension is increased and macrosomia is frequent. There is a two- to threefold increase in the rate of Caesarean sections with more complications. On obese women, anaesthesia and surgery can be problematic and special care must be taken to prevent further morbidity. Fetal morbidity does not appear to be changed when maternal weight gain is limited. With obesity, there is an increased risk for breast and endometrial cancer due to elevated levels of circulating oestrogens resulting from aromatization of male sex steroids in adipose tissue and decreased levels of sex hormone-binding globulin.

Low body weight can lead to a decrease in GnRH produced by the hypothalamus. The degree to which weight loss affects fertility will vary. In mild cases, ovulation still occurs but implantation fails. In more severe cases, there is oligo- or amenorrhoea. There is an association between low body mass index and intrauterine growth restriction. The preferred treatment would be to gain weight to restore physiological ovulation. Alternatively, treatment with GnRH or gonadotrophins will replace the missing hormones.

Ethics

In general, assisted reproduction is replete with ethical issues, either revolving around the status of the embryo or the possible conflict between the duty of care to prospective parents and the responsibility of the carer to the potential offspring. We do not intend to provide the definitive text for all ethical dilemmas faced by the clinician in assisted reproduction. Every unit will need to decide its own policy. Each couple deserves individual consideration. The ethics committee with its membership of medical and lay members may provide the forum at which the case can be discussed.

Factors that need to be taken into consideration are:

- Safety measures and the laboratory facilities necessary to store infected gametes separately.
- The health and well-being of the parents, separately and as a couple and the effect of treatment and pregnancy on any illness or chronic disease. It will be necessary to have the opinion of the caring physician.
- The effect of any illness or chronic disease on the pregnancy and any children born as a result.
- The effect of a new baby upon the family and any existing children.
- The ability of the parent(s) to care for a child.
- The right of a child to a mother or father in the case of a terminal illness or single sex relationships.
- In the UK the Human Fertilisation and Embryology Authority Act 1990 states that before offering anyone treatment, a clinic must, *'take account of the welfare of any child who may be born as a result of treatment (including the need of that child for a father) and of any other child who may be affected by the birth.'*
- If a couple is declined treatment then they should be given an explanation and the opportunity for a second opinion, if they choose.

ENDNOTE

1. ISSUE (The National Fertility Association)
   114 Lichfield Street, Walsall WS1 1SZ, UK
   Telephone 01922 722888
   Fax 01922 640070
   E-mail: webmaster@issue.co.uk
   Website at http://www.issue.co.uk

Appendix 13.1. The American Fertility Society Classification of Mullerian anomalies. (Reproduced with permission from the American Society for Reproductive Medicine, 1988.)

Patient's Name _____ Date _____ Chart _ _____

Age _____ G _____ P _____ Sp Ab _____ VTP _____ Ectopic _____ Infertile Yes _____ No _____

Other Significant History (i.e. surgery, infection, etc.) _____

_____

HSG _____ Sonography _____ Photography _____ Laparoscopy _____ Laparotomy _____

EXAMPLES

I. Hypoplasis/Agenesis
a vaginal   b cervical
c tundal   d tubal   e combined

II. Unicornuate
a communicating   b non-communicating
c no cavity   d no horn

III. Didelphus

IV. Bicornuate
a complete   b partial

V. Septate
a complete   b partial

VI. Arcuate

VII. DES Drug Related

* Uterus may be normal or take a variety of abnormal forms.
** May have two distinct cervices

Type of Anomaly

Class I	_____	Class V	_____
Class II	_____	Class VI	_____
Class III	_____	Class VII	_____
Class IV	_____		

Treatment (Surgical Procedures): _____

_____

_____

Prognosis for Conception & Subsequent Viable Infant*

_____ Excellent (> 75%)

_____ Good   (50-75%)

_____ Fair   (25%-50%)

_____ Poor   (< 25%)

*Based upon physician's judgment.

Recommended Followup Treatment: _____

_____

_____

Property of
The American Fertility Society

Additional Findings: _____

_____

_____

_____

Vagina: _____

Cervix: _____

Tubes: Right _____ Left _____

Kidneys: Right _____ Left _____

DRAWING

L   R

For additional supply write to:
The American Fertility Society
2140 11th Avenue, South
Suite 200
Birmingham, Alabama 35205

Appendix 13.2. The American Fertility Society Classification of distal tubal occlusion. (Reproduced with permission from the American Society for Reproductive Medicine, 1988.)

Patient's Name _____ Date _____ Chart # _____

Age _____ G _____ P _____ Sp Ab _____ VTP _____ Ectopic _____ Infertile Yes _____ No _____

Other Significant History (i.e. surgery, infection, etc) _____

HSG _____ Sonography _____ Photography _____ Laparoscopy _____ Laparotomy _____

		<3 cm	3-5 cm	>5 cm
Distal ampullary diameter	L	1	4	6
	R	1	4	6
Tubal wall thickness		Normal/Thin	Moderately Thickened or Edematous	Thick & Rigid
	L	1	4	6
	R	1	4	6
Mucosal folds at neostomy site		Normal/ >75% Preserved	35% to 75% Preserved	<35% Preserved Adherent Mucosal Fold
	L	1	4	6
	R	1	4	6
Extent of adhesions		None/Minimal/Mild	Moderate	Extensive
	L	1	3	6
	R	1	3	6
Type of adhesions		None/Filmy	Moderately Dense (or Vascular)	Dense
	L	1	2	4
	R	1	2	4

Prognostic Classification for Terminal Salpingostomy (Salpingoneostomy)

	LEFT		RIGHT
A. Mild	_____	1-3	_____
B. Moderate	_____	9-10	_____
C. Severe	_____	>10	_____

Treatment (Surgical Procedures):

Salpingostomy	L	R
A. Terminal	_____	_____
B. Ampullary	_____	_____

Other: _____

_____

_____

_____

_____

Prognosis for Conception & Subsequent Viable Infant*

_____ Excellent (> 75%)

_____ Good (50 - 75%)

_____ Fair (25%-50%)

_____ Poor (< 25%)

*Physician's judgment based upon adnexa with least amount of pathology.

Recommended Followup Treatment: _____

_____

_____

Additional Findings: _____

_____

_____

_____

_____

_____

DRAWING

L R

For additional supply write to:
The American Fertility Society
2140 11th Avenue, South
Suite 200
Birmingham, Alabama 35205

Property of
The American Fertility Society

Appendix 13.3

AMERICAN SOCIETY FOR REPRODUCTIVE MEDICINE
REVISED CLASSIFICATION OF ENDOMETRIOSIS

Patient's Name _____   Date _____

Stage I (Minimal) - 1–5	Laparoscopy _____ Laparotomy _____ Photography _____
Stage II (Mild) - 6–15	Recommended treatment _____
Stage III (Moderate) - 16–40	
Stage IV (Severe) - >40	
Total _____	Prognosis _____

PERITONEUM	ENDOMETRIOSIS		< 1 cm	1–3 cm	> 3 cm
		Superficial	1	2	4
		Deep	2	4	6
OVARY	R	Superficial	1	2	4
		Deep	4	16	20
	L	Superficial	1	2	4
		Deep	4	16	20
	POSTERIOR CUL-DE-SAC OBLITERATION		Partial		Complete
			4		40
	ADHESIONS		< 1/3 Enclosure	1/3–2/3 Enclosure	> 2/3 Enclosure
OVARY	R	Filmy	1	2	4
		Dense	4	8	16
	L	Filmy	1	2	4
		Dense	4	8	16
TUBE	R	Filmy	1	2	4
		Dense	4*	8*	16
	L	Filmy	1	2	4
		Dense	4*	8*	16

* If the fimbriated end of the Fallopian tube is completely enclosed, change the point assignment to 16

Denote appearance of superficial implant types as red ([R], red, red–pink, flamelike, vesicular blobs, clear vesicles),
white ([W], opacifications, peritoneal defects, yellow–brown) or black ([B], black, hemosiderin deposits, blue).
Denote percent of total described as R___%, W___% and B___%. Total should equal 100%.

Additional Endometriosis: _____   Associated Pathology: _____

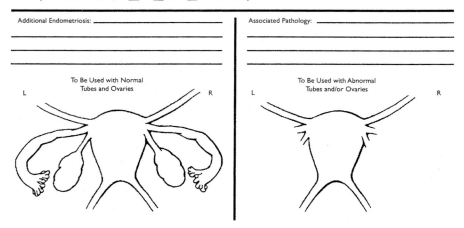

To Be Used with Normal Tubes and Ovaries   To Be Used with Abnormal Tubes and/or Ovaries

(Reproduced with permission from the American Society for Reproductive Medicine, 1998.)

REFERENCES

American Society for Reproductive Medicine (1988). The American Fertility Society classifications of adnexal adhesions, distal tubal occlusion, tubal occlusion secondary to tubal ligation, tubal pregnancies, Mullerian abnormalities and intrauterine adhesions. *Fertil. Steril.* **49**: 944–55.

American Society for Reproductive Medicine (1998). The American Society for Reproductive Medicine revised classification of endometriosis. *Fertil. Steril.* **67**: 817–21.

Azem, F., Lessing, J. B. & Geva, E. (1999). Patients with stage III and IV endometriosis have a poorer outcome of an in vitro fertilization embryo transfer than patients with tubal infertility. *Fertil. Steril.* **72**: 1107–9.

Bolumar, F., Olsen, J. & Boldsen, J. (1996). Smoking reduces fecundity: a European multicentre study on infertility and subfecundity. The European Study Group on infertility and subfecundity. *Am. J. Epidemiol.* **143**: 578–87.

Bolumar, F., Olsen, J. & Boldsen J. (1997a). Does moderate alcohol intake reduce fecundability? A European multicentre study on infertility and subfecundity. The European Study Group on infertility and subfecundity. *Alcohol. Clin. Exp. Res.* **21**: 206–12.

Bolumar, F., Olsen, J. & Boldsen, J. (1997b). Caffeine intake and delayed conception: a European multicentre study on infertility and subfecundity. The European Study Group on infertility and subfecundity. *Am. J. Epidemiol.* **145**: 324–34.

Bolumar, F., Olsen, J., Rebagliato, M., Saez-Llover, I. & Bisanti, L. (2000). Body mass index and delayed conception: a European multicentre study of infertility and subfecundity. *Am. J. Epidemiol.* **151**: 1072–9.

Bryan, E. M. (1992). *Twins and Higher Order Births. A Guide to their Nature and Nurture.* London: Edward Arnold.

Camus, E., Poncelet, C., Goffinet, F., Wainer, B., Merlet, F., Nisand, I. & Phgilippe, H. J. (1999). Pregnancy rates after in-vitro fertilization in cases of tubal infertility with and without hydrosalpinx: a meta-analysis of of published comparative studies. *Hum. Reprod.* **14**: 1243–9.

Cohen, M. A., Lindheim, S. R. & Sauer, M. V. (1999). Hydrosalpinx adversely effect implantation in donor oocyte cycles. *Hum. Reprod.* **14**: 1087–9.

Eldar-Geva, T., Meagher, S., Healy, D. L., Maclachlan, V., Breheny, S. & Wood, C. (1998). Effect of intramural, subserosal and submucosal uterine fibroids on the outcome of assisted reproductive technology treatment. *Fertil. Steril.* **70**: 687–91.

Freeman, M. R., Whitworth, C. M. & Hill, G. A. (1998). Permanent impairment of embryo development by hydrosalpinx. *Hum. Reprod.* **13**: 983–6.

Grimbizis, G., Camus, M., Clasen, K., Tournaye, H., De Munck, L. & Devroey, P. (1998). Hysteroscopic septum resection in patients with recurrent abortions or infertility. *Hum. Reprod.* **13**: 1188–93.

Human Fertilisation and Embryology Authority (2000). *The Patients' Guide to IVF Clinics.* London: Human Fertilisation and Embryology Authority. Website http://www.hfea.gov.uk

Law, P. & Regan, L. (2000). Interstitial thermo-ablation under MRI guidance for the treatment of fibroids. *Current Opinion in Obstet. Gynecol.* **12**: 277–82.

Marcoux, S., Maheux, R. & Berube, S. (1997). Laparoscopic surgery in infertile women with minimal or mild endometriosis. Canadian Collaborative Group on Endometriosis. *N. Engl. J. Med.* **337**: 217–22.

Marcus, S., Al-Shawaf, T. & Brinsden, P. (1996). The obstetric outcome of in vitro fertilization and embryo transfer in women with congentical uterine malformation. *Am. J. Obstet. Gynecol.* **175**: 85–9.

Marcus, S. F. & Edwards, R. G. (1994). High rates of pregnancy after long-term down-regulation of women with severe endometriosis. *Am. J. Obstet. Gynecol.* **171**: 812–17.

Nakamura, K., Oosawa, M., Kondou, I. et al. (1992). Menotropin stimulation after prolonged gonadotrophin releasing hormone agonist pre-treatment for in vitro fertilization in patients with endometriosis. *J. Assist. Reprod. Genet.* **9**: 113–17.

Office for National Statistics (1996). *Mortality Statistics: Childhood, Infant and Perinatal Series.* PH3, No. 37. London: HMSO.

Petterson, B., Nelson, K., Watson, L. & Stanley, F. (1993). Twins, triplets and cerebral palsy in births in Western Australia in the 1980s. *BMJ* **307**: 1239–43.

Rice, J. P., Kay, H. H. & Mahony, B. S. (1989). The clinical significance of uterine leiomyomas in pregnancy. *Am. J. Obstet. Gynecol.* **160**: 1212–16.

Scott, R. T. & Navot, D. (1994). Enhancement of ovarian responsiveness with microdoses of Gonadotrophin releasing hormone agonist during ovulation induction for IVF. *Fertil. Steril.* **61**: 880–5.

Seracchioli, R., Rossi, F., Govoni, E., Rossi, S., Venturoli, C., Bulletti, C. & Flamigni, C. (2000). Fertility and obstetric outome after laparoscopic myomectomy of large myomata: a randomized comparison with abdominal myomectomy. *Hum. Reprod.* **15**: 2663–8.

Smeenk, J. M., Stolwijk, A. M., Kremer, J. A. & Braat, D. D. (2000). External validation of the Templeton model for predicting IVF success after IVF. *Hum. Reprod.* **15**: 1065–8.

Strandell, A., Lindhard, A., Waldenstrom, U., Thorburn, J., Janson, P. O. & Hamberger, L. (1999). Hydrosalpinx and IVF outcome: a prospective randomised multicentre trial in Scandinavia on salpingectomy prior to IVF. *Hum. Reprod.* **14**: 2762–9.

Subspecialty Group in Reproductive Medicine (2000). A multicentre analysis of 1000 cycles of ovulation induction and IUI: what is the impact on multiple pregnancy rates? *Joint UK Fertility Societies meeting Edinburgh July 31st – 2nd August 2000.*

Tanbo, T., Abyholm, T., Bjoro, T. & Drake P. O. (1990). Ovarian stimulation in previous failures from IVF: Distinction of two groups of poor responders. *Hum. Reprod.* **5**: 811–15.

Templeton, A. & Morris, J. K. (1998). Reducing the risk of multiple births by transfer of two embryos after in vitro fertilisation. *N. Engl. J. Med.* **339**: 573–7.

Tinkanen, H. & Kujansuu, E. (2000). In vitro fertilization in patients with ovarian endometriomas. *Acta Obstet. Gynecol. Scand.* **2**: 119–22.

Tummon, I. S., Asher, L. J., Martin, J. S. & Tulandi, T. (1997). Randomised controlled trial of superovulation and insemination for infertility associated with minimal or mild endometriosis. *Fertil. Steril.* **68**: 8–12.

Van Voorhis, B. J., Sparks, A. E., Syrop, C. H. & Stovall, D. W. (1998). Ultrasound-guided aspiration of hydrosalpinx is associated with improved pregnancy and implantation rates after in-vitro fertilization cycles. *Hum. Reprod.* **13**: 736–9.

Vercellini, P., Bocciolone, L., Rognonoi, M. T. & Bolis, G. (1992). Fibroids and infertility. In *Uterine Fibroids: Time for Review*, ed. R. W. Shaw, pp. 47–56. Carnforth: Parthenon Publishing.

Younis, J. S., Ezra, Y., Laufer, N. & Ohel, G. (1997). Late manifestation of pelvic abscess following oocyte retrieval in vitro fertilisation, in patient with severe endometriosis and ovarian endometriomata. *J. Assist. Reprod. Genet.* **14**: 343–6.

14

Alternatives to in vitro fertilization: gamete intrafallopian transfer and zygote intrafallopian transfer

Gj c d Mg rc f c c p f Kc p E tc hv
London Gynaecology and Fertility Centre, London, UK

Assisted conception comprises techniques that allow a couple's infertility to be treated by bringing together their gametes and subsequently transferring gametes or embryos into the female reproductive tract.

Gamete intrafallopian transfer (GIFT)

GIFT involves a direct transfer of human gametes, sperm and oocytes into the fallopian tubes. The first successful pregnancy following the use of this technique was reported by Asch *et al.* in 1984, and is used to treat infertile women with patent tubes and has now become established procedure.

In the natural environment, the fertilized oocyte reaches the uterine cavity approximately five days after release from the ovary, that is, on day 19 of a 28-day menstrual cycle. The slow progress of the embryo permits progesterone-stimulated endometrial maturation. Once the embryo reaches the uterine cavity, an additional 24 to 48 hours pass before implantation occurs. The tubal and endometrial secretions, which bathe the conceptus, may promote implantation. By placing oocytes and sperm into the fallopian tube, GIFT attempts to mimic this natural state and may overcome deficiencies in the natural transport of gametes to the ampullary tube that account for the infertility.

Recent data demonstrate a 34.4% clinical pregnancy rate, with the highest pregnancy rate achieved in women who are infertile due to endometriosis or unexplained infertility (Abramovici *et al.*, 1993).

Indications

- Unexplained infertility.
- Endometriosis.
- Male factor infertility.
- Cervical factor infertility.

Good Clinical Practice in Assisted Reproduction, ed. P. Serhal & C. Overton.
Published by Cambridge University Press. © Cambridge University Press 2004.

Pre-requisite
- At least one normal patent fallopian tube on previous laparoscopy (the preferred method of pelvic assessment) or hysterosalpingogram.
- Ideally, proven fertilization either through embryos created during a previous IVF cycle or previous natural pregnancy regardless of its outcome.

Technique

Ovarian stimulation

Several regimens are used to induce controlled ovarian hyperstimulation (COH). The use of luteinizing hormone-releasing hormone (LHRH) analogues with go-nadotrophins has resulted in greater ease of planning the ovarian stimulation than was possible with the earlier use of clomiphene citrate with gonadotrophin.

Long protocol

Pituitary down-regulation is achieved using LHRH analogue (one depot injection; or daily subcutaneous injections or nasal spray), administered either in the mid-luteal phase (seven days after presumed day of ovulation) or early follicular phase (day two of the menstrual cycle). In 90% of women the process is complete in 14 days. Once the ovaries are suppressed, daily gonadotrophin injections are given until the time when human chorionic gonadotrophin (HCG) is administered.

Short protocol

This is designed to take advantage of the release of stored gonadotrophin, which occurs soon after commencing the LHRH analogue. The analogue is started on day two of the menstrual cycle and gonadotrophin added from day three. Both medications are continued on a daily basis until the ovulatory dose of HCG is given.

LHRH antagonist

The use of this protocol is particularly suitable for women who have limited ovarian reserve (poor responders). Following a baseline scan performed on day two of menstruation, gonadotrophin injections are given either daily or on alternate days. Clomiphene citrate 100 mg daily is given from day two for five days. From the sixth day of gonadotrophin stimulation (on cycle day seven) LHRH antagonist (cetrorelix) 0.25 mg daily is administered by subcutaneous injection until the day of HCG injection.

Cycle management

All patients are treated on a day case basis. Ovarian follicular response is assessed by serial ultrasound scans to determine changes in follicular diameter and growth rate. Evaluation of changes in the endometrial thickness and quality in response to increasing oestrogen production is also assessed. Serial measurements of plasma oestradiol may be undertaken to guide the adjustment of daily gonadotrophin injections. HCG 10 000 iu is administered intramuscularly near to midnight on the day in the cycle when three or more follicles are at least 18 mm in diameter and ultrasound scanning shows satisfactory development of the endometrium.

Oocyte recovery

The oocyte retrieval can be precisely timed to occur 34–38 hours after the administration of HCG. Some collect the oocytes laparoscopically, although it is our preference to perform transvaginal ultrasound-guided oocyte retrieval, because this permits a more reliable aspiration of all the stimulated follicles. However, if one or both ovaries are inaccessible for transvaginal oocyte recovery, then laparoscopic retrieval can be carried out at the same time as GIFT.

Gamete preparation and transfer

A split ejaculate is produced by masturbation some two hours before the transfer procedure. After preparing the sample by the wash, spin and swim-up technique between 50 000 and 200 000 sperm are transferred into the distal fallopian tube. The recovered oocytes are washed in Earle's culture medium (Medicult, Denmark) and those selected for transfer are inseminated with sperm. Minilaparotomy has been rendered unnecessary by special instruments for GIFT (Rocket of London, UK). The fimbrial end of the fallopian tube is held with atraumatic forceps introduced via a separate trochar and cannula. A graduated smooth stainless-steel cannula with a trochar-pointed obturator is then passed through the abdominal wall and the sharp obturator is withdrawn to allow the passage of a blunt obturator. This enables the end of the cannula to be inserted into the distal fallopian tube without trauma once the correct alignment has been achieved. The oocyte/sperm mixture is then instilled 1.5–2.0 cm within the distal end of the fallopian tube.

Luteal phase support

This is provided by progesterone pessaries (Cyclogest, Hoechst) at a dose of 400 mg twice a day. All patients have a serum β-HCG assay determined 12 days after oocyte recovery to detect pregnancy and, if positive, progesterone pessaries are continued. The first ultrasound scan is scheduled for four weeks after GIFT to detect clinical pregnancy, i.e. fetal heart seen on the scan.

One or both tubes and which tube to select

Several groups have examined the issue of unilateral versus bilateral tubal transfer during GIFT. Each group discovered there was no advantage to bilateral transfer (Haines & O'Shea, 1991). With unilateral GIFT, it is only necessary to load the gametes once and cannulate a single fallopian tube, thus avoiding additional extracorporial manipulation and handling of the gametes, and shortening operating time. Despite their apparent positive influence on fertilization rates, the fallopian tubes do not act independently. The ovaries communicate with the tubes both through their close anatomic relation to the tubes, as well as through a counter current blood flow exchange mechanism. This physical and physiological approximation allows for an ovarian contribution to fertilization even after ovulation occurs. Accordingly, some authors suggest that transfer of gametes should be performed ipsilateral to the ovary with the most follicles, as they believe this to mimic the physiological state (Ransom *et al.*, 1994). On the other hand, it is known that ectopic pregnancy can occur on the contralateral tube to the ovulating ovary, and that in women with premature ovarian failure the fallopian tube can transport gametes, and pregnancies can occur when donated oocytes are used. Also, because there are so many confounding variables that affect the outcome of GIFT treatment, we believe that this issue has not been fully examined in the available literature. Therefore, we take the view that the operating surgeon may use the healthier looking and more accessible tube without fear of compromising the patient's chance of achieving pregnancy.

Zygote intra-fallopian transfer (ZIFT)

ZIFT involves the transfer of embryos at the pronucleus stage into the fallopian tubes. The first successful use of ZIFT in humans was described in 1986 by Devroey *et al.* Proponents of tubal embryo transfer for various causes of infertility suggest that these embryos have a higher chance of implantation because the tubal environment contributes actively to embryo quality, the embryos reach the uterus at a more advanced stage of development in comparison with uterine embryo transfer, the embryos encounter a more receptive endometrium at the time of their entry, and tubal replacement is a more efficient modality of transfer than uterine transfer. Some investigators have reported considerably higher pregnancy rates following ZIFT in comparison with uterine transfer or GIFT in women with nontubal factor infertility. A clinical pregnancy rate of 40.4% and delivery/ongoing rate of 34.2% overall when using ZIFT for all nontubal infertility during a two-year period has been reported (Pool *et al.*, 1990). ZIFT, GIFT, and IVF-embryo transfer (ET) outcomes were statistically compared and the clinical pregnancy and delivery rates from ZIFT were found to be significantly higher than those from both GIFT (1.3 times higher) and IVF-ET (2.2 times higher).

Transcervical GIFT/ZIFT

A major disadvantage with GIFT and ZIFT is the need for laparoscopy with operating theatre facilities. Therefore, several techniques for transcervical tubal cannulation have been described: ultrasound guided; blind (tactile); and hysteroscopic (Abyholm & Tanbo, 1993). One centre reported a pregnancy rate between 25.5% and 29.2% with the use of hysteroscopic GIFT in a few series. This was slightly lower than their own success rate of 30.1% using laparoscopic GIFT (Seracchioli *et al.*, 1991, 1993).

In 1992, Balmaceda *et al.* summarized the data available at that time. The results of the pooled data on transcervical GIFT and ZIFT give pregnancy rates of 18.6% (24 out of 129) and 25.5% (53 out of 208) respectively. The results on GIFT are not encouraging when compared with the reported results in the World Collaborative Report on IVF-ET and GIFT (Testart *et al.*, 1989) and the 1990 results from the IVF-ET registry reporting clinical pregnancy rates of 27.5% and 29% respectively (Medical Research International Society for Assisted Reproductive Technology, 1992).

Although in principle, transcervical tubal transfer techniques seem to be more attractive than laparoscopic transfer, there are questions to be answered. Whether prolonged carbon dioxide exposure of the tubal microenvironment or direct endometrial trauma could limit the efficacy of this technique remains to be determined (Balmaceda *et al.*, 1992). Also, it has to be decided whether a rigid, semi-rigid, or flexible hysteroscopy would be best, and the type of catheter and depth of insertion into the fallopian tube are important matters to be clarified (Possati *et al.*, 1991). Therefore, in our opinion, hysteroscopic tubal transfer is not recommended as representing a reliable alternative to laparoscopy.

GIFT/ZIFT versus IVF

In IVF, the four- to eight-cell embryo is transferred 48–72 hours after oocyte collection and thus reaches the uterine cavity some two to three days earlier than would occur in a natural cycle. This alteration in environmental conditions for preimplantation growth might be expected to reduce the success rates of IVF when compared with GIFT/ZIFT. However, studies in favour of tubal transfer procedures are mostly retrospective, nonrandomized studies with improper controls, or without controls at all. The few prospective, randomized studies performed generally fail to show a higher pregnancy rate with ZIFT or GIFT compared with IVF-ET.

Nevertheless, no adequate, well-designed, prospective, randomized, study with sufficient power has compared the efficacy of IVF with GIFT/ZIFT in a well-defined infertility population. In reality, it is almost impracticable to design such a study, as it would invariably require the participation of many centres, close adherence to a standardized treatment protocol, significant logistical efforts and major research funding. Moreover, the European Society of Human Reproduction and Embryology (ESHRE) previously published a multicentre trial comparing different methods of assisted conception for unexplained infertility and highlighted the serious practical and methodological problems resulting from such an approach.

A prospective randomized study to compare GIFT and IVF in the treatment of couples with unexplained infertility who have failed to conceive after at least three cycles of ovarian stimulation and intrauterine insemination (IUI) reported a clinical pregnancy rate of 34% after GIFT and 50% after IVF-ET (Ranieri *et al.*, 1995). This difference was not statistically significant.

However, IVF pregnancy rates have risen dramatically since the early 1990s. As pregnancy rates among fertile couples rarely exceed 25% per cycle, which is comparable to IVF success rates for those suffering from infertility, one would assume that in vitro embryo culture systems might now be as nurturing as the fallopian tube itself. Consequently, fewer patients are currently undergoing GIFT and ZIFT because of the invasive nature of laparoscopy and the potential adverse effects of general anaesthesia.

Despite the lack of convincing prospective data to support the tubal transfer of gametes or zygotes over IVF, there may be clinical conditions that warrant GIFT or ZIFT treatment. These are discussed below.

Older women

In the UK, the Human Fertilisation and Embryology Authority (HFEA) *Code of Practice* (1993) insists that all fertility centres limit the number of embryos/oocytes transferred with IVF or GIFT to a maximum of three, irrespective of an individual couple's circumstances. In order to minimize the risk of high-order gestations, this guideline presumes that all women of reproductive age have the same prospects of success with fertility treatments, and the same risk of a multiple pregnancy.

The Office of Population Censuses and Surveys data clearly indicate that older women have a lower incidence of multiple pregnancy than younger women. In addition, older women produce fewer oocytes in response to gonadotrophin stimulation and have a lower success and higher miscarriage rate with assisted conception (Al-Shawaf *et al.*, 1992). It has been shown that in women aged >40 years limiting the number of oocytes transferred with GIFT actually reduces the chance of a successful outcome (Craft *et al.*, 1988; Craft & Brinsden, 1989). We have previously proven that there is a clear association between the number of oocytes transferred and the outcome of treatment. Pregnancy occurred in 21.4% of women having up to four oocytes transferred compared with 40.3% in whom five or more were transferred. However, multiple pregnancy rates were 17.3% and 32.3% respectively, of which most were twins (Craft & Brinsden, 1989). Therefore, it would appear that a flexible policy on the number of gametes and embryos transferred is essential to maximize the chance of success for older age women who, in reality, could have all available embryos/oocytes transferred with IVF/GIFT.

Repeated treatment failure

ZIFT and IVF among patients with repeated implantation failure were compared and ZIFT resulted in higher pregnancy and implantation rates at 34% and 9% respectively, compared with IVF at 17% and 4% respectively (Levran et al., 1998). The lower pregnancy rate with IVF may result from difficulty with embryo transfer, loss of embryos through the cervix, or from asynchrony between embryonic and uterine receptivity. Tubal transfer techniques can circumvent these problems. Difficulty with entry into the cervix in cases of cervical stenosis or previous in utero diethylstilbestrol exposure may mandate utilization of the fallopian tube to achieve pregnancy.

Ethical dilemmas

When GIFT is used the complex legal and ethical dilemmas related to excess human embryos and their disposal are not relevant because only gametes are transferred, not fertilized oocytes or embryos. There is *no* in vitro contact between the gametes during the course of the procedure, so there is no possibility of embryo manipulation (Abramovici et al., 1993).

Conclusion

Centres should offer comprehensive assisted conception, including IVF, GIFT and ZIFT. IVF-ET has become much more acceptable, with improvements in vaginal ultrasound, oocyte retrieval techniques and ambulant care with local sedation and analgesia. Whether IVF pregnancy rates can achieve higher levels, especially in women aged >40 years, by improvement in culture media, co-culture on feeder layers or better selection of superovulation protocols, has yet to be evaluated. Similarly, prospective studies need to be undertaken on a multicentre basis with regard to IVF-ET and transcervical gamete or embryo tubal transfer. In the meantime, conventional GIFT treatment will remain an important treatment option in assisted reproduction. Also, we advocate ZIFT for very selective cases, which may well benefit from the technique.

Key points

- GIFT and ZIFT are effective therapies for selected patients.
- Laparoscopy is the gold standard technique for pelvic assessment and tubal transfer.
- If indicated, GIFT is better reserved for couples with proven fertilization.
- In women aged >40 years, a flexible number of oocytes transferred during GIFT will maximize the chance of achieving singleton pregnancy.
- ZIFT is indicated for couples who have had repeatedly failed IVF cycles.
- GIFT/ZIFT should be considered for patients who have cervical stenosis or in utero exposure to diethylstilbestrol.

REFERENCES AND FURTHER READING

Abramovici, H., Dirnfeld, M., Bornstein, J., Lissak, A. & Gonen, Y. (1993). Gamete intrafallopian transfer, an overview. *J. Reprod. Med.* **38**: 698–702.

Abyholm, T. & Tanbo, T. (1993). GIFT, ZIFT, and related techniques. *Curr. Opin. Obstet. Gynecol.* **5**: 615–22.

Al-Shawaf, T., Nolan, A., Guirgis, R., Harper, J., Santis, M. & Craft, I. (1992). The influence of ovarian response on gamete intra-fallopian transfer outcome in older women. *Hum. Reprod.* **7**: 106–10.

Asch, R. H., Ellsworth, L. R., Balmaceda, J. P. *et al.* (1984). Pregnancy after translaparoscopic gamete intrafallopian transfer. *Lancet* **2**: 1034.

Balmaceda, J., Gonzales, J. & Bernardini, L. (1992). Gamete and zygote intrafallopian transfers and related techniques. *Curr. Opin. Obstet. Gynecol.* **4**: 743–49.

Braeckmans, P., Devroey, P., Camus, M. *et al.* (1987). Gamete intra-fallopian transfer: evaluation of 100 consecutive attempts. *Hum. Reprod.* **2**: 201–5.

Castelbaum, A. & Freedman, M. (1998). Is there a role for gamete intra-fallopian transfer and other tubal insemination procedures? *Curr. Opin. Obstet. Gynecol.* **10**: 239–42.

Cohen, J. (1991). The efficiency and efficacy of IVF and GIFT. *Hum. Reprod.* **6**: 613–18.

Craft, I., Ah-Moye, M., Al-Shawaf, T. *et al.* (1988). Analysis of 1071 GIFT procedures – the case for a flexible approach to treatment. *Lancet* **i**: 1094–8.

Craft, I. & Brinsden, P. (1989). Alternatives to IVF: the outcome of 1071 first GIFT procedures. *Hum. Reprod.* **4** (Suppl): 29–36.

Craft, I. & Al-Shawaf, T. (1992). IVF versus GIFT. *J. Assist. Reprod. Genet.* **9**: 424–7.

Crosignani, P., Walters, D. & Soliani, A. (1991). The ESHRE multicentre trial on the treatment of unexplained infertility: a preliminary report. *Hum. Reprod.* **6**: 953–8.

Devroey, P., Braeckmans, P., Smitz, J. *et al.* (1986). Pregnancy after translaparoscopic zygote intrafallopian transfer in a patient with sperm antibodies. *Lancet* **i**: 1329.

Driscoll, G., Tyler, J., Clark, L. & Bernstein, J. (1996). Transfer of gametes into the fallopian tubes – is choice of side important? *Hum. Reprod.* **11**: 1881–3.

Haines, C. & O'Shea, R. (1991) The effect of unilateral versus bilateral tubal cannulation and the number of oocytes transferred on the outcome of gamete intrafallopian transfer. *Fertil. Steril.* **55**: 423–5.

Helsa, J. & Schoolcraft, W. (1997). Treatment of idiopathic infertility with assisted reproductive technologies. *Infert. Reprod. Med. Clin. N. Am.* **8**: 665–87.

Levran, D., Mashiach, S., Dor, J., Levron, J. & Farhi, J. (1998). Zygote intrafallopian transfer may improve pregnancy rate in patients with repeated failure of implantation. *Fertil. Steril.* **69**: 26–30.

Medical Research International Society for Assisted Reproduction Technology (1992). The American Fertility Society: in vitro fertilization-embryo transfer (IVF-ET) in the United States: 1990 results from the IVF-ET registry. *Fertil. Steril.* **57**: 15-24.

Mills, M., Eddowes, H., Cahill, D. *et al.* (1992). A prospective controlled study of in-vitro fertilization, gamete intra-fallopian transfer and intrauterine insemination combined with superovulation. *Hum. Reprod.* **7**: 490–4.

Nadakarni, P., Shrivastav, P., Bharath, M. & Craft, I. (1996). What factors predetermine the risk of having a high-order multiple pregnancy with gamete intra-fallopian transfer? *Hum. Reprod.* **11**: 655–9.

Padilla, S., Smith, R., Dugan, K., Zinder, H. & Maruschak, V. (1996). Laparoscopically assisted intrafallopian transfer with local anaesthesia and intravenous sedation. *Fertil. Steril.* **66**: 404–7.

Penzias, A., Berger, M., Alper, M., Thompson, I. & Oskowitz, S. (1991). Gamete intrafallopian transfer: assessment of the optimal number of oocytes to transfer. *Fertil. Steril.* **55**: 311–13.

Pool, T., Martin, J., Ellsworth, L., Miller, S., Garza, J. & Atiee, S. (1990). Zygote intrafallopian transfer as a treatment for nontubal infertility: a 2-year study. *Fertil. Steril.* **54**: 482–8.

Possati, G., Pareschi, A., Seracchioli, R., Maccolini, A., Melega, C. & Flamingi, C. (1991). Gamete intrafallopian transfer by hysteroscopy as an alternative treatment for infertility. *Fertil. Steril.* **56**: 496–9.

Qasim, S., Shelden, R., Karacan, M., Kemmann, E. & Corsan, G. (1995). High-order oocyte transfer in gamete intrafallopian transfer patients 40 or more years of age. *Fertil. Steril.* **64**: 107–10.

Ranieri, M., Beckett, V., Marchant, S., Kinis, A. & Serhal, P. (1995). Gamete intra-fallopian transfer or in-vitro fertilization after failed ovarian stimulation and intrauterine insemination in unexplained infertility? *Hum. Reprod.* **10**: 2023–6.

Ransom, M., Doherty, K., Corsan, G., Kemmann, E. & Garcia, A. (1994). Tubal selection for gamete intrafallopian transfer. *Fertil. Steril.* **61**: 386–9.

Redgment, C., Al-Shawaf, T., Grudzinskas, J. & Craft, I. (1994). Gamete intrafallopian transfer in older women: effect of limiting number of gametes transferred. *BMJ* **309**: 510–11.

Rombauts, L., Dear, M., Breheny, S. & Healy, D. (1997). Cumulative pregnancy and live birth rates after gamete intra-fallopian transfer. *Hum. Reprod.* **12**: 1338–42.

Seracchioli, R., Possati, G., Bafaro, G. *et al.* (1991). Hysteroscopic gamete intra-fallopian transfer: a good alternative, in selected cases, to laparoscopic intra-fallopian transfer. *Hum. Reprod.* **6**: 1388–90.

Seracchioli, R., Maccolini, A., Porcu, E. *et al.* (1993). A new approach to gamete intra-fallopian transfer via hysteroscopy. *Hum. Reprod.* **8**: 2093–5.

Testart, J., Piachot, M., Mandelbaum, J., Salat-Baroux, J., Frydman, R. & Cohen, J. (1992). World Collaborative Report on IVF-ET and GIFT: 1989 results. *Hum. Reprod.* **7**: 362–9.

Tournaye, H., Camus, M., Khan, I., Staessen, C., Steirteghem, A. & Devroey, P. (1991). In vitro fertilization, gamete or zygote intra-fallopian transfer for the treatment of male infertility. *Hum. Reprod.* **6**: 263–6.

Wang, X., Warnes, G., Norman, R., Kirby, C., Clark, A. & Matthews, C. (1993). Gamete intra-fallopian transfer: outcome following the elective or non-elective replacement of two, three or four oocytes. *Hum. Reprod.* **8**: 1231–4.

Wong, P., Ng, S., Hamilton, M., Anandakumar, C., Wong, Y. & Ratnam, S. (1988). Eighty consecutive cases of gamete intra-fallopian transfer. *Hum. Reprod.* **3**: 231–3.

15

Counselling

Jennifer Clifford

London, UK

Infertility is a silent loss; generally unrecognized in our society (Applegarth, 1990). The Assisted Conception Unit can be the place where, during the process of treatment, this loss can be given a voice and a hearing. There is now increasing international recognition of the necessity to understand, encompass and make explicit the psychological and emotional dimension of the experience of impaired fertility. Good practice means that the consequent use of assisted reproductive technology should therefore be inextricably linked with counselling provision. In the United Kingdom, a licensed assisted conception unit is legally obliged to ensure that counselling is available for anybody contemplating fertility treatment. The words 'assisted conception' encapsulate a process by which procreation is replaced by reproduction. The consciousness of the possibility of the creation of life by sexual intercourse is one of the most private, primitive, internal and mysterious aspects of being human. The mystery is replaced by the 'unnatural' and public intervention of a third party – the clinician/scientist. This is a loss. The need for intervention can cause profound distress and the negative psychological impact of chronic infertility can be equally as serious as that seen in potentially fatal medical conditions (Donmar et al., 1993).

The public requirement for counselling

From the birth of the first IVF baby in 1978, there has been both intense public concern about the vulnerability of potential users, the welfare of children either created or affected by the use of ART and a real fear of uncontrolled scientific development. This led to the Warnock Report (1984), the Human Fertilisation and Embryology Act (1990), the setting up of the Human Fertilisation and Embryology Authority (HFEA), the King's Fund Centre Counselling Committee report (King's Fund, 1991) and the publication of the HFEA *Code of Practice* (5th edition, 2001).

Good Clinical Practice in Assisted Reproduction, ed. P. Serhal & C. Overton.
Published by Cambridge University Press. © Cambridge University Press 2004.

The Human Fertilisation and Embryology Act (1990) is the only legislation that has established counselling on a statutory basis and set out its duties. Counselling was required to perform a vital mediating function between rapid scientific advances and public perception of moral and social acceptability. Provision of counselling by properly qualified and trained counsellors was put in place to allow those contemplating the use of assisted reproductive technology (ART) to make informed and considered decisions (Blyth & Hunt, 1995).

Definitions of counselling

'Counselling is a contractual process undertaken by psychological therapists to enable people to identify the source of their distress, to explore ways of coping more effectively, and to implement change, and the tolerance of change, in their lives. It can be offered to individuals, couples and groups. It is about the development and maintenance of resilience, encouraging linguistic expression as the starting point of change; it is about addressing maladaptive problem-solving systems so that more efficient strategies can be developed for coping with discomfort, rather than eradicating it. Counselling is undertaken through the medium of the therapeutic relationship regardless of the model' (Counsellors and Psychotherapists in Primary Care, 2000: 5).

'Counselling is a process through which individuals and couples are given an opportunity to explore their thoughts, feelings and beliefs, in order to come to a greater understanding of their present situation, and to discover ways of living more satisfactorily and effectively. Given this opportunity, they will often change their perspectives, become less stressed and so be in a better position to make informed decisions for the future' (British Infertility Counselling Association, 1991).

'By offering an empathic, reflective, thinking relationship, counselling provides an experience that can mirror early developmental interactions and help to process and contain primitive and hitherto unmanageable feelings' (Bion, 1962; Schore, 1994).

Three types of counselling – implication, support and therapeutic – are specified in the HFEA Code of Practice.

Implications counselling

This form of counselling, which must be offered, was deemed necessary by the Warnock Report and the King's Fund Committee Report. It differs fundamentally from other forms of counselling because it is not 'client/patient led'. After the infertile couple have been given the necessary information about their treatment by the clinician and taken the time necessary for contemplation, a dedicated implications counselling session should be conducted in a properly private environment by either a nurse practitioner with counselling skills or a trained counsellor. The specific aim of this dedicated implications counselling session is to provide an opportunity for the infertile couple to:

- Give 'informed consent', by ensuring understanding of the implications of their treatment.
- Explore the meaning of the choice of treatment.
- Express how they feel about their own or their partner's infertility and the means they are using to avoid childlessness.
- Express how they feel about a child not being their own or their partner's genetic offspring.
- Be made aware of and agree on the question of whether to tell any resulting offspring about the method of their conception.
- Be made aware of and understand the significance of the Central Register. For example, from 2008 the HFEA can make available to the relevant adults who enquire, information on whether they were conceived with donor gametes. Although identifying information about the gamete donor will not be available, it is possible that this may change in the future (a precedent for this is the retrospective change in adoption law).
- Consider how they would manage in the future if they opted for secrecy. For example, who else knows of the child's method of conception and how they might deal with unplanned disclosure?
- Discuss and clarify issues of child welfare.
- Consider and agree upon the posthumous use of stored gametes or embryos.
- Express their feelings about known or unknown gamete donors.
- Discuss and understand the risks associated with multiple pregnancy.
- Discuss and understand the implications of using intracytoplasmic sperm injection.

Gamete donors should particularly be encouraged to consider the implications of their decision. Both men and women:

- Need to think about the fact that in the future there may well be children in existence that they will never know and that whatever happens to them in the future, the action they are about to take has irrevocable consequences.
- Consider that they are undergoing tests with results that could prove life-changing.
- Think about whether they are going tell any future/current partner/children.

Women:

- Need to think that they are undergoing medical intervention that will not benefit them at all and might have both short- and long-term effects on their own health.
- Should be encouraged to consider how participation will effect her partner/family.

Obviously, different treatments have different implications and it is not possible to cover them all in detail in this chapter. The cryopreservation and storage of gametes/embryos by oncology patients and their partners and the advent of pre-implantation genetic diagnosis, will involve other specialist counselling as well as the counselling available on the unit.

The counsellor and the welfare of the child

The HFEA requires all units to take account of the welfare of any child that might be born as a result of ART or any child who might be affected by this event. The counsellor might on occasion assess and report on the suitability of the potential patient. It is absolutely imperative that the patient be informed before the session that it is an assessment and that confidentiality rests not just with the counsellor but also with the ART team and possibly an ethics committee. This is not strictly a counselling session but is similar to the psycho-social evaluations that are undertaken in clinics in the United States. Providing knowledgeable and compassionate care is essential (Klock, 1998).

Support counselling

All staff working with people with infertility problems will be offering support. Support counselling will be different in so far as both parties know that it is going on. (It is not just a cheery greeting.) Also, it is conducted in a dedicated location for a reasonable length of time either by a nurse practitioner with counselling skills or a trained counsellor. Additional support can be provided by a client self-help group organized within the ART unit. Regularly up-dated information on helpful agencies, self-support groups, self-help organizations, Internet sites and public bodies concerned with fertility should be clearly displayed in the client waiting area to convey the image of an understanding and supportive unit culture.

Therapeutic counselling

'Therapeutic counselling' might seem a tautology – all counselling is therapeutic (in that it strives to alleviate suffering); or meaningless – it is either therapy *or* counselling. However, the ART unit has a responsibility to recognize that people may experience longer term or more profound problems caused or exacerbated by their infertility, and facilitate appropriate counselling. A regularly up-dated list of experienced and approved therapists and counsellors should be available to clinicians and patients.

How the client gets to the first counselling session

The offer of the opportunity to use a counselling service should be presented positively, and clearly endorsed by all clinic staff as an integral part of client care. This could be reinforced if at least some counselling charges were included in the cost of the treatment on private units. Most NHS units offer counselling as part of the treatment.

   Implications counselling should be routine, perceived by staff and clients alike as part of the treatment process, particularly when gametes are being donated or donated gametes used. For support and therapeutic counselling, clients should have clear opportunities to self-refer. In this way their autonomy is respected. Written information about counselling needs to be clearly available, with the telephone number of an independent counsellor to facilitate this process. If staff are concerned about clients, the careful suggestion that 'more time and space might be helpful' may be more effective than 'you are being referred for counselling' as this can be perceived by clients as being 'sent' because they are not coping adequately. They may be very eager to do the right thing for the specialists who will help them have a child and an insensitive referral can reinforce a sense of powerlessness. If the offer can be made sensitively, the client will feel empowered and supported.

The counsellor and the counselling session

- Most people have only one or two counselling sessions.
- A counselling session usually lasts between 45 and 60 minutes.
- A counselling session should be conducted in a comfortable, quiet and dedicated time and space.
- Issues of confidentiality should be made explicit.
- The counsellor must be accredited to a recognized counselling or psychotherapy training association with a code of ethics and a complaints procedure, and should also have up-to-date knowledge of ART.
- As client is the word most frequently used by counsellors, this is the word used in this chapter. Significantly 'client' implies a proactive participant, with no particular health or status connotations.

For once, in their infertility experience, the client is the expert

Whether the client is the couple, or a man or woman alone, only the client knows what it feels like to be them. Counselling takes place, optimally, when there is a 'therapeutic alliance' between the counsellor and the client. Whatever the theoretical background or model used by the counsellor (psychodynamic, humanistic, existential, integrative, cognitive, solution focused, person centred, bereavement, transpersonal or transactional analysis) there are certain common features. These might be:
- Careful observation.
- Close attention.

- Listening empathically.
- Learning from the client.
- Using the way a client makes one think or feel as a means of understanding them.
- Nonjudgemental responses.
- Acknowledgement and normalization of feelings and thoughts.
- Sensitive and cautious articulation of unexpressed thoughts and feelings.
- Mirroring or reflecting back to the client, so that they have a sense of being understood and their feelings contained and processed.
- Facilitating exploration of previously difficult issues by providing a safe space.
- Clarification of issues.
- Self-awareness.
- Cultural awareness.
- That the client experiences they are with somebody who has them in mind.

Counselling for ART

The ART unit is the last stop for many men and women in their quest for a child. At this stage most people will not have received counselling and may not be able to see how counselling can help. However, infertility treatment is generally so stressful and intrusive that the acknowledgement of the psychological and emotional aspects is invaluable in helping patients cope with the experience. Infertile couples may express a variety of thoughts and emotions to each other and to ART unit staff:

- *Ambivalence*

  'Its really confusing, I've ostensibly got what I always wanted, but I don't feel over the moon. I sort of got used to just wanting and now I'm going to get it, I'm scared.'

- *Anger*

  'Why me? Why us? Why not those people who shout at their kids in supermarkets?'

- *Anxiety*

  'How can I cope? What shall we do? Where shall we go? I just tremble all the time, I can't think about anything else.'

- *Blame*

  'Why can't you understand, it's perfectly OK for you, you've already got kids from your first marriage!'
  'Those doctors were just incompetent, and that stupid counsellor didn't help at all.'

- *Confusion*

  'I just don't know what to feel or think any more; sometimes the hope really buoys you up, and then the treatment fails and I'm just devastated; I can't decide whether to go on or stop.'

- *Couple problems*

  'He doesn't seem to care, just says it'll work the next time.' 'She's driving me crazy, I try and stay at the office around the time she's due to get her period, she's completely hysterical.'

- *Cultural pressure*

  'It's just not thought about at all in my culture, everybody just thinks a young couple will do the normal thing after marriage and start a family. I don't know what will happen to me now.'

- *Denial*

  'Of course its my baby, so there's just no point telling it anything. The fact it's not my own egg is not relevant.'

- *Depression*

  'I don't seem to want to do anything now, just stay inside, don't answer the phone, don't bother to wash, eat or even get up some days.'

- *Despair*

  'It's just hopeless, I can't go on like this. I'd rather die than not have a baby.'

- *Envy*

  'I feel terrible, I could almost wish something would happen to my friend's baby.'

- *Ethical dilemma*

  'How are we meant to cope with deliberately killing babies we've longed for. Calling it fetal reduction is just avoiding the issue.'

- *Existential anxiety*

  'What is the point of anything now? Work, love, life even.'

- *Family pressure*

  'I'm an only child, so the family name ends with me. My parents would be completely devastated if they thought there were not going to be any grandchildren.'

- *Fatigue*

  I'm just so tired of this roller-coaster ride of emotions, of the waiting, of the anxiety. I'd just love to sleep for days.'

- *Fear and panic*

  'It just terrifies me, to contemplate the implications for our life together, the treatments I've got to endure and whether I'll be left for somebody who can give him a child. This just can't be happening to me.'

- *Feelings of abnormality*

  'Why can't we do what the whole of nature does so easily?'

- *Feeling infantilized and helpless*

  'I'm completely dependent on the doctor if I'm to become a father' 'I just have to lie here, with my legs in the air, exposed and vulnerable.'

- *Financial difficulties*

  'We've got to stop now, we've run out of money. All those years, those thousands of pounds, for nothing.'

- *Grief*

  'It feels like somebody's died, except this child never existed and nobody has a clue what we're going through.'

- *Guilt*

  'I did lead a bit of a rackety life when I was younger, and I did have a termination. I can't forgive myself for destroying that life. I almost deserve this as a punishment.'

- *Hope*

  'Every treatment just lifts me up, I start sniffing and everything seems possible; but you hardly dare feel like that for fear of the next blow.'

- *Invasion of privacy*

  'I've had my insides probed, looked at on a television screen, commented on so often, I hardly feel I own my body anymore.' 'It's a nightmare, I find myself leafing through a porn. mag. with my wife, a nurse and a doctor standing outside waiting for me to masturbate!'

- *Jealousy*

  'I can't bear to look at my sister now she's pregnant.'

- *Loneliness*

  'I can't contact my friends anymore, they've got kids which hurts and I know I'm a real bore.'

- *Loss of control over one's life*

  'We just don't want to commit ourselves to anything that might interfere with treatment. Career, holidays, moving, staying with friends even.'

- *Loss of a developmental stage in life*

  'I feel I'll always be a child to my parents, having a family is part of becoming a mature adult.'

- *Loss of faith in the body*

  'I suppose I always took it for granted, but now anything could go wrong.'

- *Loss of libido*

  'It doesn't work anyway; besides I can't perform to a timetable any longer.'

- *Loss of potency*

  'I know sterility and impotency aren't the same, but I just couldn't get an erection for weeks after my sperm count result.'

- *Loss of self-esteem*

  'I feel a complete failure as a human being.'

- *Loss of sense of identity*

  'I've grown up always believing I'd become a parent, I don't know quite who I'll be as a childless woman.'

- *Loss of sense as a gendered and sexual being*

  'When we thought there was always the possibility of conception when making love, however unwelcome or remote, it made us feel more male, more female. Now we feel sort of neuter and asexual.'

- *Magical thinking*

  'If I wear the same clothes that I passed my driving test in, then it's bound to work this month.'
  'I feel now my friend's had a baby, she's sort of depleted the supply and I'll be deprived.'

- *Obsessional*

  'I can't think about anything else, it consumes my every waking thought, my dreams too.'

- *Peripherality and redundancy*

  'I might as well go out and get drunk for all the use I am. It's not even going to be my own child.' 'You feel you don't belong anywhere any more. There's a sort of 'parent club' that we're not ever going to belong to.'

- *Rage*

  'I'm just paralysed by this sense of outrage. I just can't deal with having to go to a bloody hospital to get a baby. If I believed in God, I'd have become an atheist.'

- *Self-blame*

  'If only I'd not had the vasectomy.'
  'Why did I wait so long? I shouldn't have put my career first.'

- *Stigmatized*

  'Everybody just thinks you're selfish.'

- *Weakness*

  'I feel so weak, I do nothing but cry; he's so much stronger than me.'

- *Withdrawal and isolation*

'We don't go out much any more, it's too painful to answer those questions about children. We don't want everybody knowing our business.'

(Murray-Parkes, 1991; Raphael-Leff, 1991; Kerr *et al.*, 1999.)

Staff anxiety

Constantly dealing with heightened emotions can take its toll and working with distressed clients for whom failure may be more likely than success is bound to cause stress and anxiety. The cheery injunction to 'Keep cheerful, don't get so anxious, it will improve your chance of getting pregnant', is not only virtually impossible for the client to obey and thus reinforces their feelings of contributing to their own failure, but is an unconscious plea not to be made anxious themselves by the person who says it. One of the best defences against being overwhelmed is a kind of emotional withdrawal; a sense of 'us' and 'them'; 'they' are 'desperate, not coping, dependent, demanding and unreasonable'. The team meeting, which includes the counsellor, can be an important forum for mutual support, reflection, discussion and shared acknowledgement of difficulties.

'Major tasks in infertility counselling involve examining personal motivation, deepening understanding, mobilizing personal resources to cope with a heightened sense of vulnerability and making extremely difficult decisions with indeterminate consequences' (Bond, 2000).

It is a fact that more people will leave the ART unit without a baby than with one. If the holistic culture that a good counselling service fosters and good practice prevails, clients should leave (maybe having even been helped to stop treatment) knowing they have given it their best shot (Mander, 2000). With understanding and helpful support and possibly therapeutic counselling, through mourning the child they will never have, they will start moving towards acceptance and a fruitful journey towards different ways of being creative or founding a family (Bryan & Higgins, 1999).

Acknowledgements

Christa Drennan, Sue Mack, Alexina McWhinnie, Jim Monach, Antonia Murphy, Sheila Naish, Jane Read, Julie Tucker, Robert and Elizabeth Snowden.

REFERENCES

Applegarth, L. (1990). Individual counselling and psychotherapy. In *Infertility Counselling. A Comprehensive Handbook for Clinicians*, pp. 85–101. ed. L. Hammer Burns & S. A. Covington, p. 87. New York: Parthenon Publishing Group.

Bion, W. R. (1962). *Learning from Experience*. London: Maresfield Reprints.

Blyth, E. & Hunt, J. (1995). A history of infertility counselling in the United Kingdom. In *Infertility Counselling*, ed. Sue Emmy Jennings, pp. 175–91 Oxford: Blackwell.

Bond, T. (2000). Issues of confidentiality in fertility counselling. *Hum. Fertil.* **3**. 259–64.

British Infertility Counselling Association (1999). *Guidelines for Practice* (1990). Website: www.bica.net

Bryan, E. M. & Higgins, R. T. (1999). *Infertility. New Choices, New Dilemmas*. London: Penguin.

Counsellors and Psychotherapists in Primary Care (2000). *Professional Counselling and Psychotherapy, Guidelines and Protocols*. Website: www.cpc-online.co.uk

Donmar, A. D., Zuttermeister, P. C. & Froedman, R. (1993). The psychological impact of infertility: a comparison with patients with other medical conditions. *J. Psychosom. Obstet. Gynaecol.* **14**: 45–52.

Human Fertilisation and Embryology Act (1990). London: HMSO.

Human Fertilisation and Embryology Authority (2001). *Code of Practice*, 5th edn. London: Human Fertilisation and Embryology Authority.

Kerr, J., Balen, A. & Brown, C. (1999). The experience of couples in the United Kingdom who have had fertility treatment: the results of a survey performed in 1997. National Infertility Awareness Campaign. *Hum. Reprod.* **14**: 934–8.

King's Fund (1991). *Counselling for Regulated Infertility Treatments. A Report of the King's Fund Centre Counselling Committee*. London: King's Fund.

Klock, S. C. (1998). Psychosocial evaluation of the infertile patient. In *Infertility Counselling. A Comprehensive Handbook for Clinicians*, ed. L. Hammer Burns & S. N. Covington, pp. 49–63. New York: Parthenon Publishing Group.

Mander, G. (2000). *A Psychodynamic Approach to Brief Therapy*. London: Sage.

Murray-Parkes, C. (1991). *Bereavement. Studies of Grief in Adult Life*, pp. 34–107. Harmondsworth: Penguin.

Raphael-Leff, J. (1991). *Psychological Processes of Childbearing*, pp. 29–41. London: Chapman and Hall.

Schore, A. N. (1994). *Affect Regulation and the Origins of the Self. The Neurobiology of Emotional Development*. Hove: Lawrence Erlbaum Associates.

Warnock Report (1984). *Report of the Committee of Inquiry into Fertilisation and Embryology*. Cmnd no. 9314. London: HMSO.

16

Good nursing practice in assisted conception

Kathy Boon, Leigh Oliphant and Elizabeth Fleming

Assisted Conception Unit, UCLH, London, UK

The specialist nurse in assisted conception

Because of the rapidly developing and expanding nature of reproductive medicine and assisted reproductive technology (ART), the role of the nurse working in this area initially developed and expanded in parallel without any real plan or guidance, dependent primarily on the needs of individual centres. In 1987, The Royal College of Nursing, Fertility Nurses Group (RCN/FNG) was established after a small group of nurses working in assisted conception expressed concern about the lack of specific training and professional guidance. In 1990, the RCN/FNG circulated a questionnaire to 100 assisted conception centres and the results were indicative of the great diversity in the role of the nurse in these centres and in training and experience. For example, it was apparent that in the absence of formal training or previous experience, doctors were largely providing ad hoc hands-on training, and the urgent need for professionally recognized training, practical guidelines and support was highlighted (Royal College of Nursing, Fertility Nurses Group, 1990).

In 1993, the RCN/FNG published *Standards of Care for Fertility Nurses* and in 1994 ran its first course: RCN Institute of Advanced Nursing Education Assisted Conception Nursing Care. This course covered reproductive physiology, ethics, research and issues in nursing practice, sociology, political and legal perspectives, psychology and issues relating to counselling. Subsequently other courses have been developed with the aim that nurses will meet the requirements for qualification as specialist infertility nurse practitioners.

In 1996, Castledine *et al.* undertook a survey for the provision of guidelines for nurses practising as either specialists or advanced practitioners, and the attributes required by the nurse working in assisted conception can be identified within this framework. Many of these nurses have a multifaceted role and require a wide range of skills in both clinical practice and leadership. They require a depth knowledge

Good Clinical Practice in Assisted Reproduction, ed. P. Serhal & C. Overton.
Published by Cambridge University Press. © Cambridge University Press 2004.

and experience of the specialty and often have experience in related areas such as midwifery and gynaecology. Many of these nurses are expanding their role to meet the changing needs of assisted conception treatment, but it is important that nursing in this field continues to develop within guidelines for safe clinical practice (Barber, 1997).

Factors influencing the role of the nurse in assisted reproduction

Clinics licensed by the Human Fertilisation and Embryology Authority (HFEA) are obliged to comply with its code of practice (HFEA 1990) and the individual nurse with the Nursing and Midwifery Council (NMC) code of professional conduct (NMC, 2002a) and the scope of professional practice (NMC, 2002b), with the issues encompassing accountability as the basis for their actions. Although the HFEA stipulates that each centre must employ a nurse or midwife with current effective UKCC registration, the doctor:nurse ratio varies from centre to centre, with some providing a doctor-led service and others a higher proportion of nursing input. Some factors that influence the role of the nurse in assisted conception are:

- Size of clinic
  - patient turnover;
  - number of treatment cycles per year;
  - constraints of resources/time.
- Services offered
  - private or NHS funding;
  - specialist services, e.g. preimplantation genetic diagnosis (PGD);
  - links with other hospitals or centres.
- Previous experience
  - previous employment duties;
  - additional training;
  - individual requirements of clinic.
- Staffing levels
  - nursing and medical;
  - administrative and clerical.
- Geographical factors
  - city-based or rural;
  - proximity of other treatment centres.

The nurse as treatment program co-ordinator

The role of the nurse in assisted conception is really that of treatment program co-ordinator and as such the nurse plays an important role within a multidisciplinary team, liaising closely with the other specialties involved. Further, the intense and stressful nature of the treatment requires the nurse to provide emotional support to the couples undergoing treatment in a caring and sensitive manner, whilst imparting a vast amount of new and often complex information. Within the multidisciplinary team, good communication is essential to ensure that information is appropriately and effectively given and received (Muirhead, 1997). The pre-eminent role of the nurse in caring for an infertile couple seeking assisted conception is to provide support, education and counselling (Garner, 1991).

Planning

Each couple should receive holistic care, be satisfied with their involvement in discussing and planning their care and be able to express anxieties. They should feel fully involved from the outset and feel that they are fully informed about their circumstances and planned treatment or management. The role of the nurse in caring for the infertile couple is to support them whether or not a pregnancy is achieved. Therefore, as treatment programme co-ordinator, the nurse in assisted conception requires a high level of communication, teaching and primary counselling skills to provide the best possible care.

Understanding the infertile couple

Nurses working in assisted conception often have more contact with patients and develop a closer relationship with them than other members of the assisted conception team. Therefore, to provide effective nursing care, nurses working in assisted conception must clearly understand the emotional aspects of infertility (Millard, 1991).

It has been suggested that most couples follow a similar pattern in their emotional response to infertility and that this is similar to the five-stage response to bereavement described by Kubler-Ross (1969). It must be recognized that along with these stages of shock, denial, anger, guilt and acceptance, infertile couples may be experiencing other complex emotions specific to infertility such as, isolation and low self-esteem (Marshak, 1993). Further, it must be recognized that at the time of seeking treatment for infertility patients may be at any of the following emotional stages either as a couple or individually.

Shock and denial

For example, a man or woman may be shocked when confronted by his or her infertility and display ambivalence or denial as a defensive reaction, thereby providing protection from further emotional turmoil. This ambivalence and denial may serve only to delay treatment in circumstances where delay is problematic.

Anger

This may manifest itself in unreasonable expectations of the professionals involved in the treatment and in anger directed to those in the wider community such as men and women with large families or women who undergo termination of pregnancy.

Guilt

Feelings of guilt may develop if, for example, a woman previously had a termination of pregnancy or if starting a family was delayed in favour of a high-powered career, when the infertility may be perceived as a cause and effect punishment.

Isolation

Couples often decide not to confide their infertility in family, friends or colleagues, so that when they are undergoing treatment for assisted conception a personal support network is not in place. This can place them under additional pressure with the need for a degree of deception, for example to explain excessive time off work for investigations and treatment. This may lead to feelings of isolation, and the stressful nature of fertility treatment is known to cause difficulties in relationships (Boxer, 1996). In these circumstances, women are thought to respond differently to men, with women finding social support more important and men more likely to take comfort from their work.

Low self-esteem

Many infertile men and women feel that they are inadequate or 'defective' leading to low self-esteem. This can interfere with the pursuit of professional, personal and social goals.

Depression

The despair felt with every menstrual cycle without pregnancy and reinforcing their feelings of inadequacy may lead to depression. Symptoms may include tearfulness, gastro-intestinal disturbances, insomnia, weight loss and an inability to cope with day-to-day life.

Acceptance

This is the stage at which the individual accepts the fact of his/her infertility and regains energy and self-esteem, with a shifting of focus away from their infertility. However, difficulties can arise if there is wide disparity between partners reaching this stage. Acceptance can be made more difficult by constant advances in assisted conception seeming always to offer a glimmer of hope.

The nurse as counsellor

For many years it has been acknowledged that involuntary childlessness and fertility treatment causes a great deal of stress for the vast majority of couples (Royal College of Obstetricians and Gynaecologists, 1992). It is a legal requirement that everyone seeking treatment for assisted conception or considering gamete donation is offered formal counselling and given sufficient information to enable an informed decision. The Royal College of Obstetricians and Gynaecologists' *The Management of Infertility in Tertiary Care* (2000) states:

Infertility and its investigation and treatment can cause significant psychological stress. Counselling decreases stress and may also alter the outcome of treatment though this is not yet proven. Counselling should be offered to all patients.

The HFEA has emphasized the importance of counselling in assisted conception. The HFEA (1990) *Code of Practice* states:

Centres should ensure that, as part of their training, all staff are prepared to offer appropriate emotional support at all stages of their investigation, counselling and treatment to clients who are suffering distress.

From the first consultation most often it is the nurse who is the primary contact for couples. It is the nurse who co-ordinates the treatment programme and provides information and support either face-to-face, via the telephone or in writing. It is preferable to provide continuity of care with the same doctor or nurse seeing the couple at each visit. A good understanding of the type of emotional process the couple may be experiencing and continuity of care enables the nurse to build rapport and trust with the couple and constantly to assess their interaction with each other and their level of anxiety. Effective communication will help reduce feelings of isolation and anxiety and encourage the expression of confidences and concerns, thus facilitating the provision of support.

Ingis & Denton (1992) suggest that support by the nurse aims to:

- Enable people to retain a feeling of control.
- Include them in decision-making and treatment plan.
- Acknowledge the sensitive nature of the investigations and treatment.
- Acknowledge the invasiveness of treatments.
- Acknowledge the success, failure rates and uncertainty of outcome.
- Facilitate the grieving process when appropriate.
- Offer counselling when appropriate.

Referring from nurse to counsellor

The nurse has a comprehensive role to play by using her interpersonal and counselling skills, but it is essential that the nurse understands his/her limitations and when it is appropriate to refer to a professional counsellor. The nurse must recognize that, for example, a woman may not want to disclose her psychological or marital problems to the nurse as she may feel this could jeopardize her continuing treatment. Also, the conditions for counselling may not be ideal. For example, there may be a lack of privacy in the nurses' room, and organizing the time for a 'counselling' session in the middle of a busy clinic may not be feasible.

Nurses must recognize that any feelings of failure in having to refer to a professional counsellor are unwarranted and that while referral is necessary, the couple may not want to discuss their problems with anyone other than the nurse with whom they have built a relationship of trust. It is well documented that there is poor uptake of psychosocial counselling (Boivin *et al.*, 1999). Therefore, careful explanation of the role of the professional counsellor and the assistance they can provide may be necessary. Further, the decision as to whether referral is required may need to be a team decision.

Referral to a counsellor may be required when:

- The patient mentions isolation, and cannot communicate effectively with or confide in their partner.
- Experiencing marital or sexual problems.
- The patient frequently requires *extra* time for support, showing signs of not coping.
- The patient mentions feelings of despair or panic, or may describe symptoms of anxiety attacks.
- The patient mentions feelings of overwhelming anger, or is inappropriately aggressive with clinic staff.
- Any signs of depression (e.g. unkempt or poor standard of hygiene).
- A previous history of needing psychological help, or a concern about their psychological stability.
- Couples contemplating receiving donor gametes or surrogacy.
- Issues about the patient's own parenting or childhood that feel unresolved or problematic.
- When the nurse feels she is out of her depth or overwhelmed by the feelings of the session.

Financial implications

Most assisted conception centres refer to specialist counsellors outside the centre and sometimes the additional cost could deter an infertile couple from proceeding with counselling. This is another reason for why the nurse in assisted conception should be able to provide a high standard of counselling skills.

The nurse as educator

Patient education is central to the nursing role regardless of the clinical setting (Rankin & Stallings, 1996). However, this is not merely to provide the facts but to facilitate learning and engage and empower the patient. The infertile couple are learning new and complex information at a difficult and stressful time (Balen & Jacobs, 1997). It is vital that the nurse encourages the couple as much as possible to increase their knowledge, thereby helping to reduce feelings of anxiety and increasing feelings of control.

Health education

All nurses have an obligation to advise patients to strive for good physical and psychological health, and thus it is possible to prevent, promote, maintain or modify health-related behaviours (Redman, 1993). There are specific aspects on which couples aiming to conceive should concentrate:
- Maintenance of a healthy balanced diet.
- Reduction or omission of alcohol.
- Smoking cessation.
- Practice of stress-relieving techniques.
- Prevention of neural tube defects by taking a folic acid supplement.
- Rubella immunization and infection screening.

The risks of alcohol consumption and smoking in the general population are common knowledge but their effect on fertility cannot be underestimated. Couples who smoke have elevated cadmium levels. Cadmium is a heavy toxic metal that can stop the utilization of zinc, which is required for both male and female fertility (Glenville, 2000). A study reported by Hakim *et al.* (1998) concluded that women should abstain from consuming alcohol due to its link with failure to conceive.

Informed choice

Information enables relevant questioning and independent access of resources, thus facilitating informed choice. The right to know applies to all patients but is especially relevant for infertile couples (Zion, 1988). In Scotland, a Gynaecology Audit Project study in 1995/96 identified a need for more information for infertile patients, particularly in relation to the possible cause of infertility and explanation of drug treatments (Souter *et al.*, 1998). Information about fertility treatment must be comprehensive enough to ensure informed consent and this increased knowledge can help make expectations about treatment more realistic.

The Internet is an important resource as it allows access to an infinite amount of information previously unavailable to the general public. Weissman *et al.* (2000) found that a large proportion of infertile couples are actively using the Internet to obtain information and to seek support. Furthermore, health care providers should consider the Internet an important tool for communication with the infertile population.

Assessment

Prior assessment of the infertile couple is essential to understand what they need to be taught and to what extent, and their preferred learning methods. It is imperative that assumptions about existing skill levels are not made as this can lead to misunderstandings that could affect the outcome when dealing with complex treatment. As the learning process can be stressful in itself, the nurse should enquire about the coping mechanisms and support network of the patient. When discussing patient education Rankin & Stallings (1996) state that it is important to acknowledge each patient's support needs and his or her anxiety about learning new health behaviours. Barriers to learning are revealed by effective assessment. In the infertile couple these can be numerous but can include:

- Physical – pain, drug side-effects, fatigue.
- Emotional – stress, anxiety, fear, mood swings, depression.
- Social – family/peer pressure, lack of understanding, work commitments, financial worries.
- Cultural – communication/language difficulties, conflict with religious beliefs.

Planning

Before initiating teaching, the nurse should establish learning priorities based on the assessment. Planning should follow a logical sequence of conveying the most essential information first and progressing from the straightforward to the complex with the aim that the couple will feel as motivated as possible during and after learning. Zion (1988) states that infertile couples are usually highly motivated and this could be due to their dedication to the desired outcome. The nurse should aim to create a learning environment as far as possible and give consideration to privacy and time constraints. Matters such as comfort, lighting and ventilation should also be taken into account.

Liaison with other members of the team is also important and the nurse should ensure that methods of teaching a particular topic do not vary diversely between colleagues. Efficient teaching depends on teamwork and each team member builds on the teaching of others (London, 1999). Sharing insights on teaching avoids confusion for patients.

Implementation

Patient stress levels often run high at teaching sessions and information retention may not be optimal. Therefore, teaching sessions should be arranged with both partners present so that subsequently they can remind each other of points that they may have missed. Enthusiasm and interest from the nurse can help the couple to relax and become more receptive to learning. If appropriate, some humour can be therapeutic. If the general atmosphere of the session remains positive and the nurse teaches with a sense of fun, the information may be associated with positive emotions (London, 1999).

Quinn (1997) describes memory as three stages: encoding or putting representations into the memory system; storage; and retrieval. The nurse should pause, repeat and question throughout the teaching session to assist the couple in remembering what is taught. The use of repetition within the session will reinforce ideas. The aim should be to increase the understanding by offering the information again, but changing the projection slightly to get the point across. This repetition helps the patient to process the information in order to commit it to memory. Patient responses and nonverbal signals should be noted for signs of misunderstanding. Facial expressions of boredom, interest or confusion will give clues about understanding (Redman, 1993). Jargon and excessive use of medical terminology are best avoided.

The use of learning aids, such as videos and leaflets, is important to reinforce knowledge, and nurses can develop education materials they find effective or to suit the individual (Zion, 1988). People learn better and faster using active rather than passive participation (London, 1999). For example, when teaching self-injection, the patient should handle the equipment from the beginning while the nurse talks them through it.

Evaluation

To ascertain whether teaching has been effective it is vital to have a period of evaluation. It is important to summarize the main points and ask the couple to demonstrate their understanding, either verbally or physically. Misinterpretation can then be identified and addressed. Most couples worry about what to do if something goes wrong or if they make a mistake which could jeopardise the treatment. This reflective period provides an opportunity for the nurse to highlight common obstacles and suggest problem-solving tactics.

The nurse can maintain good communication within the team by carefully documenting in the patient notes the topics covered. Protocols should be developed and used to ensure uniformity of practice within the team (Meerabeau & Denton, 1995).

The couple should be encouraged to provide regular feedback so that any knowledge gaps are highlighted. Evaluation is a continuous process and the nurse should be aware that what has been taught may not necessarily be practised.

The clinical role of the nurse

The role of the nurse in assisted conception has been described as pivotal (Meerabeau & Denton, 1995) as, apart from their role as treatment program co-ordinator, educator and counsellor, they are required to carry out a variety of clinical procedures:

- Venepuncture.
- Administration of hormone injections.
- Ultrasonograghy (abdominal and vaginal).
- Follicular tracking.
- Scrubbing and circulating in theatres.
- Cervical and intrauterine inseminations.
- Semen analysis and preparation.
- Post coital tests.
- Pregnancy testing.
- Participation in decisions regarding drug dosages and protocols.

Key points for good practice:
- Understanding the diverse emotional responses to infertility.
- Excellent communication and interpersonal skills.
- Knowing your own limitations and when to refer.
- Continuous professional development.

Professional development

As consumer expectations of professional care increase, the acquisition of further skills and knowledge becomes necessary (Phillips *et al.*, 1985). High expectations from professionals and patients lead to additional pressure on nurses in a medical area fraught with moral and ethical dilemmas to challenge even the most experienced nurse.

Assisted reproduction clinics usually work independently as a small team of nurses, doctors, embryologists and administration staff, and the lack of opportunity to interact professionally outside that team has led nurses to report a sense of isolation (Denton, 1998). Therefore, it is important that nurses regularly interact with nurses outside their team to share experience and attend study days and courses that will contribute towards their professional development. To this end, the RCN/FNG provides written guidelines for ART procedures, holds frequent study days and has a telephone advice line for immediate queries.

REFERENCES AND FURTHER READING

Bakpa, P. (1995). The nurse and infertility counselling. In *Infertility Counselling*, ed. S. E. Jennings, Ch. 2. Oxford: Blackwell Science.

Balen, A. H. & Jacobs, H. S. (1997). *Infertility In Practice*, pp. 259–60. Edinburgh: Churchill Livingstone.

Barber, D. (1997). Research into the role of fertility nurses for the development of guidelines for clinical practice. *Hum. Reprod.* **12**: 195–7.

Blenner, J. L. (1990). Passage through infertility treatment: a stage theory. *IMAGE J. Nurs. Schol.* **22**(3). Fall.

Boivin, J., Scanlan, L. C. & Walker, S. M. (1999). Why are infertile patients not using psychosocial counselling? *Hum. Reprod.* **14**: 1384–91.

Boxer, A. S. (1996). Images of infertility. *Nurs. Pract. For.* **7**: 60–3.

Castledine, G., Brown, R. & McGee, P. (1996). A survey of specialist and advanced nursing practice in England. *Brit. J. Nurs.* **5**(11): 682–6.

Denton, J. (1998). The nurses role in treating fertility problems. *Nurs. Times* **94** (Jan. 14):

Garner, C. (1991). *Principles of Infertility Nursing*, pp. 155–6. Florida: C.R.C Press.

Glenville, M. (2000). *Natural Solutions to Infertility*, p. 75. London: Judy Piatkus (Publishers) Ltd.

Hakim, R., Gray, R. H. & Zacur, H. (1998). Alcohol and caffeine consumption and decreased fertility. *Fertil. Steril.* **70**: 632–7.

Human Fertilisation and Embryology Authority (2000). *Ninth Annual Report and Accounts 2000*. London: HFEA

Human Fertilisation and Embryology Authority (1990). *Code of Practice*. London: HFEA.

Inglis, M. M. & Denton, J. (1992). Infertility nurses and counselling. In *Infertility*, ed. A. Templeton & Drife, J., ch. 24. Berlin: Springer-Verlag.

Kennedy, H. P., Griffin, M. & Frishman, G. (1998). Enabling conception and pregnancy – midwifery care of women experiencing infertility. *J. Nurse-Midwifery* **43**: 197–203.

Kerr, J., Brown, C. & Balen, A. H. (1999). The experiences of couples who have had infertility treatment in the United Kingdom: results of a survey performed in 1997. *Hum. Reprod.* **14**: 934–8.

Kubler-Ross, E. (1969). *On Death and Dying*. MacMillan: New York.

London, F. (1999). *No Time To Teach?*, pp. 4, 37, 115–129, 328. Philadelphia: Lippincott.

Marshak, L. S. (1993). The role of the female doctorally prepared nurse in caring for infertile women. *Can. Nurse Spec.* **7**: 8–11.

Meerabeau, L. & Denton, J. (Eds). (1995). *Infertility Nursing and Caring*, p. 121. London: Scutari Press.

Millard, S. (1991). Emotional responses to infertility. *AORN J.* **54**: 310–5.

Muirhead, M. A. (1997). Nursing Care in an assisted conception unit. In *In Vitro Fertilization and Assisted Reproduction*, ed. P. R. Brinsden, p. 391. New York: The Parthenon Publishing Group Inc.

Nursing and Midwifery Council (NMC) (2002a). *Code of Professional Conduct for Nurse, Midwife and Health Visitor*, 3rd edn. London: NMC

Nursing and Midwifery Council (NMC) (2002b). *The Scope of Professional Practice*. London: NMC.

Olshansky, E. F. (1996). A counselling approach with persons experiencing infertility: implications for advanced nursing. *Adv. Pract. Nurs. Q.* **2**: 42–7.

Phillips, S. E., Wood, B. A. & Brennan, J. (1985). Infertility therapy – the genesis of a course? *Aust. Nurs. J.* **15**: pp. 49–51.

Quinn, F. M. (1997). *The Principles and Practice of Nurse Education*, 3rd edn. p. 43. Cheltenham: Stanley Thornes.

Rankin, S .H. & Stallings, K. D. (1996). *Patient Education – Issues, Principles, Practices*, 3rd edn. pp. 4, 175–179. Philadelphia: Lippincott.

Redman, B. K. (1993). *The Process of Patient Education*, 7th edn. pp. 5, 226–65. Missouri: Mosby-Year Book Inc.

Royal College of Nursing (1991). *Standards of Care for Gynaecological Nursing* – RCN *Standards of Care Project–1991*. London: Royal College of Nursing.

Royal College of Nursing, Fertility Nurses Group (1990). *Report of a Professional Survey*. London: Royal College of Nursing.

Royal College Nursing, Fertility Nurses Group (1993). *Standards of Care for Fertility Nurses*. London: Royal College of Nursing.

Royal College of Obstetricians and Gynaecologists (1992). *Infertility Guidelines for Practice*. London: Royal College of Obstetricians and Gynaecologists.

Royal College of Obstetricians and Gynaecologists (2000). *The Management of Infertility in Tertiary Care: Evidence-Based Clinical Guidelines*, No. 6. London: Royal College of Obstetricians and Gynaecologists.

Sherrod, R. A. (1998). Infertility education in baccalaureate schools of nursing. *J. Nurs. Ed.* **37**: 412.

Souter, V .L., Penney, G., Hopton, J. L. & Templeton, A. A. (1998). Patient satisfaction with the management of infertility. *Hum. Reprod.* **13**: 1831–6.

Weissman, A., Gotlieb, L., Ward, S., Greenblatt, E. & Casper, R. F. (2000). Use of the Internet by infertile couples. *Fertil. Steril.* **73**: 1179–82.

Zion, A. B. (1988). Resources for Infertile Couples and "The process of Developing Patient Education Materials for Infertile Couples". *J. Obstet. Gynaecol. Neo-nat. Nurs.* **17**: 255–63.

17

Setting up an IVF unit

Alpesh Doshi[1] and Caroline Overton[2]

[1]Assisted Conception Unit, UCLH, London, UK
[2]St Michael's Hospital and the Bristol Royal Infirmary, Bristol, UK

The aim of this chapter is to guide the clinician in the steps necessary to set up and run a successful IVF unit. This involves planning, clinical aspects and laboratory set up.

Planning

Before setting up it is necessary to identify the need for the service. This will involve the identification of the population base that the unit will serve, the demographic details of that population and the aetiology of infertility. If an infertility clinic already exists it is possible to extrapolate the demographic details and aetiology from clinic statistics. There may be other IVF units already established in the area and it will be necessary to assess whether an additional unit will have a place. If treatment is only available privately there may already be a waiting list for state funded treatment. It may be possible to apply for state funding to assist these patients.

There are few data on the extent of subfertility. Approximately 80% of couples are pregnant after a year of trying, rising to 95% after two years. Failure to conceive after two years is a useful definition for health service planning because of the high spontaneous conception rate before one year. However, earlier access to specialist services may be indicated for some individuals where an underlying cause has been identified or because of increased age (Templeton *et al.*, 1991).

The prevalence of subfertility is between 9% and 14%, of whom 70% will have primary infertility and 30% secondary infertility. A health authority (e.g. with a population of 250 000 with 46 000 women aged 20–44 years) with an established subfertility service can expect around 230 (0.5%) new consultant referrals each year. The need for subfertility services is likely to grow towards later pregnancies and an increasing number of remarriages, and will be sensitive to changes in incidence of some sexually transmitted diseases.

Good Clinical Practice in Assisted Reproduction, ed. P. Serhal & C. Overton.
Published by Cambridge University Press. © Cambridge University Press 2004.

Demand is increasing because of raised public awareness of treatment possibilities. The estimate of the need is higher than the historical demand of 0.37% per year. If services are expanded, planning should take into account hitherto unexpressed demand and the possible effect on demand from women with secondary infertility and increased access to treatment (Effective Health Care, 1992).

In setting up a new unit it is necessary to convince others that there is an economical need for one to be established. This will involve discussion with consultant colleagues, hospital management and those who commission health care. It will also involve talking to patient welfare groups. The local press may be helpful in publicizing the need for a new unit and providing advertisement.

A business plan is essential if you hope to secure capital or development money. This informs the executives of the key facts and figures in terms of income and expenditure to enable them to make a decision. The help of an accountant is essential.

The plan should include a mission statement; a vision of what you are trying to achieve and how you intend to achieve it. Outline the need and demand for the service and the five-year plan. Include a SWOT analysis of the internal strengths, weaknesses, external opportunities and threats. There are key considerations such as external factors that will impact on the business plan, such as pay awards and a contingency plan if there is under recovery of income, for example bad debt provision.

Procedure costing

This must be carried out for your own service, although there are some reasonably accurate costings available. There are two methods. The *top-down approach*, where the total budget for the unit is divided by the realistically achievable workload and the *bottom-up approach*. Here a detailed breakdown of the costs of the procedure is produced. This is far more time consuming and can only be achieved by the finance person having sufficient familiarity with all aspects of the treatment to be able to cost the treatment down to the last detail. However, it will be more accurate and auditable. It is important that there is an element of all aspects of the service included in the costing. This cost is then multiplied by the activity to obtain the overall income and expenditure.

Activity levels

The calculation of likely activity is based on a number of factors that include market research, existing waiting lists, referral base and the currently available service in the area and their activity. It is most important to plan conservatively by underestimating the likely activity and planning accordingly. Mounting referrals and lengthening waiting lists can be used as a powerful tool to present a case for expansion in the future.

Financial status of the unit

Assisted conception services fall into three categories: wholly private and independent; state funded units; and part academic (university), part patient funded units. Unit costs in private units need to be higher because of higher capital set up costs and higher wages. Financial systems for invoicing and accounting should be no different.

Clinical set-up

Location

Location should ideally be close to or within an existing obstetrics and gynaecology department, being sensitive to the particular needs of these patients (i.e. away from the labour ward). Emergencies arising during oocyte recovery are rare but easy access to an emergency theatre is reassuring. Close proximity to the gynaecology ward is helpful as admission is occasionally needed for patients with ovarian hyperstimulation, nonviable pregnancy and suspected ectopic pregnancy. This also facilitates the exchange of nursing staff into the unit to acquire knowledge that may be useful when dealing with complications. Furthermore, out-of-hours injections may need to be given on the gynaecological ward.

Anatomy of the assisted conception unit

This list is not exhaustive, but certain principles apply:
- Reception and waiting area.
- Consultation room.
- Nurses room.
- Scanning room.
- Dedicated theatre for oocyte recovery/ embryo transfer.
- Embryology laboratory and theatre in close proximity.
- Clearly defined access to ultrasound for monitoring.
- Quiet, undisturbed rooms for counselling.
- Secure sensitive room for obtaining semen samples.
- Separate patient records and secure storage.

Staffing requirements

The absolute minimum staff requirements to provide assisted conception services including IVF are a:

- whole time experienced fertility nurse (with experience in IVF);
- whole time experienced embryologist with at least two years experience in human embryology/IVF;
- clinician with five sessions devoted to infertility;
- supporting clinician who can share on-call/holidays;
- independent counsellor;
- secretary/administrator/personal assistant.

Additional staff in all areas will be based on the activity levels, the range of treatments offered and whether a seven-day a week service is to be offered.

Practice considerations

In order to avoid unnecessary duplication of diagnostic testing and treatment and to reduce the stress experienced by patients it is important that the unit agrees and adheres to a common management philosophy and framework. Guidelines are available from the Royal College of Obstetricians and Gynaecologist[1] and the American Society for Reproductive Medicine[2] that could form the basis of such guidelines. This is likely to optimize the continuity of care for individuals as they move between primary, secondary and tertiary levels of care.

There are particular questions that need to be decided:

- Which patients will be eligible for treatment?
- What baseline investigations will be provided?
- What are the treatment options prior to IVF?
- Which techniques for IVF?

Protocols

Written protocols for both laboratory and clinical practice are required. IVF is now a well established treatment and protocols are common in many respects from one unit to another but need to be modified for a particular unit. Clinical protocols should include, for example, pre-treatment work-up, ovarian stimulation regimes, management of ovarian hyperstimulation. Laboratory procedure should be clearly defined to outline standards and expectations and to minimize interstaff variation. Consent forms will also need to be produced and agreed with hospital's solicitors. The Human Fertilisation and Embryology Authority (HFEA)[3] produce consent forms for long-term storage of gametes and embryos but may not be sufficient.

Emergency cover

How will your emergency cover be provided? Your patients will require an out-of-hours telephone contact number for problems or queries that may arise outside office hours.

Patient information

Written patient information is essential throughout the health service and more so in this area. It must be clear, understandable by the lay person and in appropriate languages. Among the many details, the information needs to include:

- Up-to-date pregnancy rates for all licensed treatments.
- Most recent live birth rate data for all licensed treatments.
- Complications of IVF and related treatments.
- Legal information (storage of embryos and donor gametes).
- Multiple pregnancy rates in your unit for the treatments proposed.
- Complications of multiple pregnancy.
- Information on ovarian hyperstimulation syndrome.
- Costs of treatment.
- Availability of counselling.
- Emergency telephone contact numbers.

Audit/data collection

This is a vital part of the work and is essential for research, training and service development. There is a statutory requirement in the United Kingdom (UK) to return data to the HFEA on every cycle of a licensed treatment carried out. There should be an effective and reliable computer database of which there are a few commercially available. With large throughput of patients it will be necessary to employ someone to manage the data collection and returns.

Quality control

In the UK licensed treatment (IVF, donor insemination, ICSI, storage of gametes and embryos, oocyte donation) cannot be carried out without application to the HFEA and agreement of the local ethics committee. The HFEA produce a guide that is a useful starting point when planning a unit. There is a statutory requirement for all units providing these treatments to be inspected before treatment is carried out and then on an annual basis. In addition there are National External Quality Assurance schemes that monitor performance on a rolling programme basis.

Laboratory set-up

A well planned laboratory is the foundation of a successful IVF practice. There are several factors that should be taken into consideration when designing the laboratory. Work stations need to be positioned sensibly and logically to make working more practical and accident free. Efficiency and safety should be considered when positioning incubators, centrifuges, flow cabinets and cryopreservation equipment. In addition, local health and safety guidelines must be complied with. A sterile environment should be maintained in the laboratory with rigorous daily cleaning of floors and surfaces. This is of particular importance in areas where tissue culture techniques are applied, such as media making, to prevent any microbial contamination. If the andrology and embryology areas are within a single setting it is advisable to allocate separate incubators for each to prevent temperature and pH fluctuations every time the incubator door is opened.

The IVF laboratory should be located in a low traffic area and entry restrictions should apply (discussed later in the chapter). Careful attention has to be paid to the type of paint used as the use of solvent-based paints is lethal to embryos. Low fume or water-based paint should be used on the walls and surrounding area. It is recommended that the paintwork should be completed at least two weeks before starting laboratory work involving oocytes and embryos. The use of strong adhesives also should be avoided for the same reasons. It is best to have vinyl or single layered flooring which is antistatic. Wooden or tiled floors should be avoided as their crevices and ridges can trap dirt and they are more difficult to clean. The benches should be of an adequate height to enable comfortable working. Adjustable height chairs are quite useful. These should be PVC or leather coated to avoid the accumulation of dust in fabric covers.

The laboratory should ideally be located next to the theatre where oocyte recovery and embryo transfers are carried out. The size of the laboratory depends on several factors, such as the number of embryologists, equipment, number of cycles performed and whether any specialized treatments are performed (such as preimplantation genetic diagnosis on sperm washing for HIV positive patients). The laboratory should have adequate space to ensure aseptic and optimal handling of gametes and embryos at all times.

Entry restriction

Entry into the laboratory should be restricted to laboratory personnel only. This not only helps to maintain a sterile environment but also prevents disruption of positive air flow. There should be a designated separate changing area for theatre and laboratory staff and a set of clean theatre clothes, disposable cap, mask and antistatic shoes should be worn. Antimicrobial adhesive mats attract dirt from shoes and should be placed at the laboratory entrance. All staff entering the laboratory should have hand washing facilities, which should be near the entry/exit door and all personnel must wash their hands with Hibiscrub (or an antibacterial fragrance free soap) on both entry to and exit from the laboratory. Laboratory staff should not wear any nail varnish, perfume/after shave or any alcohol-based deodorants. These have been known to be embryo toxic.

It is preferable to have a separate office area for computerized data entry and paper work. Patient files and extraneous papers should not be taken into the laboratory as they can be a source of infection and contamination. Laboratory staff should be encouraged to wear nontoxic powder-free gloves for procedures and these should be changed frequently.

Air filtration in the laboratory

Awareness about air quality has increased in the last few years. Air contaminants include: volatile organic compounds (VOCs) such as aldehydes; small organic molecules such as nitric oxide, sulphur dioxide and carbon monoxide (from exhaust fumes); and liquids such as floor wax that contain heavy metals. The degree of pollution depends on the location of the IVF unit. Urban laboratories are more likely to have higher pollution. Any contaminants in the ambient air will also be circulating through the incubators. Cohen *et al.* (1997) showed that certain adhesives arrested >90% of mouse embryos at the 2-cell stage with very low blastocyst formation. Brand new incubators emit >100 times higher concentrations of VOCs than used ones (Cohen *et al.*, 1997).

Many laboratories have a positive pressure hepa filtration system to extract inorganic contaminants (e.g. dust, bacteria). Additional absorption systems containing activated carbon and potassium permanganate are required to remove VOCs. Air conditioning systems should recirculate hepa-filtered air rather than drawing air from the outside.

The University College London Hospital (UCLH) laboratory is maintained at a temperature of 28–30 °C to prevent temperature shocks when removing oocytes and embryos from the incubators. Air conditioning is only switched on when the laboratory gets too warm to maintain adequate incubator function (there needs to be a 7–8 degree difference between the laboratory temperature and the incubator temperature).

Coda air filtration system

The incubator filter contains activated carbon and conveniently fits into an incubator compartment. It purifies the air by reducing VOCs, heavy metals and chemical air contaminants. The filters are changed monthly or every time the incubators are cleaned.

The filtration towers incorporate a four-stage filter, which contains a unique blend of activated carbon, alumina impregnated with potassium permanganate for absorption and oxidation of a wide variety of gases and particulate contaminants. It removes up to 99% of all contaminants by filtration through 0.2 μm filters and performs 12–15 air exchanges per hour. The number of Coda Towers (Figure 17.1a) needed depends on the size of the laboratory (one tower for 300 square feet). The filters are changed quarterly with a yearly general service.

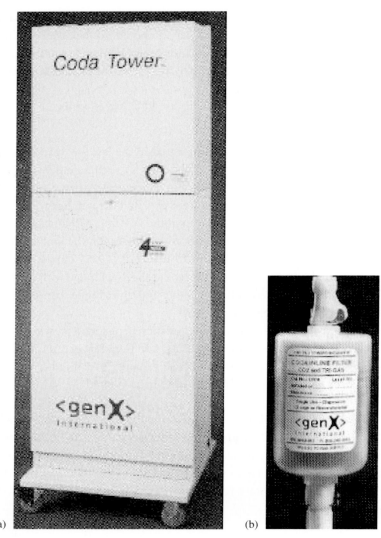

Figure 17.1. (a) Coda tower; (b) coda in line filter.

In line CO_2 filters (Figure 17.1b) are installed in the tubing between the CO_2 tanks and the incubator. This filter is suitable for tri-gas as well as pure CO_2. These filters can also be attached to CO_2 controlled environmental chambers used for routine embryology.

Laboratory lighting

Laboratory lighting is important. There is very little known on the detrimental effects of light on human gametes and embryos. However, studies carried out on other mammalian oocytes have shown that visible light has deleterious effects on the cleavage patterns of the resulting embryos (Hirao *et al.*, 1978; Fisher *et al.* 1988). Minimum indirect lighting is best. The use of UV light (white fluorescent lights) should be avoided since these are thought to be mutagenic to the DNA. Microscopes should be set with the minimum amount of light exposure. Culture media has also been shown to be light sensitive and should be stored in the dark.

Laboratory safety

A well equipped laboratory should have fire extinguishers and fire blankets. There should be evacuation schedules clearly displayed in the laboratory. A general wet area for washing and sterilizing of equipment should be well away from the main embryology area. The use of strong chemicals such as fixatives should be confined to a fume cupboard in a separate room. Incubators and other electrical equipment should be switched off and unplugged from their sockets before cleaning. A spill kit as well as a first aid kit should be available for emergencies.

Laboratory security

The laboratory should be secure with locks or security codes on the main doors.

Generator back-up

There should be emergency generator back-up systems in the event of power failure and regular checks of the back-up system.

Cryostorage room

The cryostorage room should be close to the main laboratory with an adequate built-in ventilation system. The cryo dewars containing sperm and embryos must be locked for security. The liquid nitrogen level is monitored electronically and will alarm if it drops below a pre-determined level. There should be separate dewars for hepatitis B, hepatitis C and HIV patients.

Laboratory equipment

Laminar flow cabinets

There are two types of air flow cabinets commonly used. These are the horizontal flow (Class I) and the vertical flow (Class II) (Figure 17.2a, b). The former only

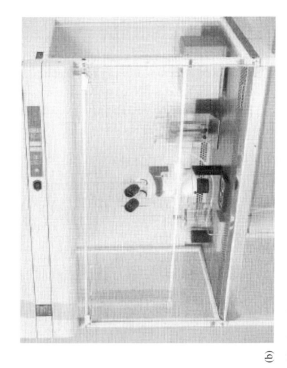

(b)

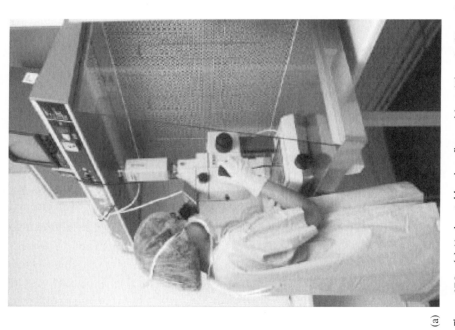

(a)

Figure 17.2. (a) Horizontal laminar flow cabinet (Class I); (b) vertical laminar flow cabinet (Class II).

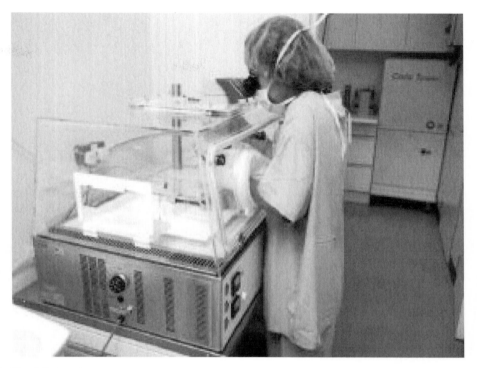

Figure 17.3. The IVF chamber.

protects the sample whereas the latter protects the operator and the sample. Recent guidelines suggest that vertical flow cabinets should be used to handle samples from patients with HIV or hepatitis B or C. They should be kept clean at all times and the number of items inside the flow hood minimized to ensure that air flow is not disrupted. The flow cabinets should be serviced annually with filter changes every six months.

The IVF chamber

This is a controlled environmental chamber (Figure 17.3) which is mobile and is specifically designed to maintain ideal temperature and pH during the handling of gametes and embryos. The working chamber is maintained at a temperature of $37\,^{\circ}$C with 5–6% CO_2 in air. Temperature is monitored by a thermostat and CO_2 levels by an infra-red sensor. A dissecting microscope is needed for egg collections, inseminations, fertilization checks, denuding eggs for ICSI (intracytoplasmic sperm injection), normal evaluation and grading of embryos and embryo transfers. Several studies have shown that prolonged temperature fluctuations can be very detrimental to the meiotic spindle in human oocytes. This can lead to chromosomal aberrations in the resulting embryo with a reduced chance of implantation

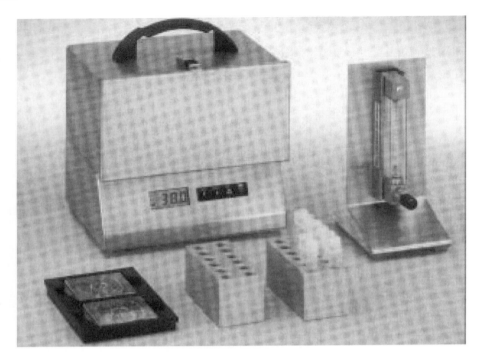

Figure 17.4. A transport incubator.

(Almeida & Bolton, 1995). The IVF chamber is ideal for training embryologists as temperature fluctuations are minimized if the manipulation takes longer than expected.

Heated stages

Prolonged exposure of oocytes and embryos to temperatures below 37 °C can disrupt their cytoskeleton. All microscopes used for gametes and embryos should have heated stages. Heated stages can be installed on most brands of dissecting microscopes (Nikon, Hunter Scientific). A heated surface with a wide working area can also be incorporated in a Class II flow cabinet.

It is suggested that the stage temperature is set slightly higher than 37 °C so that the drops of media with the embryos or oocytes are maintained at 37 °C. It is advisable to experiment with a dish without embryos (in the system that you intend to use) to determine the ideal temperature setting. At UCLH we set the stages at around 40 °C to achieve the right temperature in our culture system.

Transport incubators

Transport incubators (Figure 17.4) are essential where oocyte retrievals and/or micro manipulations are performed away from the main laboratory. The oocytes

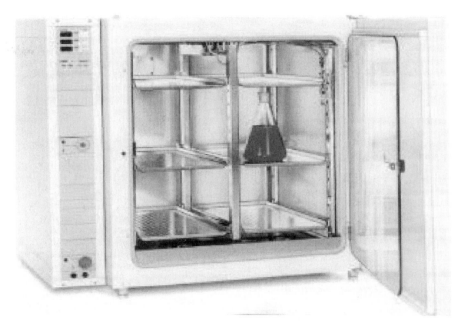

Figure 17.5. A conventional incubator.

can be collected in tubes or dishes. Within the transport incubator temperature is maintained between 37–38 °C with 5% CO_2.

Incubators

The right choice of an incubator is crucial. The principal function of an incubator is to maintain controlled pH and temperature allowing fertilization and cleavage. A gas phase of 5–6% CO_2 is needed to maintain the pH of bicarbonate buffered culture media at around 7.3–7.4. A good IVF laboratory should have at least two incubators. One is used for oocytes and embryos only and the other one for andrology, pH equilibration and warming of tubes and dishes of media. More than two incubators may be required in a unit performing over 300 IVF cycles per year.

Conventional CO₂ incubators

The most commonly used incubators for IVF are manufactured by Heraeus and are available in sizes ranging from 60 to 220 litre volumes (Figure 17.5). Depending on the brand, extra accessories can be included such as six-door screens and oxygen control. The six-door screen is beneficial for culturing oocytes and embryos as this will minimize the rate of CO_2 loss and rapid drops in temperature when the door is opened. Oxygen control is beneficial if the laboratory performs blastocyst transfers, as current literature suggests the use of 5% O_2 for extended culture (Dumoulin *et al.*,

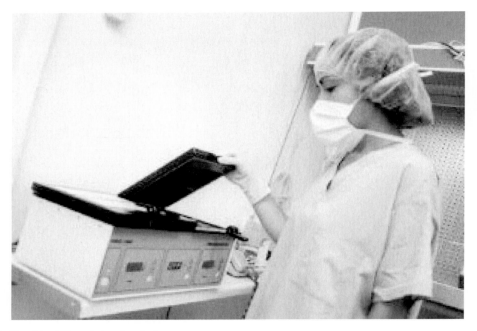

Figure 17.6. The 'Cook' bench top incubator.

1999). However, studies with mouse ova have shown spindle damage and unaligned chromosomes in low oxygen tensions (Hu *et al.*, 2001).

Incubators can be run either dry or humid. If a culture system incorporates the use of oil overlay, then humidity is irrelevant. Humidity also poses the risk of fungal and bacterial contamination. Some incubators come with a built in 'disinfection routine' module which is useful for cleaning (the walls and plates heat up to 90 °C). Otherwise incubators should be cleaned at least once a month with 70% ethanol (analar grade) and flushed out with one litre of sterile water (tissue culture grade non-pyrogenic). They should be left running overnight after cleaning before culturing gametes or embryos.

Bench top incubators (MINC-Cook)

These are the new generation incubators and are compact with a very small chamber volume (Figure 17.6). Their main advantage is the rapid recovery of CO_2 and temperature within three minutes of opening the chamber lid. It does this by purging the gas at a rate of 25 ml/min in the chamber. It uses a tri gas mixture of 5% O_2, 6% CO_2 and 89% nitrogen, which is quite expensive compared to pure clinical grade CO_2. They can be used for conventional IVF. However, at UCLH we tend to use them when performing embryo biopsy for preimplantation genetic diagnosis when embryos are frequently moved in and out of a conventional incubator. This can in turn jeopardize other patients' embryos or oocytes within the incubator due to sub-optimal temperature and pH.

The bench top incubator is much easier to clean than the conventional one. It uses 150 ml of water as opposed to 5 l with the conventional one. However they can only contain a maximum of eight dishes which means that bigger laboratories may need three to four MINC incubators. The cost effectiveness has to be borne in mind.

Bench top incubators have to be installed with auto diallers that will dial out in cases of incubator emergencies. In case of a power cut or CO_2 depletion the chamber will maintain its pH and temperature for about an hour if unopened which gives the embryologist some time to rectify the problem. Incubators should also have two tanks of CO_2/mixed gas attached to a change-over unit, in case one runs out so that the other is activated immediately. All fittings and silcone tubing should be checked for leaks. Incubators should be fully serviced twice yearly.

Microscopes

Good microscopes are required for routine embryological and andrological procedures. A dissecting microscope is essential to score oocyte cumulii complex, pronuclei and embryos for transfer. The range of its magnification should be between 20 and 160×. A phase contrast microscope is needed to score detailed semen parameters such as morphology. Some clinics use the computer aided semen analysis system (CASA) to reduce inter-observer variation.

Micromanipulation

A micromanipulator is necessary for ICSI and embryo biopsy for preimplantation genetic diagnosis. In addition, a good inverted microscope with a heated stage and a magnification of up to 400× is needed. The controls can either be pneumatic or hydraulic. Although hydraulic syringes have more effective control and movement, it can be fairly time consuming and messy to prime the tubing with oil every time there is air trapped within the system. The micromanipulation system should be placed in a vibration free environment. Hydraulically controlled anti-vibration tables are commercially available. If there is limited air filtration in the laboratory, the micromanipulator system can be placed within a class II flow hood. When choosing the manipulators it is very important to consider the ease of manoeuvrability. Some systems have automated and complicated electrical controls whereas some are more manual. The simpler the system, the easier it is to rectify problems in an emergency without the need to call in a technician. For units performing embryo biopsy, a triple tool holder may be necessary to breach the zona. However, if an infra-red laser system is installed then a dual tool holder should be sufficient to perform the procedure. For teaching purposes it is advisable to have a video-linked camera mounted on the micromanipulator. This is also useful to record embryo biopsies and look back to detect any contamination of cumulus cells. Commonly

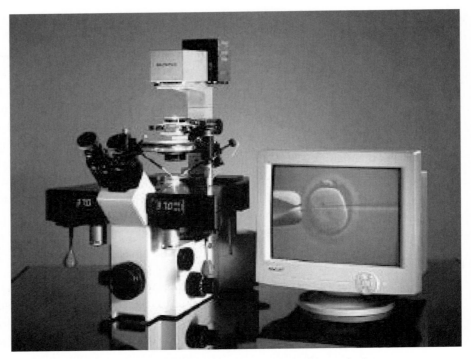

Figure 17.7. The Research Instruments micromanipulator with Olympus inverted microscope.

used micromanipulator systems are Research Instruments (Figure 17.7), Narashige and Eppendorf. Disposable micropipettes are available commerically from Cook, Humagen, the Pipette Company, Conception Technologies and Research Instruments.

Controlled rate embryo freezing machine

Any surplus good quality embryos can be cryopreserved. The choice of a freezing machine depends on whether straws or ampoules are used. Portable freezers have been recently introduced and are very economical on the liquid nitrogen consumption but can only be used for straws. For laboratories freezing in glass ampoules, cryo vials and straws, larger freezers such as Planar are more practical. The viability of frozen embryos is greatly dependent on the freezing machine as well as the freezing method.

General equipment

- Centrifuge for density gradient semen preparation.
- Refrigerator/freezer to store culture media and other media used for embryology and andrology. Culture media are very temperature sensitive. Certain amino acids

and proteins in the media can be inactivated by extreme temperatures and hence should be kept at 2–8 °C.

- Dry heat oven for sterilizing. For drying and sterilizing glass pipettes and other nondisposable items such as tweezers, spatulas and media-making glass ware.
- A four digit accurate weighing scale to weigh salts for making any kind of medium.
- A pH meter and an osmometer for laboratories making their own media.
- All laboratory equipment should be easy to use and maintain, but also have good service and repair facility. A log of servicing and maintenance should be kept.

Culture systems

There should be a separate designated sterile area for preparation of culture media. The reagents used should be of the highest purity. It is good practice to discard batches of reagents annually before the manufacturer's expiry date.

Glassware used for preparation should be well washed and sterilized (foil wrapped) and stored in a clean separate cabinet. All glass ware should be used within one month of the sterilization date or re-sterilized. Only tissue culture grade glassware that is boro silicate should be used in media preparation. The water used should also be of ultra pure quality (endotoxin free, low in ion content and free of organic molecules). This can either be purified in-house using a well maintained and serviced filtration unit (e.g. millipore) or bought commercially. Batch numbers of all reagents, water and disposables used in media making should be recorded. This aids trouble shooting and batch-to-batch variation. Home-made media should be subject to stringent quality control checks before use. Media should be stored in small aliquots (maximum 30–40 ml) at between 2 °C and 8 °C after preparation.

Commercially prepared media may be preferable for laboratories not equipped for quality control checks and the time required for preparation. The benefits of using commercially available media are that all the quality control testing has been done and mouse embryo assays have been carried out. All the certificates of analysis supplied by the manufacturer should be checked and kept for future reference.

Many laboratories are changing to use stage specific or 'sequential' media designed to meet the changing nutritional and metabolic requirements of the embryo during development. Sequential media has been used to achieve successful embryo culture up to day 5 (blastocyst stage) in vitro (Gardner 2000).

When using commercially prepared media it is important to follow the manufacturer's guidelines for use in order to obtain optimum results. For example, the Cook sequential medium works best at a 6% CO_2 concentration rather than 5%. When choosing the brand of commercially prepared culture medium, attention should be paid to the stringency of the quality control, cost and most importantly the reliability of supply. Other products commercially available, which have all undergone toxicity testing and are ready to use, are:

- Hyaluronidase (enzyme for denuding oocytes for ICSI).
- Poly vinyl pyrollidone (PVP to enable sperm immobilization).
- Paraffin/mineral oil (pre washed).
- Acid tyrodes.
- Embryo freezing and thawing media.
- Sperm freezing media.
- Sperm washing (hepes buffered) medium.
- Embryo biopsy medium.
- Blastocyst freeze/thaw medium.
- Follicle flushing media (heparinized saline can also be used).

When choosing a supplier of culture medium, importance should be given to the source of albumin in it. Most commercial suppliers use virology screened human serum albumin (HSA). However, culture media with recombinant HSA or synthetic serum substitute are also available. The use of maternal serum is slowly disappearing because of the risks associated with blood products. If laboratories do use maternal serum in home-made media then this should be strictly patient specific and not used as 'donor serum'.

The use of hepes in the culture system is also a concern since hepes is known to alter ion channel activity in the plasma membrane. This could be potentially toxic to embryos. However, consideration has to be given to the speed with which procedures are carried out and whether avoiding hepes may cause more damage in terms of pH imbalance. If hepes is used, the gametes or embryos must be thoroughly washed in hepes-free medium before returning them to culture.

Laboratory consumables

All plastic ware that is used in the laboratory should be proven to be nonembryo toxic. The most commonly used plastic ware in IVF laboratories are supplied by Falcon or Nunc. These brands have been extensively tested for their safe use in clinical IVF. All the plastic ware should be disposable and not re-used under any circumstances. All new batches should undergo in-house quality control testing before use. Batches that fail in-house checks should be returned. If possible new packs of dishes should be opened for each patient or each working day to keep the contents sterile. Resealing opened packs should be kept to a minimum. It is strongly recommended to use individually wrapped sterile pipette tips and plastic pipettes for inseminations and sperm preparation. This will minimize the potential risk of any cross-contamination.

Glass pipettes used for routine embryology should be boro silicate and not the cheaper soda glass since these are thought to leach minerals into the culture media. The pipettes should be double washed and sonicated in sterile water before being plugged with cotton wool and sterilized at 100 °C. Glass pipettes should be stored in special metal canisters and the number of pipettes in each should be kept to a minimum so that a new sterile can is opened each day. All pipettes should be flame polished before use. Pre-sterilized (gamma irradiated) and plugged pipettes are also commercially available.

Sterile nontoxic powder-free latex gloves should be worn during embryo transfer. The powder can be embryo toxic if it enters the dish. Gloves minimize the introduction of for example, contaminants and skin flora, into the incubator or culture system.

The choice of embryo transfer catheter is a joint decision between the clinician and the embryologist. Several factors have be taken into account when deciding which catheter to use. These are:

- The material used in making the catheter (embryo safe).
- Packaging/sterility.
- The lumen diameter of the inner sheath and the ease of loading the embryos.
- Embryos should be released in a minimum amount of medium.
- The ease of canulating the cervix.
- Cost.
- Any clinical trial results.

Quality control in the laboratory

All products that are used in clinical embryology should have undergone a quality control check by the manufacturer or be done in-house. Bacterial endotoxin levels, pH, osmolality, HSA virology screen and mouse embryo assay (MEA) should be checked.

In-house quality control testing can be done by the following methods. The sperm survival test is the most common in-house quality control test. A normal sample is prepared by either density gradient centrifugation or by swim-up method. An analysis is carried out after preparation and an equal amount is divided into two aliquots. The test and the control material (or new and old batch of medium/oil/ plastic ware) are added to the two aliquots and kept in the incubator. The samples are re-analysed for the percentage motility and progression after 24 and 48 hours. If results in both the groups are comparable with less then 3–5% variance then the test material is good enough for clinical use. If this test is satisfactory, further tests such as culturing of multi-pronucleate embryos or a blastocyst assay can be carried out and the embryonic development compared between batches of medium or oil. The quality of embryos and blastocyst formation rates are recorded on file. Batch-to-batch variation is common in paraffin/mineral oil and is cited as causing human embryo toxicity (Miller *et al.*, 1994). Each batch should be tested according to the above methods. Some laboratories prefer to eliminate the use of oil in their culture systems. However, the benefit of using an oil-based system is that oil acts as preventative barrier for the entry of any air borne pathogenic contaminants in the atmosphere.

Paraffin/mineral oil reduces the loss of pH and heat whilst the gametes and embryos are being manipulated thus preventing any form of thermal, osmotic or pH fluctuations. In addition, pre-equilibrated oil is thought to remove lipid soluble toxins from the culture medium thus enhancing embryonic development. It also prevents any evaporation of medium and allows the use of nonhumidifying incubators.

In addition to the quality control of new batches, it is also important to check regularly the performance of laboratory equipment, especially the incubators. There can be considerable fluctuations in temperature and CO_2 levels and the display may be inaccurate. It is therefore crucial to have additional referencing equipment to cross check the readings and adjust the incubators accordingly. Such equipment includes certified reference thermometers. Daily temperature logs should be taken of water baths, travel incubators, incubators and IVF chambers. This is best done first thing in the morning before any embryology work begins and record keeping is very essential to trouble-shoot cases of low or failed fertilization and retarded cleavage rates.

CO_2 analysers such as Anagas or Fyrite kits are useful to monitor daily CO_2 concentrations in the incubators and IVF chambers. If the analyser reading does not correlate with the display then the setting should be adjusted to set up perfect culture conditions. pH meters should be used weekly to countercheck the pH of equilibrated culture media. Media pH should be between 7.3 and 7.4. If the pH does not lie within this range, then the CO_2 levels in the incubators should be adjusted to achieve the correct pH.

The ultimate success of an IVF unit lies in its implantation, multiple pregnancy and live birth rates. The laboratory should also monitor fertilization rates, embryo quality and number of immature oocytes so that critical evaluation of laboratory and clinical practices can be regularly undertaken.

Laboratory procedures and policies

All the procedures carried out in the laboratory should be according to written protocols. These protocols should be evaluated and updated monthly and a copy kept in the reference manual for laboratory staff.

It is crucial to ensure patient details on dishes, tubes and laboratory forms are correct. Patient details should include name, medical number and date of birth. It is good practise that every procedure undertaken in the laboratory such as semen preparation, inseminations and embryo transfers should be witnessed by another member of the laboratory team.

ENDNOTES

Further information can be obtained from:
1. Royal College of Obstetricians and Gynaecologists, 27 Sussex Place, Regents Park, London NW1 4RG.
2. American Society for Reproductive Medicine, 1209 Montgomery Highway, Birmingham, Alabama 35216-2809, USA. Email asrm@asrm.com
3. Human Fertilisation and Embryology Authority, Paxton House, 30 Artillery Lane, London E1 7LS. www.hfea.gov.uk

REFERENCES

Almeida, P. A. & Bolton, V. N. (1995). The effect of temperature fluctuation on the cytoskeletal organisation and chromosomal constitution of the human oocyte. *Zygote* **3**: 357–65.

Effective Health Care (1992). *The Management of Subfertility*, No. 3. York: Centre for Health Economics, University of York.

Cohen, J., Gilligan, A., Esposito, W., Schimmel, T. & Dale, B. (1997). Ambient air and its potential effects on conception in vitro. *Hum. Reprod.* **12**: 1742–9.

Dumoulin, J. C., Meijers, C. J., Bras, M., Coonen, E., Geraedts, J. P. & Evers, J. L. (1999). Effect of oxygen concentration on human in-vitro fertilization and embryo culture. *Hum. Reprod.* **14**: 465–9.

Fisher, B., Schumacher, A., Hegele-Hartung, C. & Beier, H. M. (1988). Potential risk of light and room temperature exposure to preimplantation embryos. *Fertil. Steril.* **50**: 938–44.

Gardner, D. K. (2000). Blastocyst culture. Towards single embryo transfers. *Hum. Fertil.* **3**: 229–37.

Hirao, Y. & Yanagimachi, R. (1978). Detrimental effect of visible light on meiosis of mammalian eggs in vitro. *J. Exp. Zool.* **206**: 365–9.

Hu, Y., Betzendahl, I., Cortvrindt, R., Smitz, J. & Eichenlaub-Ritter, U. (2001). Effects of low O_2 and ageing on spindles and chromosomes in mouse oocytes from pre antral follicle culture. *Hum. Reprod.* **16**: 737–48.

Menezo, Y., Veiga, A. & Benkhalifa, M. (1998). Improved methods for blastocyst formation and culture. *Hum. Reprod.* (Suppl 4): 256–65.

Miller, K. F., Goldberg, J. M. & Collins, R. L. (1994). Covering embryo cultures with Mineral oil alters embryo growth by acting as a sink for an embryo toxic substance. *J. Assist. Reprod. Genet.* **11**: 342–5.

Templeton, A., Fraser, C. & Thompson, B. (1991). Infertility – epidemiology and referral practice. *Hum. Reprod.* **6**: 1391–4.

18

Information technology aspects of assisted conception

René van den Berg

Infertility Database Ltd, London, UK

Introduction

In general practice and in hospitals, computerized clinical records have been available for many years, but in assisted conception units information technology has been generally neglected. Until recently no commercial software specifically developed for assisted conception units has been available, probably because it is highly specialized with a relatively small market and there has been a lack of expertise in this area amongst commercial software suppliers. As clinicians strive to provide the best possible care to patients, information technology should be an integral part of that care and as important to the assisted conception unit as the latest intracytoplasmic sperm injection (ICSI) machine or microscope.

- Good software can increase the efficiency of all aspects of an assisted conception unit.
- The more efficient the processing of information, the more time can be spent on quality care.
- Data recording and analysis through computerized systems enhances the capability for quality control, thereby facilitating better success rates.
- Data recording and analysis through computerized systems enhances the capability for research, thereby facilitating progress in the speciality.

The ideal information technology solution

The ideal information technology solution is a totally integrated system, encompassing all areas of the daily clinical and administrative work routine.

The hardware infrastructure is important and computer workstations should be adequate and appropriately sited for easy access during the daily work routine. For example, if clinic staff must share workstations or if workstations are not sited conveniently, efficiency will be reduced.

Good Clinical Practice in Assisted Reproduction, ed. P. Serhal & C. Overton.
Published by Cambridge University Press. © Cambridge University Press 2004.

The ideal software integrates all aspects of the processing of information. There is little point in having a collection of databases, for example one to store laboratory details and another for patient demographics, because this leads to duplication of tasks with the increased margin for error inherent in the duplication process, and limits the capacity for cross-referencing information. The ideal software for an assisted conception unit should integrate:

- Patient appointments.
- Patient demographics.
- Contacts and correspondence.
- Patient general medical history.
- Previous treatments and investigations.
- Current treatment:
  - progress notes;
  - investigations, semen analyses;
  - drugs;
  - ultrasound follicle tracking;
  - laboratory data, egg collection, embryo transfer;
  - outcomes.
- Image recording and display.
- Drug prescriptions.
- Semen and embryo storage recording.
- Treatment cycle outcome and other statistics.
- Standard letters and reports.
- Integration with laboratory equipment.
- Billing.
- Government required reporting facilities, such as SART (North America), NPSU (Australia) and HFEA (UK).
- Web-based and multi-site capabilities.
- Voice recognition.
- Bar coding facilities.
- E-mail integration.

Where patients are registered through a central hospital system, interaction with existing hospital systems is sometimes appropriate, and seamless interfacing between the clinic software and the hospital system should be achieved. This may also apply to billing systems, particularly in North America.

The assisted conception unit and information technology: a scenario

The following scenario is intended to give the reader an overview of the possible application of information technology in an assisted conception unit. At the end of each section the advantages of a computerized system over a paper-based system are listed.

The scenario
Clinic statistics

A prospective patient rings the assisted conception unit for information. She knows that she needs fertility treatment and is particularly interested in the unit's pregnancy rates. Because the nurse taking the call has access to computer records, within seconds the prospective patient can be given up-to-date pregnancy rates.

- Software can provide 'instant' access to information and the individual assisted conception unit statistics.

Demographic details, contacts and correspondence log

The prospective patient asks for more information to be sent. Using the computer, the nurse records the prospective patient's basic demographic details (name, address, telephone number, e-mail address) and subsequently selects from the computer the appropriate information pack from a number of standard letters, reports and information sheets. A covering letter is automatically created with the prospective patient's demographics and stored in the contact and correspondence log, which contains details of all the contacts between the patient and assisted conception unit. The nurse enters a short summary of the conversation and a follow-up date to contact the prospective patient to confirm that the information has been received. The information is e-mailed to the prospective patient (or printed and posted).

- Computerized standard letters and reports linked to other parts of the database facilitate streamlined 'customer service'.
- E-mail direct to the patient eliminates the need for printing and posting.
- A computerized contact log records all patient contacts and facilitates follow-up.
- A computerized contact log can be used as a medico-legal tool.

Appointment scheduling and e-mail integration

A few days later, the prospective patient again rings the assisted conception unit. The nurse of previous contact is unavailable. The receptionist accesses the computerized contact log with the details of all previous contacts with the caller. An appointment is made in seconds by using the 'next available appointment' feature. An e-mail confirming the appointment details is sent to the patient.

- The computerized contact log provides continuity of 'client care' regardless of the member of staff available.
- A central computerized appointment booking system is efficient and eliminates the confusion/duplication often caused by noncentralized paper-based appointment booking.

Consultation, diagnosis, image recording and internal messaging

On arrival for the appointment, additional demographic details are entered on the computer by the receptionist. During the initial consultation the clinician enters details of the past medical history and other relevant medical information. Pre-constituted adaptable lists minimize the keyboarding required. Images of previous investigations performed elsewhere, for example ultrasound or laparoscopy, can be scanned into the computer and stored in the patient's personal image library.

Meanwhile, in the laboratory the embryologist enters the result of a basic semen analysis into the laboratory computer and by internal messaging this is received on the clinician's computer in the consulting room. (At a later stage, the embryologist may record semen preparations, detailed morphology, immunological parameters, etc., or record the freezing and storage of the sample.)

Although the ultimate goal is a 'paperless office', at the end of the consultation a printout of the medical history and examination findings can be generated if desired.

- Computerized pre-constituted formats reduce keyboarding (which can be done from written copy immediately following the consultation, if desired).
- The 'paperless office' is possible, but a legible printed copy is always an option.
- The computer ability to record images facilitates a comprehensive record of investigations.
- Computerized internal messaging streamlines the sharing of information.

Treatment plan and protocol

An individual treatment plan for IVF/ICSI is established and recorded on the computer. A computerized treatment protocol automatically assigns blood tests, ultrasound scans and drug schedules for down-regulation, stimulation and luteal support. This information can be accessed from the nurse's computer to initiate ovarian down-regulation and stimulation.

- Standard treatment protocols in assisted conception are particularly suited to computerization.
- Computerized, pre-defined standard treatment protocols dramatically reduce keyboarding.

Drug prescriptions, dispensing and investigations

Drug prescriptions are generated through the software using the pre-defined treatment protocols and, if dispensed in-house, a computerized stock list tracks the dispensing of drugs.

Results of hormone screening and ultrasounds are recorded on the computer. Follicle numbers and sizes are recorded graphically on the computer on a standardized form that also displays hormone levels and drugs, giving a snapshot overview of key details of the treatment cycle.

- Computerized prescribing and dispensing facilitates tracking of drug stores.
- Investigation results can be 'instantly' imported from the laboratory or equipment.
- Capability for on-screen 'snapshot' including graphics of key details of the treatment cycle.
- Data can be accessed from any workstation, thereby eliminating search for paper-based records.

Progress notes

During the treatment cycle, various members of staff are updating the patient record as part of the daily work routine and this complete record is instantly available at other workstations for access by other staff members at any given time.

- The computerized patient record is always completely up-to-date.

Billing

All items and procedures are automatically linked to the patient's billing record as they are entered into various areas of the computer system, and up-to-date accounts can be generated when required. In North America, insurance billing packages can be integrated with clinic management software, thereby preserving the ultimate aim of integrated software.

- Integrated software, linking patient records with billing, facilitates 'instant' accounting.

Laboratory details

During the egg collection, fertilization and embryo tracking, data is constantly entered onto the patient's computerized record as part of the daily work routine. Digital image capture devices and other integrated equipment (e.g. laser zona drilling devices) allows the import of embryo images and associated data. For good quality control embryos are tracked individually so that blastocyst culturing, media changes and handling by different embryologists can all be recorded.

- Integrated software linking patient records with laboratory procedures and the capacity for storing images facilitates quality control and research.

Embryo and semen storage

Some of the embryos are frozen for later use and the computer system records, for example, storage location, consent, expiry. With the use of standard letters, patients can be notified of consent expiry and charges for storage are generated through the integrated billing.

- A computer-based system allows much more effective checking of stored embryos and semen.

Treatment cycle, pregnancy outcome and reporting

Two weeks later, the patient has a positive pregnancy test and this is recorded on the system. A treatment summary report is submitted online to a government body (or printed if required). Government reporting of assisted reproductive treatment is compulsory in a number of countries and software is able to generate the reports or files in the required format to allow this reporting without duplication of work.
- Computerized record-keeping enhances the recording of outcomes.
- Computerized record-keeping facilitates mandatory reporting.

Audit trail and security

An audit trail logs all changes made to data, so that one can always identify who has made what changes. In addition, general password security and different security levels can be set to allow or deny users access to particular parts of the system.
- Security is enhanced by audit trail tracking changes and setting access rights.

Software: buy or DIY?

Basically, there are two options for acquiring the ideal software: develop your own or buy a commercially available package. Due to the lack of commercially available software, in the past a number of clinics have resorted to creating their own software package. For example, a member of staff who is either proficient or not in database design may set about writing the program, but the latter seems usually to have been the case.

Designing your own software

Designing a database system in-house has a number of *apparent* advantages:
- Tailor-made to individual needs
  Advantage: software tailor-made to meet the requirements of the individual assisted conception unit is probably the greatest apparent advantage. Although it may closely match a unit's requirements, commercially available software is often less specific to individual user needs.
  Disadvantage:
  – developing software is extremely time-consuming and this could compromise the usual work of the assisted conception unit;
  – the programming skills of staff members are probably inadequate and may result in severe design flaws that only come to light after some time;

- implementing new software is temporarily disruptive and time and data can be lost to 'teething' problems that need to be dealt with promptly and effectively. Some aspects of the software may need to be rewritten;
- technical documentation may be inadequate and this can be disastrous when trying to recover or retrieve data;
- what happens when the in-house software 'expert' moves on?

- Economical

  Advantage: if a staff member develops a system in-house, there is no payment required for professional programmers and commercial software. Commercial software can cost around US$25 000.

  Disadvantage: it is likely that the total cost of in-house software, in terms of disruption, lost time, lost data, workplace tensions and general aggravation, will exceed the cost of professional programmers and commercial software that has a proven track record.

- Software source code ownership/flexibility

  Advantage: if the software is written in-house, then the software ownership and source code are in-house. Any modifications specific to the assisted conception unit can be easily applied and the fate of the software is determined by the unit, rather than relying on the continued existence of an outside company.

  Disadvantage: the greatest pitfall is that the software ownership and source code belong to the person who wrote the software, unless a specific agreement to the contrary was signed. Many assisted conception units are not aware of this and when the writer of the program moves on the software can be taken with them.

- On-site support

  Advantage: having the writer of the program on-site means instant availability to deal with problems arising.

  Disadvantage: unless the clinic employs the writer of the program solely for this purpose, he/she may be performing other duties or be on leave when problems arise. With remote access support, the trained and help-desk dedicated staff of commercial suppliers can analyse and rectify problems more quickly, assuming that the supplier of the commercial software provides good support services with remote access capability.

Commercially available software

The cost of commercial software for the assisted conception market generally starts at around US$1000 per month, or US$25 000 to purchase outright, mainly due to its specialized nature. However, it is possible for an assisted conception unit a good commercial software package to recoup the cost within six months of installation by increased efficiency and productivity and a reduction in ongoing expenses.

Which software to buy?

Although it may closely match a unit's requirements, commercially available software is often less specific to individual user needs but should be flexible enough to accommodate individual variations, or the supplier should be able to provide customization at a reasonable rate. The best guide to good commercial software is a proven track record of effective use by a number of clients. Software with a large user base is more likely to be consistently improved and developed based on user input. The supplier organization should be sound and able to provide ongoing software support, preferably via toll free numbers.

Characteristics of good commercially available software:

- Software must have proven track record
- Supplier must have proven track record
- Software must have a large client base
- Supplier must be able to provide satisfactory references to established users
- Telephone and remote access software support should be available.

The UCH Infertility Database Systems Ltd provides all the above characteristics.

Implementation

Taking an integrated approach to the installation and implementation of your computer system will ensure that maximum advantage is gained. For example, one area that is often neglected is staff orientation and training that can overcome any fears the staff may have of change and of new technology. If a positive attitude to the installation of a new computer system is engendered, efficient use of the system will be maximized. A number of conditions must be met for successful installation and implementation and your software supplier should make you aware of these.

- A computer network should have hardware with sufficient power to run the software at satisfactory speed.
- Computer monitors must be of adequate size. Most software is written for screen resolutions of at least 800 × 600 pixels. Although this resolution is compatible with 14-inch screens, technically a 14-inch screen is too small for comfortable use. Computer monitors should be at least 15-inch but preferably 17-inch or larger. Space restrictions are often an issue, particularly in ultrasound scanning rooms and laboratories. LCD monitors are the ideal solution, as they take up less space and emit less radiation.
- To optimize efficiency, the number of workstations must be adequate. Wherever there is a desk and a telephone, there should be a workstation. Additionally, there should be workstations in any areas where data is collected, for example the laboratory and operating theatre.

- Multiple or branch clinics should be linked. Using wide area networks or the Internet, it is possible to link multiple clinics, and your software supplier must be able to advise you on this.
- If you have existing electronic data, it is advisable to ask your supplier to transfer these into your new software. Your software supplier must be able to advise you on the various options available to reduce costs.
- Staff orientation and training is extremely important to achieve a positive attitude to changes and ultimately to optimize efficiency. Your software supplier should be able to organize on-site visits to other users for the purpose of orientation and to advise you on and organize comprehensive staff training.

19

Assisted reproductive technology and older women

Paul Serhal

Assisted Conception Unit, UCLH, London, UK

The life expectancy of women has increased significantly over the past century and the advent of efficient contraception has given women the opportunity to choose when to have children. At present many women delay childbearing for a variety of social and economic reasons, including higher education, a career and economic pressure to remain at work, that have contributed to a constant increase in older women seeking treatment for infertility (Medical Research International, 1990). The trend towards older parenting is evident in the general population (Baldwin & Windquist Nord, 1995) and the number of births for every thousand British women in their early 30s has exceeded that of women in their early 20s (Office of Population Censuses and Surveys, 1994).

Fecundity

Female fecundity is generally acknowledged to decrease by the age of 30 years (van Noord-Zaadstra *et al.*, 1991; Leridon, 1977). The decline is gradual until a rapid decline from the age of 35 years and by the age of 45 years fecundity is almost lost (Navot *et al.*, 1987). Women aged over 35 years take longer to conceive and a higher proportion will never achieve a pregnancy when compared to younger women (Navot *et al.*, 1991). This decline is related to a process of follicular depletion and diminished oocyte quality.

Follicular depletion

The ovarian function is limited by the size of the follicular store laid down pre-natally. Approximately seven million human germ cells are formed in fetal ovaries, with only two million remaining at birth and around 300 000 remaining at the menarche (Gosden, 1987). The reduction in the number of oocytes is a dynamic process that continues throughout a woman's premenarcheal and menstrual life.

Good Clinical Practice in Assisted Reproduction, ed. P. Serhal & C. Overton.
Published by Cambridge University Press. © Cambridge University Press 2004.

Further, it has been reported that with advanced age there is a decreased ovarian response to an increased amount of gonadotrophin stimulation, measured by follicle recruitment and steroidogenesis (Sharma *et al.*, 1988; Hughes *et al.*, 1989; Jacobs *et al.*, 1990). The rate of oocyte depletion varies with the genetic line (Faddy *et al.*, 1983) and this variability manifests itself in assisted reproductive technology (ART) programs when some young women respond unexpectedly poorly to ovarian stimulation and some older women respond unexpectedly well.

Oocyte quality

Fertility is markedly compromised several years before the menopause, suggesting that factors other than complete depletion of the follicular store play a role in the loss of oocyte competency in ageing women (Wu *et al.*, 2000). The reduced reproductive potential of older women is related to the functional and structural qualities of the oocytes (Navot *et al.*, 1991).

Using high resolution confocal microscopy, the effects of maternal ageing on the meioitic apparatus in young (20–25 years) and older (40–45 years) women were examined (Battaglia *et al.*, 1996) and it was demonstrated that the meiotic spindle in older women is frequently abnormal with regard to both chromosomal alignment and the microtubule matrix that comprise the meiotic spindle. In 79% of the oocytes from older women, the spindle exhibited abnormal tubulin placement and one or more chromosomes were displaced from the metaphase plate during the second meiotic division. In contrast, in young women the majority of the oocytes had well-ordered meioitic spindle-containing chromosomes that were fully aligned within a distinct metaphase in the spindle, and only 17% exhibited aneuploid conditions. Maternal ageing is associated with an increased incidence of nondysjunction or aneuploidy (autosomal trisomy) in the offspring (Hassold & Jacobs, 1984). The rate of early pregnancy loss increases significantly for those in their 30s and is >50% after the age of 40 years (Navot *et al.*, 1991).

It has been suggested that poor embryonic development and implantation failure in some patients (Brenner *et al.*, 2000) may be related to mitochondrial dysfunction and/or reduced metabolic activity. Older women have fewer intact, nondeleted copies of mitochondrial DNA (mtDNA) in their oocytes resulting from mtDNA susceptibility to the ageing process (St John & Barrat, 1997). A recent investigation of a point mutation (T414G) in the control region of the mtDNA showed that the oocytes of young patients (26–36 years) exhibited this mtDNA mutation in only 4.4% of oocytes compared to 39.5% in the older age group (37–42 years) ($P < 0.01$). It was suggested that since this mutation exists in the control region of the mtDNA it may affect the regulation of mtDNA transcription and replication during oocyte and post-embryonic development (Barritt *et al.*, 2000).

Other factors affecting fertility in older women

Older women are more likely to be affected by a number of pathologies that can reduce their fertility potential.

Menstrual cycle and ovulation

In older women the follicular phase is significantly shorter (Sherman *et al.*, 1979) but the luteal phase is not affected and, if anything, can be longer (Gindoff & Jewelewicz, 1986). Increasing maternal age is also associated with an increase in ovulatory dysfunction (Doring, 1969).

Uterine receptivity

A number of physiological and molecular markers of normal implantation have been developed (Edwards, 1995) but the application of probes for specific endometrial markers in the assessment of endometrial receptivity in a clinical setting is still a long way off. Consequently, reduction in uterine receptivity as a possible contributing factor to the decline in fertility with age has been difficult to ascertain. However, from studies using the oocyte donation model and comparing pregnancy, implantation and abortion rates in young and older oocyte recipients, there is increasing evidence of an age-related decrease in uterine receptivity (Flamigni *et al.*, 1993; Cano *et al.*, 1995; Borini, *et al.*, 1996) and reduced vascular perfusion of the uterus is demonstrated by Doppler ultrasound scan studies (Goswamy *et al.*, 1988).

Other contributing factors

Uterine fibroids are thought to occur in 30% of women over the age of 30 years (Anderson & Barbieri, 1995) and fibroids that distort the uterine cavity can significantly reduce the chances of successful implantation (Farhi *et al.*, 1995). Endometriosis is more commonly diagnosed in older women and the association of endometriosis with infertility is well documented. Further, deciliation of the fallopian tubal endothelium may increase with age (Crow *et al.*, 1994).

Predictors of outcome of assisted reproduction treatment

The prediction of outcome is important because it gives the clinician and patient realistic expectations of the chances for pregnancy, and can identify women who are destined for failure and who should not undergo treatment (Licciardi *et al.*, 1995).

It is well established that age is the main determinant of the success of fertility treatment. The presence of a regular ovulatory cycle does not preclude the possibility of a poor response to gonadotrophin stimulation, because the ovary has the ability to maintain a surprisingly constant frequency and number of ovulations whilst follicle reserve continuously dwindles (Gosden, 1987).

Elevated basal follicle stimulating hormone (FSH) (>15 iu/l) is associated with poor IVF performance (Scott *et al.*, 1989). Basal FSH and chronological age in combination have been shown to be good predictors of IVF outcome (Toner *et al.*, 1991) and for controlled ovarian stimulation (COS) combined with intrauterine insemination (IUI) (Pearlstone *et al.*, 1992). However, women with normal basal FSH levels do not always respond well to ovarian stimulation (Farhi *et al.*, 1997).

The clomiphene citrate challenge test and the gonadotrophin-releasing hormone agonist (GnRHa) test have been proposed as dynamic or provocative tests to un-mask poor ovarian reserve in women with normal basal FSH (Navot *et al.*, 1987; Muasher *et al.*, 1988; Galtier-Dereur *et al.*, 1996). Because GnRHa is routinely used in combination with gonadotrophins for ovarian stimulation in IVF treatment, the GnRHa test performed during the IVF treatment cycle is practical and convenient. The administration of a GnRHa induces an initial surge of FSH, luteinizing hormone (LH) and 17-β oestradiol (E2) flare-up, followed by pituitary desensitization. The E2 response (ΔE2) to stimulation reflects the functional integrity of the follicles and it has been demonstrated that the simultaneous evaluation of basal FSH and E2 response to ovarian stimulation is the most sensitive predictor available for response to ovarian stimulation (Ranieri *et al.*, 1998). The result of the GnRHa test and the basal FSH can be used to counsel patients in the older age group before starting treatment.

Controlled ovarian stimulation with intrauterine insemination

It has been demonstrated that COS/IUI can be an effective first-line treatment for women with unexplained infertility and is less invasive and less expensive than IVF (Serhal *et al.*, 1988). However, the efficacy of COS/IUI in the management of women aged 40 years and over is significantly reduced. A 5.6% cycle fecundity was reported in women aged 40 years or over (Legro *et al.*, 1997) and 5% in women aged over 40, compared to 21% in women aged under 30 years (Dodson & Haney, 1991). A pregnancy rate of 3.5% and live birth rate of 1.2% was reported from 402 cycles in 85 women aged 40 years or older, using a variety of stimulation regimens and medications (Pearlstone *et al.*, 1992).

Regardless of age, with COS/IUI treatment most pregnancies will occur in the first four treatment cycles.

IVF/gamete intrafallopian transfer (GIFT)

It is now well recognized that with increasing maternal age there is a substantial drop in live births per IVF treatment cycle. In 1999, national data statistics on 21 733

IVF cycles over all maternal age groups show a live birth rate per cycle of 7.3% at aged 41–42 years, 3% at 43–44 years and 0.5% at >45 years (Human Fertilisation and Embryology Authority, 1999). These statistics clearly illustrate that biological ageing of the oocytes is a physiological process that cannot be reversed with IVF.

Ovarian stimulation for IVF/GIFT

An important determinant of success with IVF is the ovarian response to go-nadotrophin stimulation resulting in an optimal number of good-quality eggs and embryos (Roest *et al.*, 1996). It is well recognized that advanced age is correlated with a low response to ovarian stimulation and to a poor prognosis for IVF (Licciardi *et al.*, 1995). With increasing maternal age the ovaries became more resistant to exogenous gonadotrophin stimulation. Increased maternal age is associated with a progressive decline in the ovarian response to gonadotrophin treatment in terms of the number of oocytes retrieved and cancelled treatment cycles (Sharma *et al.*, 1988; Hughes *et al.*, 1989). Receptors for the GnRH have been found in ovarian gran-ulosa cells (Liscoviych & Amsterdam, 1989). In addition, it has been shown that women undergoing ovarian stimulation using the long GnRHa down-regulation drug regimen had a high dose of gonadotrophin and a lower number of oocytes retrieved (Hazout *et al.*, 1993). Excessive down-regulation can be detrimental to ovarian response in patients with reduced ovarian reserve. Such patients may ben-efit from cessation of GnRHa upon down-regulation combined with high-dose gonadotrophin stimulation (Faber *et al.*, 1998; Dirnfeld *et al.*, 1999). Alternatively, a gonadotrophin releasing hormone antagonist can be used (see Chapter 14).

Our pre-stimulation protocol includes a basal FSH assessment and GnRHa test to predict the response pattern and facilitate individualizing the ovarian stimula-tion regimen (Ranieri *et al.*, 1998). Women with diminished ovarian reserve ($\Delta E2$ <180 pmol/l and/or FSH >9.5 iu/l but not >15 iu/l) may benefit from com-mencing down-regulation in the mid-luteal phase, followed by cessation of GnRHa administration on the first day of menstruation. This protocol, in combination with gonadotrophin 375 IU daily for ovarian stimulation, rescued some treatment cycles that would otherwise have been cancelled if a conventional drug regimen was used, and a satisfactory pregnancy rate was achieved (Ranieri *et al.*, 2001).

It is suggested that women aged >40 years with FSH >15 iu/l and $\Delta E2$ <180 pmol/l have a very poor prognosis with ART and should be advised not to undergo IVF treatment.

Donor insemination

The chances of success with donor insemination are well known to decrease with age. In France, a CECOS (Centre d'Etude et de Conservation du Sperme Humain) study of the results of donor sperm insemination in over 2000 nulliparous women with azoospermic husbands shows a significant decrease in the cumulative success rate for women aged >30 years (Schwartz et al., 1982). The mean success rate per cycle was 10.5% aged 26–30 years, 9.1% aged 31–35 years and 6.5% aged >35 years. In the United Kingdom, the Human Fertilisation and Embryology Authority database on donor insemination shows 10–12% live births per treatment cycle in women aged <30 years, 9% at 35–39 years and 3–4% at >40 years (Human Fertilisation and Embryology Authority, 1999).

Oocyte donation

As many as 10% of women have ovarian failure by the age of 40 years (Leridon 1977). Serhal & Craft (1989) introduced the notion that reproductive potential might be extended to women aged >40 years who have already entered the menopause. Menstrually cyclic women with poor response to gonadotrophin stimulation or repetitive IVF failure can also benefit from egg donation (see Chapter 10).

Assisted hatching

Embryo hatching is a fundamental requirement for implantation. The zona pellucida is the glycoprotein layer just external to the oolemma. It has been suggested that in humans, zona hardening can be induced by the in vitro culture conditions (Cohen et al., 1990) and increased maternal age. The hypothesis of assisted hatching (AH) is that an alteration of the zona pellucida, either by drilling a hole through it or by thinning it, will promote hatching of embryos otherwise entrapped within the zona pellucida (Cohen et al., 1990).

A randomized controlled trial (Cohen et al., 1992) demonstrated that AH was most efficient in women aged >38 years and in those with elevated FSH levels, indicating a possible correlation between age, basal FSH and physical or chemical changes in the zona pellucida. Other studies have reported the benefits of AH in women with repetitive IVF failure (Schoolcraft et al., 1994) and in women aged >40 years (Schoolcraft et al., 1995).

Controversy regarding AH arose when some centres failed to derive the same benefits from AH and prospective randomized trials showed no benefit from AH in all patients (Hellebaut et al., 1996; Edirisinghe et al., 1999) and in patients >38 years (Lanzendorf et al., 1998).

Blastocyst transfer

For optimal growth, human embryos require a very specific environment that varies through the different stages of development and standard IVF culture media cannot meet these specific demands. Consequently, embryo transfers have been traditionally performed two days after insemination, at the 2- to 4-cell stage, whilst in a natural cycle the embryo reaches the uterine cavity on the fourth or fifth day after ovulation at the blastocyst stage (Croxatto *et al.*, 1972). With the introduction of sequential culture media designed to meet the changing physiological and metabolic need of developing embryos (Gardner *et al.*, 1996), it is now possible to culture fertilized oocytes successfully up to the blastocyst stage.

The ability to develop to the blastocyst stage can be a good indicator of oocyte developmental competence in older women and can facilitate diagnosis in women who produce oocytes that consistently fail to reach the blastocyst stage after fertilization (Jones *et al.*, 1998). Moreover, whilst development to the blastocyst stage does not necessarily exclude the possibility of chromosomal abnormality, the inability to do so excludes a substantial proportion of chromosomally abnormal embryos (Jones & Trounson, 1999). However, not all women are suitable for blastocyst transfer (Sholtes & Zeilmaker, 1996; Coskun *et al.*, 2000) and, rather than growth to the blastocyst stage, some may benefit from an early transfer (Tsirigotis, 1998).

Published data on the effect of maternal age on blastocyst transfer is limited and inconclusive. While some studies report reduced blastocyst development with increasing maternal age (Janny & Menezo, 1996; Sholtes & Zeilmaker, 1996; Pantos *et al.*, 1999) others have found that maternal age did not have any effect on blastocyst formation (Schoolcraft *et al.*, 1999; Coskun *et al.*, 2000). Rather than maternal age, the chance of successful blastocyst transfer seems to depend on the number of oocytes retrieved (Sholtes & Zeilmaker, 1996; Schoolcraft *et al.*, 1999), but the pregnancy rate with blastocyst transfer remains significantly lower in women aged >40 years.

Preimplatation genetic diagnosis (PGD) of aneuploidies

It has been demonstrated that aneuploidy in morphologically and developmentally normal embryos markedly increases with maternal age (Munne *et al.*, 1995). Consequently, it has been suggested that the use of PGD in older women could improve the success of IVF (Gianaroli *et al.*, 1999). PGD requires IVF, 1- or 2-cell biopsy on the third day after fertilization and genetic analysis of the cell(s), followed by selective transfer of euploid embryos. The biopsy does not interfere with in vitro embryo development (Hardy *et al.*, 1990). Fluorescent in situ hybridization (FISH) is the preferred method for sexing of embryos (Delhanty, 1994) and for testing different autosomes (Munne *et al.*, 1993; Harper *et al.*, 1995). This technique involves in situ hybridization of the embryonic cell nucleus with fluochrome-labelled chromosome-specific probes producing different colour signals for each chromosome tested (Harper *et al.*, 1994).

Although PGD seems an attractive idea for older women undergoing IVF, it has certain clinical and technical limitations. It is well established that the success of IVF with PGD is very much dependent on the number of oocytes/embryos available for transfer (Vandervorst *et al.*, 1998) and a significant number of women aged >40 years produce a limited number of oocytes/embryos. Consequently, PGD may not be an option for a significant number of women aged >40 years as there may be insufficient embryos for biopsy or transfer. In addition, FISH is subject to technical difficulties that limit the number of chromosomes to be analysed simultaneously in a single cell. Consequently, fewer than half the chromosome complement can be analysed in any one cell (Wells & Delhanty, 2000). A full analysis of the copy number of all 24 chromosome cell types is mandatory to ascertain the incidence of aneuploidy and mosaicism in human embryos.

Comparative genomic hybridization (CGH) is a revolutionary technique that allows a full analysis of all chromosomes (Kallioniemi, 1992) and has been successfully applied on single cells of human preimplantation embryos (Wells & Delhanty, 2000). Although the early data are promising, the major drawback of CGH is the long hybridization time and more work needs to be done to reduce this before applying the technique to PGD. Alternatively, the biopsied embryo can be transferred at the blastocyst stage or cryopreserved allowing extra time for the diagnosis.

Pregnancy complications in older women

Maternal mortality is closely related to both maternal age and parity. The mortality rate for women over 40 is now higher than the rate for grand multiparous women. Maternal death rates rise from 7.6 per 100 000 maternities in women <20 years to 30.3 in women of 40 years and older (Department of Health, 1988).

Obstetric complications such as gestational diabetes, hypertension, placenta praevia, abruptio placenta and preterm delivery are more common in women aged >40 years (Naeye, 1983; Tuck *et al.*, 1988).

Co-existing medical problems are more common in women >40 years. Pre-pregnancy counselling should include a general health check in order to optimize maternal health prior to pregnancy.

REFERENCES

Anderson, J. & Barbieri, R. L. (1995). Abnormal gene expression in uterine leiomyomas. *J. Soc. Gynecol. Invest.* **2**: 663–72.

Baldwin, W. H. & Winquist Nord, C. (1995). Delayed childbearing in the United States: fact and fictions. *Popul. Bull.* **39**: 14–23.

Barritt, J. A., Cohen, J. & Brenner, C. A. (2000). Mitochondrial DNA point mutation in human oocytes is associated with maternal age. *Reprod. Biomed.* **1**: 96–100.

Battaglia, D. E., Goodwin, P., Klein, N. A. & Soules, M. R. (1996). Influence of maternal age on meiotic spindle assembly in oocytes from naturally cycling women. *Hum. Reprod.* **11**: 2217–22.

Borini, A., Bianchi, L., Violini, F. *et al.* (1996). Oocyte donation program: pregnancy and implantation rates in women of different ages sharing oocytes from a single donor. *Fertil. Steril.* **65**: 94–7.

Brenner, C., Barritt, J., Willasden, S. & Cohen, J. (2000). Mitochondrial DNA heteroplasmy after human ooplasmic transplantation. *Fertil. Steril.* **74**: 573–8.

Cano, F., Simon, C. & Remohi, J. (1995). Effect of ageing on the female reproductive system: evidence for a role of uterine senescence in the decline in female fecundity. *Fertil. Steril.* **64**: 584–9.

Cohen, J., Elsner, C., Kort, H., Malter, H., Mayer, M. P. & Weimer, K. (1990). Impairment of hatching process following IVF in the human and improvement of implantation by assisted hatching using micromanipulation. *Hum. Reprod.* **5**: 7–13.

Cohen, J., Alikani, M., Trowbridge, J. & Rosenwaks, Z. (1992). Implantation enhancement by selective assisted hatching using zona drilling of human embryos with poor prognosis. *Hum. Reprod.* **7**: 685–91.

Coskun, S., Hollanders, J., Al-Hassam, S., Al-Sufyan, H., Al-Mayman, H. & Jaroudi, K. (2000). Day 5 versus day 3 embryo transfer: a controlled randomised trial. *Hum. Reprod.* **15**: 1947–52.

Crow, J., Amso, N. A., Lewin, J. *et al.* (1994). Morphology and ultrastructure of the fallopian tubes epithelium at different stages of the menstrual cycle and menopause. *Hum. Reprod.* **12**: 2224–33.

Croxatto, H. B., Fuentealba, B., Diaz, S. *et al.* (1972). A simple non-surgical technique to obtain unimplanted eggs from human uteri. *Am. J. Obstet. Gynecol.* **112**: 662–8.

Delhanty, J. D. A. (1994). Preimplantation diagnosis. *Prenat. Diagn.* **14**: 1217–27.

Department of Health (1988). *Why Mothers Die. Report on Confidential Enquiries into Maternal Deaths in the United Kingdom* London: Department of Health.

Dirnfeld, M., Fruchter, O. & Yshai, D. (1999). Cessation of gonadotrophin-releasing hormone (GnRH analogue) upon down-regulation versus conventional long GnRH analogue protocol in poor responders undergoing in vitro fertilisation. *Fertil. Steril.* **72**: 406–11.

Dodson, W. C. & Haney, A. F. (1991). Controlled ovarian hyperstimulation and intrauterine insemination for treatment of infertility. *Fertil. Steril.* **55**: 457–67.

Doring, G. K. (1969). The incidence of anovulatory cycles in women. *J. Reprod. Fertil.* **6** (Suppl.): 77–81.

Edirisinghe, W. R., Ahnonkitpanit, V., Promviengchai, S. *et al.* (1999). A study failing to determine significant benefits from assisted hatching: patients selected for advanced age, zonal thickness of embryos, and previous failed attempts. *J. Assist. Reprod. Genet.* **16**: 294–301.

Edwards, R. G. (1995). Physiological and molecular aspects of human implantation. *Hum. Reprod.* **10**: 1–13.

Faber, B. M., Mayer, J. & Cox, B. (1998). Cessation of gonadotropin-releasing hormone agonist therapy combined with high-dose gonadotropin stimulation yields favourable pregnancy results in poor responders. *Fertil. Steril.* **69**: 826–30.

Faddy, M. J., Gosden, R. G. & Edwards, R. G. (1983). Ovarian follicle dynamics in mice; a comparative study of three inbred strains and an F1 hybrid. *J. Endocrinol.* **96**: 23–33.

Farhi, J., Ashkenazi, J., Feldberg, D., Dicker, D., Orvieto, R. & Ben Rafael, Z. (1995). Effect of uterine leiomyomata on the results of in vitro fertilisation treatment. *Hum. Reprod.* **10**: 2576–8.

Farhi, J., Homburg, R., Ferber, A., Orvieto, R. & Ben Rafael, Z. (1997). Non-response to ovarian stimulation in normogonadotrophic, normogonadal women: a clinical sign of impending onset of ovarian failure pre-empting the rise in basal follicle stimulating hormone levels. *Hum. Reprod.* **12**: 241–3.

Flamigni, C., Borini, A. & Violini, F. (1993). Oocyte donation: comparison between recipients from different age groups. *Hum. Reprod.* **8**: 2088–92.

Galtier-Dereur, F., De Bouard, V., Picot, M. C. *et al.* (1996). Ovarian reserve test with gonadotrophin-releasing hormone agonist buserelin: correlation with in vitro-fertilisation outcome. *Hum. Reprod.* **11**: 1393–8.

Gardner, D. K., Lane, M., Calderon, I. & Leeton, J. (1996). Environment of the preimplantation human embryo in vivo: metabolic analysis of oviduct and uterine fluids during the menstrual cycle and metabolism of cumulus cells. *Fertil. Steril.* **65**: 349–53.

Gianaroli, L., Magli, M. C., Ferrareti, A. P. & Munne, S. (1999). Preimplantation diagnosis for aneuploidies in patients undergoing in vitro fertilisation with a poor prognosis: identification of the categories for which it should be proposed. *Fertil. Steril.* **72**: 837–44.

Gindoff, P. R. & Jewelewicz, R. (1986). Reproductive potential in the older woman. *Fertil. Steril.* **46**: 989–100.

Gosden, R. G. (1987). Follicular status at the menopause. *Hum. Reprod.* **2**: 617–21.

Goswamy, R., Williams, G. & Steptoe, P. C. (1988). Decreased uterine perfusion – a cause of infertility. *Hum. Reprod.* **3**: 955–9.

Hardy, K., Martin, K. L., Leese, H. J., Winston, R. M. & Handyside, A. H. (1990). Human preimplantation development in vitro is not adversely affected by biopsy at the 8-cell stage. *Hum. Reprod.* **5**: 708–14.

Harper, J. C., Coonen, E., Handyside, A. H. *et al.* (1995). Mosaicism of autosomes and sex chromosomes in morphologically normal, monospermic preimplantation human embryos. *Prenat. Diagn.* **15**: 41–9.

Harper, J. C., Coonen, E., Ramaekers, F. C. S. *et al.* (1994). Identification of the sex of human preimplantation embryos in two hours using an improved spreading method and fluorescent in-situ hybridisation (FISH) using directly labelled probes. *Hum. Reprod.* **9**: 721–4.

Hassold, T. J. & Jacobs, P. A. (1984). Trisomy in man. *Ann. Rev. Genet.* **18**: 69–88.

Hazout, A., De Ziegler, D., Cornel, C. *et al.* (1993). Comparison of short 7-day and prolonged treatment with gonadotrophin-releasing hormone agonist desensitization for controlled ovarian hyperstimulation. *Fertil. Steril.* **59**: 596–60.

Hellebaut, S., DeSutter, T. & Dozortov, D. (1996). Does assisted hatching improve implantation rates after in vitro fertilisation or intracytoplasmic sperm injection in all patients? A prospective randomised study. *J. Assist. Reprod. Genet.* **13**: 19–22.

Hughes, E. G., King, C. & Wood, E. C. (1989). A prospective study of prognostic factors in in vitro fertilisation and embryo transfer. *Fertil. Steril.* **51**: 838–44.

Human Fertilisation and Embryology Authority (1999). *Ninth Annual Report*, pp. 14–15. London: Human Fertilisation and Embryology Authority.

Jacobs, L., Metzger, D. A., Dodson, W. C. & Haney, A. F. (1990). Effect of age on Response to human menopausal gonadotrophin stimulation. *J. Clin. Endocrinol. Metab.* **76**: 1525–30.

Janny, L. & Menezo, Y. J. (1996). Maternal age effect on early human embryonic development and blactocyst formation. *Mol. Reprod. Dev.* **6**: 31–7.

Jones, G. & Trounson, A. O. (1999). Blastocyst stage transfer: pitfalls and benefits. *Hum. Reprod.* **14**: 1405–9.

Jones, G. M., Trounson, A. O., Kausche, A., Vella, P., Lotalgis, N. & Wood, C. (1998). Blastocyst culture and transfer. In *Treatment of Infertility: The New Frontiers*, ed. M. Flicori & C. Flamigni, pp. 191–202. Communication Media for Education Inc.

Kallioniemi, A., Kallioniemi, O. P., Sudar, D. *et al.* (1992). Comparative genomic hybridisation. *Proc. Natl. Acad. Sci. USA* **91**: 2156–60.

Lazendorf, S., Nehchiri, F., Mayer, J. F., Oehninger, S. Muasher, S. J. (1998). A prospective randomised, double-blind study for the evaluation of assisted hatching in patients with advanced maternal age. *Hum. Reprod.* **13**: 409–13.

Legro, R., Shackelford, D., Moessner, J., Gnatuc, C. & Dodson, W. (1997). ART in women 40 and over. Is cost worth it? *J. Reprod. Med.* **42**: 76–83.

Leridon, H. (1977). *Human Fertlity: The Basic Components*, p. 107. Chicago: University of Chicago Press.

Licciardi, F. L., Liu. H.-C. & Rosenwacks, Z. (1995). Day 3 estradiol serum concentration as prognosticator of ovarian stimulation response and pregnancy outcome in patients undergoing in vitro fertilization. *Fertil. Steril.* **64**: 991–4.

Liscoviych, M. & Amsterdam, A. (1989). Gonadotrophin-releasing hormone activates phospholipase D in ovarian granulosa cells. Possible role in signal transduction. *J. Biol. Chem.* **264**: 11762–7.

Medical Research International, Society for Assisted Reproductive Technology & The American Fertility Society (1990). In vitro fertilisation: embryo transfer in the United States: 1988 results from the IVF-ET Registry. *Fertil. Steril.* **53**: 13–20.

Muasher, S. J., Oehinger, S., Simonetti, S. *et al.* (1988). The value of basal and/or stimulated serum gonadotrophin levels in the prediction of stimulation response and in vitro fertilisation outcome. *Fertil. Steril.* **50**: 298–307.

Munne, S., Lee, A., Rosenwaks, Z. *et al.* (1993). Diagnosis of major chromosome aneuploidies in human preimplantation embryos. *Hum. Reprod.* **8**: 2185–92.

Munne, S., Alikani, M., Tomkin, G. *et al.* (1995). Embryo morphology, developmental rates, and maternal age are correlated with chromosome abnormalities. *Fertil. Steril.* **64**: 382–91.

Naeye, R. L. (1983). Maternal age, obstetric complications and the outcome of pregnancy. *Obstet. Gynecol.* **61**: 210–16.

Navot, D., Rosenwaks, Z. & Acosta, A. (1987). Prognostic assessment of female fecundity *Lancet* **2**: 645–7.

Navot, D., Bergh, P. A., Williams, M. A., Garrish, G. J., Guzman, I., Sandler, B. & Grunfeld, L. (1991). Poor oocyte quality rather than implantation failure as a cause of age-related decline in female fertility. *Lancet* **2**: 1375–7.

Office of Population Censuses and Surveys (1994). *Birth Statistics 1992 Annual Reference Volume Series FM1 No 21*. London: HMSO.

Pantos, K., Athanasiou, V., Stefanidis, K., Stavrou, D., Vaxevanoglu, T. & Chronopoulou, M. (1999). Influence of advanced age on the blactocyst development rate and pregnancy rate in assisted reproductive technology. *Fertil. Steril.* **71**: 1144–6.

Pearlstone, A. C., Fournet, N., Gambone, J., Pang, S. & Buyalos, R. (1992). Ovulation induction in women age 40 and older: the importance of basal follicle-stimulating hormone level and chronological age. *Fertil. Steril.* **58**: 674–9.

Ranieri, D. M., Quinn, F., Makhlouf, A. *et al.* (1998). Simultaneous evaluation of basal follicle stimulating hormone and 17 β-estradiol response to gonadotrophin-releasing hormone analogue stimulation: an improved predictor of ovarian reserve. *Fertil. Steril.* **70**: 227–33.

Ranieri, D. M., Phophong, P., Khadum, I., Meo, F., Davis, C. & Serhal, P. (2001). Simultaneous evaluation of basal FSH and oestradiol response to GnRH analogue (F-G test) allows effective drug regimen selection for IVF. *Hum. Reprod.* **16**: 673–5.

Roest, J., van Heusden, A. M., Mous, H., Zeilmaker, G. H. & Verhoeff, A. (1996). The ovarian response as a predictor for successful in vitro fertilisation treatment after the age of 40 years. *Fertil. Steril.* **66**: 969–73.

Schoolcraft, W., Gardner, D., Lane, M., Schlenker, T., Hamilton, F. & Meldrum, D. (1999). Blastocyst culture and transfer: analysis of results and parameters affecting outcome in two in vitro fertilisation programs. *Fertil. Steril.* **72**: 604–9.

Schoolcraft, W., Schlenker, T., Gee, M. *et al.* (1994). Assisted hatching in the treatment of poor prognosis in vitro fertilisation candidates. *Fertil. Steril.* **62**: 551–4.

Schoolcraft, W., Schlenker, T., Jones, G. & Jones, W. (1995). In vitro fertilisation in women age 40 and over: the impact of assisted hatching. *J. Asst. Reprod. Genet.* **12**: 581–3.

Schwartz, D. Mayaux, M. J. (1982). CECOS. Female fecundity as a function of age. *N. Engl. J. Med.* **306**: 404–6.

Scott, R. T., Toner, J. P., Muasher, S. J., Oehinger, S., Robinson, S. & Rosenwaks, Z. (1989). Follicle stimulating hormone levels on cycle day 3 are predictive of in vitro fertilisation outcome. *Fertil. Steril.* **51**: 651–3.

Serhal, P. F. & Craft, I. L. (1989). Oocyte donation in 61 patients. *Lancet* I: 1185–8.

Serhal, P. F., Katz, M., Little, V. & Woronowski, H. (1988). Unexplained infertility – the value of pergonal superovulation combined with intrauterine insemination. *Fertil. Steril.* **49**: 602–6.

Sharma, V., Riddle, A. & Mason, B. A. (1988). An analysis of factors influencing the establishment of a clinical pregnancy in an ultrasound-based ambulatory in vitro fertilisation program. *Fertil. Steril.* **49**: 468–510.

Sherman, B., Wallace, R. & Treolar, A. (1979). The menopausal transition: endocrinologic and epidemiologic considerations. *J. Biol. Sci.* **6**: 19.

Sholtes, M. & Zeilmaker, G. (1996). A prospective randomised study of embryo transfer results after 3 or 5 days of embryo culture in in vitro fertilisation. *Fertil. Steril.* **65**: 1245–8.

St John, J. C. & Barrat, C. L. (1997). Use of anucleate donor oocyte cytoplasm in recipient eggs. *Lancet* **350**: 961–2.

Toner, J. P., Philiput, C. B., Jones, G. S. & Muasher, S. J. (1991). Basal follicle-stimulating hormone level is better predictor of in vitro fertilisation performance than age. *Fertil. Steril.* **55**: 784–91.

Tsirigotis, M. (1998). Blastocyst stage transfer: pitfalls and benefits. Too soon to abandon current practice? *Hum. Reprod.* **13**: 3285–9.

Tuck, S. M., Yudkin, P. L. & Turnbull, C. (1988). Pregnancy outcome in elderly primigravida with and without a history of infertility. *Br. J. Obstet. Gynaecol.* **95**: 230–7.

Van Noord-Zaadstra, B. M., Looman, C. W. N., Alsbach, H., Habbema, J. D. F., TeVelde, E. R. & Karbaat, J. (1991). Delaying childbearing: effect of age on fecundity and outcome of pregnancy. *BMJ* **302**: 1361–5.

Vandervorst, M., Liebars, I., Sermon, K., Staessen, C., De Vos, A., Van de Velde, H., Van Assche, E., Joris, H., Van Steirteghem, A. & Devroey, P. (1998). Successful preimplantation genetic diagnosis is related to the number of available cumulus-oocyte complexes. *Hum. Reprod.* **13**: 3169–76.

Wells, D. & Delhanty, J. D. A. (2000). Comprehensive chromosomal analysis of human preimplantation embryos using whole genome amplification and single cell comparative genomic hybridisation. *Mol. Hum. Reprod.* **6**: 1055–62.

Wu, J., Zhang, L. & Wang, X. (2000). Maturation and apoptosis of human oocytes in vitro are age related. *Fertil. Steril.* **74**: 1137–41.

20

Ethical aspects of controversies in assisted reproductive technology

Françoise Shenfield

Reproductive Medicine Unit, Elizabeth Garrett Anderson and Obstetric Hospital, London, UK

Many ethical dilemmas are raised by assisted reproduction as we are confronted by our intuitive understanding of whether it is right or wrong to offer treatment, refuse treatment or perform research, often in a context of possibilities that could barely have been contemplated in the recent past. This chapter is intended to give an overview of just some of the ethical aspects of controversies in assisted reproductive technology (ART) and hopefully to enable insight into others arisen and those yet to arise.

Issues in gamete donation

The two main issues are payment or donation (a misnomer if indeed payment is offered) and the question of donor's anonymity. The interests of the donors of gametes are also an ethical issue (Shenfield, 1998).

Payment or compensation to donors

The semantic argument (Shenfield & Steele, 1995) is that a donation of gametes and embryos should be free, otherwise the term 'donation' would be 'sale'. The counter-argument is that in practice there are difficulties matching supply to demand, especially in the case of oocytes, and should pragmatism not prevail in a scarce supply environment? In the United Kingdom (UK), the law states that 'no money or other kind of benefit shall be given or received in respect of any supply of gametes or embryos unless authorised by directions' (Human Fertilisation and Embryology Act 1990)[1]. The notion of a gift is also enshrined in law in France and Spain (Shenfield, 2001).

The ethical argument against payment might be Immanuel Kant's assertion that one must 'treat all humanity always at the same time as an end and never merely as a means' (Kant, trans. 1993). In modern terms this represents the respect for

Good Clinical Practice in Assisted Reproduction, ed. P. Serhal & C. Overton.
Published by Cambridge University Press. © Cambridge University Press 2004.

autonomy in this case of the donors. The ethical argument for payment might be of utilitarianism; that in a scarce supply environment donors should be paid in order to create more happy families with 'donated' gametes. However, Titmuss (1971) identifies negative consequences of payment in the context of blood donation. For example, the discouragement of voluntary supply and the potential exploitation of society's weakest socio-economic groups, an argument that could well be used in the context of gamete donors.

In the case of donation of supernumerary oocytes as part of an IVF treatment cycle (known as egg sharing), exploitation has many guises. Of special concern is coercion, however subtle. In Denmark, egg sharing is the only method of oocyte donation permitted and in the UK the Human Fertilisation and Embryology Act 1990 allows 'benefits' for female donors, for example a sterilization procedure following oocyte donation. It could be argued that these are forms of coercion to donate, and that the latter is also a form of payment, or perhaps just an acceptable 'exchange'.

Arguably, donation of supernumerary oocytes as part of an IVF treatment cycle is easier to contemplate, as both the donor and recipient are suffering difficulties with their fertility and the exchange seems more balanced than, say, in the case of oocyte donation in exchange for female sterilization. Also, egg-sharers are more likely to be well informed, having trodden the sometimes difficult path of fertility treatments and for whom IVF is often the only remaining option for achieving a long awaited pregnancy. In such a case, consent is more likely to be very well informed, thus enabling the donor's autonomy.

The Human Fertilisation and Embryology Authority (HFEA) *Code of Practice* (2001) includes a section on how to implement a fair approach to both donors and recipients. General advice is given that 'the treatment offered should be the most suitable to suit the medical needs of both the egg provider and the egg recipient . . . who . . . should have access to an individual, such as a nurse, who should be available to provide impartial support'. More detailed advice includes that usually given on obtaining informed consent, including 'alternative treatment available'.

Of course, one alternative to egg sharing is not to share. It might be argued that egg sharing is not a therapeutic option for the egg donor, or is a lesser option if one considers for example that the donor may compromise her chances of success by not having frozen embryos in storage. Alternatively, a young fertile donor with polycystic ovaries and a male factor problem may have a very good chance of success that will not be compromised if she shares her supernumerary eggs. Published reports from units practising egg sharing are needed in order to assess better and to inform women considering egg sharing.

A harsh dilemma involves the potential egg sharing donor who is refused because she is too old or has a prejudiced ovarian reserve. If she had planned to subsidize the cost of her treatment with egg sharing she may be economically precluded from treatment, and thus we have another dilemma in the realm of justice and equitable access for all to ART.

Counselling is necessary in all cases of gamete donation and this is even more complex, time consuming and essential in egg sharing. The HFEA *Code of Practice* stresses that implication counselling 'must . . . cover . . . the implications of not knowing whether the recipient has succeeded or not, if the provider remains childless, (and) the implications for the recipient of using a sub-fertile egg provider, and . . . of there possibly being half siblings (to the donor's offspring) of a similar age resulting from treatment.'

Anonymity and secrecy in gamete donation

There is wide variation in the attitude to anonymity in gamete donation in Europe, with the contrasting examples of Sweden and France who respectively enshrine known donors and anonymity in their legislation (Shenfield & Steele, 1997; Shenfield, 2001).

In the UK the HFEA *Code of Practice* provides the guidance that 'where people seek licensed treatment using donated gametes, a child's potential need to know about his or her origins . . . should be considered'. Some offspring of sperm donation argue that they have been deprived of specific knowledge, the identity of the genetic sperm provider (avoiding the legal and emotional term father), without which their sense of identity is incomplete (Gollancz, 2001). In most cases the interests of children and parents seem to coincide as several studies have already shown that children conceived by 'assisted reproduction' fare very well in the measured personal and social criteria, when compared to children conceived 'naturally' or who are adopted (Golombok *et al.*, 1996).

Is knowing one's genetic background a human right and should policy and law reverse the traditional anonymity of oocyte and sperm donation, as was done in Sweden in 1985 (Gottlieb *et al.*, 2000)? The European Convention on Human Rights,[2] recently integrated in UK legislation (Human Rights Act 1998), refers to the right to respect for private and family life, home and correspondence (Art. 8). The International Declaration of Children's Rights alludes to the right of children to know their family, which begs interpretation within the political context of kidnapped children adopted in Argentina without familial consent. But what is a right, or at least a negative right? Usually, when we say that someone has a 'right' to do something, we are implying that it would be wrong to interfere with his or her doing it, or that special grounds would be needed to justify interference (Dworkin, 1991). Here the conflict of interests may be between the privacy interest of parents and donors, and other interests claimed by the offspring.

In 1995, Cook *et al.* compared 45 families who had a child conceived by donor insemination (DI) with 55 families who had an adopted child and 41 families who had a child conceived by IVF. At the time the children were aged between four and eight years. None of the DI parents had told their children of the means of their conception; but all of adopted families and most of the IVF parents had told their children. Interestingly, a year later a comparison of single and married recipients of donor insemination showed no significant difference in attitudes towards disclosure at the time of recruitment, but more single women said they intended to tell the child of the means of his or her conception. This makes sense as there is little option other than telling the child of the means of conception for a single mother, whilst the mother with a male partner will tend to emphasize the psychosocial side of paternity in their 'story telling' to the child. A New Zealand study (Daniels & Taylor, 1993) found that 30% of 181 DI parents/respondents gave their children information about their conception. Of the parents who had not, 77% intended to tell their child later.

There are few systematic studies of children's attitudes to anonymity or disclosure of the donor's identity with regard to their method of conception by donor insemination or oocyte donation, although we do become aware of specific cases where the frustration of not knowing the donor's identity has led to a strong feeling of deprivation in the child.

Children resulting from gamete donation and children who are adopted are intrinsically different in their origins. Gamete donation children are raised by at least one genetic parent and were desired and sought for by extraordinary means, even before they are conceived. Adopted children are first 'abandoned' by their genetic parents, though also desired and sought for through a usually complex process by their legal parent(s). A fascinating study, which could be used as a model when children resulting from ART seek information from the HFEA in the future, shows sex differences in the attitudes of adopted searchers and nonsearchers (Howe & Feast, 2000).

A study of oocyte donors in Finland showed that 59% thought that children ought to be told of their origin and 33% thought they should be given identifying information (Soderstrom-Antilla, 1995). In the UK, another study showed that 8.9% of anonymous donors provided the optional 'pen portrait' of themselves by answering questions on the HFEA registration forms (Abdalla *et al.*, 1998).

The major question is, what future legal changes are contemplated with regard to the amount of information about anonymous donors that should be given to their offspring and whether donor anonymity should eventually be dispensed with. In December 2001 in the UK a consultation document was issued, and according to the Human Fertilisation and Embryology Act 1990, 'any child who thinks he/she may be the product of assisted reproduction (licensed) treatment may at 18 or younger (16) if about to marry find out from the HFEA whether he/she is not about to marry a half sibling, or request the anonymous information as per the directions yet to be implemented'. A double track policy may be the ideal compromise to satisfy donors, recipients and offsprings interests (Pennings, 1997).

Preimplantation genetic diagnosis

The discussion on preimplantation genetic diagnosis (PGD) has been inspired largely by the preparatory work of the European Society of Human Reproduction and Embryology (ESHRE) ethics and law taskforce on PGD (ESHRE, 2002). Originally PGD was developed as an alternative to prenatal diagnosis for couples at high risk of transmitting a genetic defect. PGD allows scientists to check for specific genetic defects of an embryo obtained through IVF so that only embryos nonaffected for the tested defect, or balanced for the tested chromosomes, can be replaced. PGD is also used for sex determination in cases of X-linked disease, and enumeration of chromosomes for couples at low risk to transmit a genetic disease within the frame of their ART treatment, for example aneuploidy.

Fundamental ethical principles

The two main ethical principles of PGD are: increasing the welfare of the future child by avoiding a known potential harm; and enabling the autonomy of the potential parents to choose a technique with which they feel more comfortable, for example PGD rather than the possible prospect of termination of pregnancy. Informed consent that promotes autonomy is essential in PGD and the information given should include genetic counselling and details of the IVF treatments and procedures involved. As with all new techniques, PGD has to be demonstrated to be safe and at this stage there is no evidence to show that the removal of one or two cells affects the embryo. Nevertheless, it would be wise to prospectively assess this by monitoring children born following PGD.

Specific ethical considerations in PGD

The selection of healthy, unaffected embryos for replacement has been viewed as a type of eugenics (Milliez & Sureau, 1997), but the rationale for PGD arises from a desire to spare future children suffering and the possible burden of making similar decisions with regard to their own future children. As pointed out in the Dutch Health Council report (Health Council of the Netherlands, 1998), the risks to these future children are largely a function of the type of disease. For example, if the child resulting from PGD is a carrier of an autosomal recessive disease (like cystic fibrosis), the risk that his or her children will be affected is <1%, whilst for X-linked diseases like Duchenne's muscular dystrophy the risk of a female carrier transmitting the disease is 50% for each son. Individual risk assessment is best addressed through genetic counselling.

It seems in the best interests of all that, if available, healthy embryos should be replaced first, whilst carrier embryos are cryopreserved in case the initial embryo transfer fails. If there are only carrier embryos available, the parent couple should be counselled regarding the risk involved for the offspring with the relevant disease. Ultimately, the parent couple should decide whether the carrier embryos will be replaced, or if they wish to proceed to another IVF cycle in an attempt to produce unaffected embryos.

The case for late onset diseases is more difficult to analyse if there are uncertainties concerning therapy in the time gap between birth and the onset of the disease, for example if there was progress in the treatment of breast cancer in a case of *BCR1* diagnosis. Because of the lack of available treatment there are fewer uncertainties with other late onset diseases like Huntington's disease. Therefore, a multidisciplinary approach including genetic counselling is essential.

PGD for aneuploidy screening (PGD/AS)

There are data supporting the notion that the application of PGD/AS has some advantages, for example in women aged over 37 years and in cases of recurrent miscarriage or multiple failed IVF cycles. This advantage is achieved by reducing the miscarriage rate and consequently by improving live birth rate per transfer with healthy embryos. Recently PGD/AS has been approved in principle for licensing by the HFEA and can be ethically justified because it enables the autonomy of the parent couple, who may choose not to risk the potential distress of early pregnancy loss.

PGD for human leukocyte antigen typing (PGD/HLA)

PGD/HLA is a recent development in PGD and concerns an existing child affected by a terminal disease whose parents request HLA typing of embryos for replacement. This is to facilitate the possibility of having another child who will be genetically suited to donate haematopoietic stem cells or other tissues to his or her sibling – the existing sick child – and who will be free of the same genetic disease (Pennings & Liebaers, 2002).

In the case of PGD/HLA, the welfare of the future child and of the existing child are the primary concern and it has to be shown that the benefits for the recipient sibling outweigh the disadvantages, if any, for the future child. It is generally felt that this solution is morally acceptable if the use as a donor is not the only motive for the parents to have the child. This condition obviates the Kantian argument against using someone as a mere instrument, with the word 'mere' being of great importance here.

Also of importance is the planned operation for the future child. For example, the creation of a child for the purpose of harvesting nonregenerating organs seems extremely difficult to justify in view of the risks to the donor child. However, if the future child's operation involves minimal risk, for example cord blood or bone marrow donation, then the concept seems more acceptable. Benefits would also include family welfare in a broad sense, where family solidarity is enhanced and considered positive for all members, both donors and recipients.

PGD for sex-selection for non-medical reasons

PGD is not the only method for sex selection but is more reliable than the more innocuous sperm sorting. In the most recent ESHRE PGD taskforce (ESHRE, 2000) results, social sex selection cases were reported for the first time, leading to much debate.

Sex selection for nonmedical reasons is regarded as intrinsically sexist and can be argued as an issue of human rights, as nondiscrimination on the grounds of sex is enshrined in both the Universal Declaration of Human Rights (1948) and the European Convention of Human Rights (1950)[2]. It might also be argued that if it were acceptable to select by PGD one sex in preference to another for nonmedical reasons, antidiscriminatory measures in other areas of life may be difficult to promote (M. Strathern, pers. comm., 1993) at a time of world-wide discrimination that is often against females.

PGD arises from a desire to prevent disease and suffering; to be perceived as of the 'wrong' sex, whether male or female, cannot be defined as a disease. The possible compromise of family balancing (Pennings, 1996) may also be regarded as inherently sexist. Its promoters argue that the application for family balancing differs from unrestricted application, because the parents could not choose a child of a certain sex but a child of the other sex and that this would not be expressing a hierarchy or inequality between the sexes.

Refusing treatment

Physicians have a duty of care, both legally and morally, to their patients and can justify refusing treatment only if this avoids harm of a certain magnitude with a high degree of probability. This often very difficult dilemma is clearly outlined in the case of ART for HIV patients (Pennings, 2002).

The premise is that the fertility specialist collaborates with the potential parents who are the primary decision makers. The specialist is not a mere instrument of their will but a moral agent and must make judgements about the right or wrong of the collaboration. The specialist must decide whether the action of helping a couple to accomplish their reproductive plans is morally permissible when there is a danger of the birth of a child who is HIV+. The fertility specialist must decide whether to participate in the intentional parental project and this decision mostly depends on the potential risk to the most vulnerable party in the equation – the future child. In the UK this decision is made within the context of the statutory duty to 'take into account the welfare of the child, as well as of other children who may be affected by the treatment' (Human Fertilisation and Embryology Act, 1990).

The fertility specialist has a medical and legal duty to help with the disease infertility and to protect a future child from the risk of a possible (or probable) serious disease. The specialist's choice to help may be only morally blameworthy if this risk-taking is unjustified and unreasonable (Pennings, 2002).

- If the female partner alone is HIV+ and all measures are taken to reduce the risk of transmission, the risk to the child is now estimated at <2%. This risk seems acceptable, but there must be collaboration with HIV specialists to ensure compliance with medication and counselling on the need for Caesarean section delivery and against breast-feeding.
- If the male partner alone is HIV+ and the female partner is inseminated the probability of creating an infected child is extremely small and almost negligible. Therefore, the risk is acceptable and there should be no objection to providing treatment.
- If both partners are HIV+, the risk to the child being HIV+ and of being orphaned at an early age on the death of his or her HIV+ parents is unacceptable and treatment should be refused.

Conclusion

ART is an area of medicine fraught with controversy and ethical dilemmas.

It is the role of the fertility specialist to respect the autonomy of the potential parents and balance this with the very special responsibility towards future children. Further, the specialist must avoid doing harm whilst mindful of the macro ethical context of justice and fair access to treatment, and of human rights. This does not necessarily mean universal agreement on particular issues, as exemplified by the internationally different attitudes to gamete donor anonymity. When confronted with an ethical dilemma in the context of assisted reproduction, for example whether to treat the widowed, the single, or a lesbian couple, the fertility specialist must analyse his or her intuitive understanding of right and wrong, mindful that evidence helps to avoid prejudice and rigorous analysis enables us to best accomplish our duty of care.

ENDNOTES

1. Human Fertilisation and Embryology Act 1990. London: HMSO.
2. Council of Europe Convention for the Protection of Human Rights and Fundamental Freedoms, Strasbourg, 1950.

REFERENCES

Abdalla, H. I., Shenfield, F. & Latarche, E. (1998). Statutory information for the children born of oocyte donation: what will they be told in 2008? *Hum. Reprod.* **13**: 1106–9.

Cook, R., Golombok, S., Bish, A. *et al.* (1995). Disclosure of donor insemination: parental attitudes. *Am. J. Orthopsychiatry* **65**: 549–59.

Dworkin, G. (1991). *Taking Rights Seriously*. London: Duckworth.

Daniels, K. R. & Taylor, K. (1993). Secrecy and openness in donor insemination. *Polit. Life Sci.* **12**: 200–3.

ESHRE (2002). Law and Ethics Taskforce No. 5 PGD. *Hum. Reprod.* **18**: 1–3.

Gollancz, D. (2001). Donor insemination: a question of rights. *Hum. Fertil.* **4**: 164–7.

Golombok, S., Breaways, A., Cook, R. *et al.* (1996). The European study of assisted reproduction families: family functioning and child development. *Hum. Reprod.* **11**: 2324–31.

Gottlieb, C., Lalos, O. & Lindblad, F. (2000). Disclosure of donor insemination to the child: the impact of Swedish legislation on couple's attitudes. *Hum. Reprod.* **15**: 2052–6.

Health Council of the Netherlands (1998). Sex Selection for Non-medical Reasons. Report of a committee of the Health Council of the Netherlands 1995/Ne. The Hague: Gezondheidsraad.

Howe, D. & Feast, J. (2000). *Adoption, Search and Reunion*. London: The Children's Society Publishing Department.

Human Fertilisation and Embryology Authority (2001). *Code of Practice* London: Human Fertilisation and Embryology Authority.

Kant, I. (1993). *Critique of Pure Reason*, trans. Lewis White Beck, 3rd edn., p. 30. London: Library of Liberal Arts.

Milliez, J. & Sureau, C. (1997). PGD and the eugenic debate: our responsibility to future generations. In *Ethical Dilemmas in Assisted Reproduction*, ed. F. Shenfield & C. Sureau, pp. 51–6. London: Parthenon.

Pennings, G. (1996). Ethics of sex selection for family balancing: family balancing as a morally acceptable application of sex selection. *Hum. Reprod.* **11**: 2339–43.

Pennings, G. (1997). The double track policy for donor anonymity. *Hum. Reprod.* **12**: 2839–44.

Pennings, G. (2002). Providing infertility treatment to HIV positive people: considerations regarding the moral responsibility of the physician. In *Ethical Dilemmas in Human Reproduction*, ed. F. Shenfield & C. Sureau, pp. 35–50. London: Parthenon.

Pennings, G. & Liebaers, I. (2002). Creating a child to save another: HLA matching of siblings by means of preimplantation diagnosis. In *Ethical Dilemmas in Human Reproduction*, ed. F. Shenfield & C. Sureau, pp. 51–66. London: Parthenon.

Shenfield, F. (1998). Gamete donation: ethical implication for donors. *Hum. Fertil.* **2**: 98–101.

Shenfield, F. (2001). To know or not to know the identitity of one's genetic parent(s): a question of human rights? In *Human Reproduction in the 21st Century*, ed. P. L. Healy, G. L. T. Kovaks, R. McLachlan & O. Rodriguez-Armes, pp. 78–84. London: Parthenon.

Shenfield, F. & Steele, S. J. (1995). A gift is a gift is a gift, or why gametes donors should not be paid. *Hum. Reprod.* **10**: 253–5.

Shenfield, F. & Steele, S. J. (1997). What are the effects of anonymity and secrecy on the welfare of the child in gamete donation? *Hum. Reprod.* **12**: 392–5.

Soderstrom-Antilla, V. (1995). Follow up of Finnish volunteer oocyte donors concerning their attitudes to oocyte donation. *Hum. Reprod.* **10**: 3073–6.

Titmuss, R. (1971). *The Gift Relationship: From Human Blood to Social Policy*. London: Allen and Unwin.

Index

acrosome 22
adenomyosis 229
adnexal adhesions 106
adoption 335
age, maternal *see* maternal age
air filtration 295–6
albumin
  in culture media 306
  prevention of OHSS 156–7
alcohol 30, 248, 283
allele dropout (ADO) 216
amenorrhoea 2, 5–6, 104
American Society for Reproductive Medicine (ASRM)
  embryo transfer 140
  reproductive tract anomalies 250–2
  sperm donation 88
anabolic steroids 39
androgen receptors 32, 83
anembryonic pregnancy 177
aneuploidy
  diagnosis 210, 217–21, 222, 325–6, 337
  and miscarriage 170, 171
angiogenin 148
anonymity, gamete donation 87–8, 268, 334–6
anovulation 5–8, 103–5
anti-oestrogens *see* clomiphene citrate
antisperm antibodies 38, 42–3, 69–71, 101
assisted conception centres
  capital equipment 295–6, 297–305, 317
  human resources 277–8, 291–2, 318
  IT systems 310–18
  laboratory consumables 305–7
  physical infrastructure 131, 291, 293–7, 310, 317–18
  planning 289–91
  protocols and procedures 292–3, 294–5, 297, 308–9
  quality control 293, 305, 307–8
asthenospermia 33–4, 47–8
audit 293, 315
azoospermia
  algorithm 40
  non-obstructive 30–3, 38, 41, 44, 54–6, 79–80
  obstructive 28–30, 41, 44–6, 49–56, 80, 82

basal body temperature (BBT) charts 4
biopsy
  embryos 210, 212–14
  testes 23–4, 41, 44, 55–6, 79–80
blastocysts
  biopsy 214
  transfer 139, 247, 324–5
blastomeres 213–14
bromocriptine 9, 47
buserelin 115, 116

Caesarean sections 231, 339
caffeine 248
catheters 137, 307
CBVAD *see* vas deferens, absence of
CD45 antigen 62
cerebral palsy 245–6
cervix
  cervical mucus and sperm 66–9, 70
  embryo transfer 138, 139, 141
  infertility 105
chemotherapy 30, 242
child welfare 205, 249, 269, 335
chlamydia infections 11
choriocarcinoma 169, 170
chromosome abnormalities
  embryonic: diagnosis 210, 217–21, 222, 325–6, 337; and miscarriage 170, 171
  maternal 7, 221
  paternal 31–2, 43, 77, 80–2
cleavage stage embryos
  biopsy 213–14
  chromosome abnormalities 218–19
clinical workup 1–13, 37–46
clomiphene citrate
  clomiphene challenge test (CCT) 10, 322
  COS 108, 109
  induction of ovulation 104
  male infertility 47
COMET assays 76–7
comparative genomic hybridization (CGH) 222, 326
computer-aided sperm analysis (CASA) 64–5
computers *see* information technology
conception, natural 1, 106–7, 194

contraception 2
  oral contraceptives 113, 191, 240–1
controlled ovarian stimulation
  and DI 95
  and GIFT 257, 323
  and IUI 100–3, 106, 108–9, 322
  and IVF: endometriosis 239–40; older women
    323; PCO 8, 118–19, 123; poor ovarian reserve
    242–4; pregnancy rates 117–18; treatment
    regimes 112–24, 239–40, 257,
    323
  treatment regimes: clomiphene 108, 109; GnRH
    agonists 113, 114–19, 239–40, 257, 323;
    GnRH antagonists 114, 119, 257;
    gonadotrophins (FSH) 108–9, 119–23, 323;
    timing 279
  see also ovarian hyperstimulation syndrome
corpus luteum, steroid production 194
counselling
  concerning child welfare 269
  concerning gamete donation 268, 334
  concerning genetic issues 82, 211, 220, 337
  concerning maternal age 244
  concerning surrogacy 201–2, 205
  definition 267
  formal requirement 266–7, 281
  procedure 267–75
  referral to 3, 269–70, 282
cryopreservation
  cryo-protectants 89
  embryos 140, 156, 191, 194, 246
  equipment 91, 297, 304
  miscarriage rates 171
  sperm 88–93
cryptorchidism 37
culture media 297, 305–6, 308, 325
cystic fibrosis 82
cytomegalovirus 88

density gradient centrifugation (DGC) 93–4
diabetes 38, 248
diathermy 155, 230
disseminated intravascular coagulation 182
DNA
  analysis 210, 215–17, 218, 221–2
  damaged sperm 75–7
  mitochondrial 320
donation
  oocytes see oocytes, donation
  sperm see donor insemination
donor insemination (DI)
  American Society of Reproductive Medicine
    (ASRM) 88
  anonymity 87–8, 334–6
  British Andrology Society (BAS) 88
  counselling 268
  donor recruitment 86–8
  donor screening 88
  France 87
  insemination methods 94–5
  in research 96

sperm cryopreservation 88–93
sperm preparation 92–4
success rates 86, 95–6, 323–4
Sweden 88
Switzerland 88
Doppler imaging
  miscarriage 178–9
  oocyte retrieval 130
down-regulation 113, 116–19
  low ovarian reserve 323
  oocyte donation 191–2

early pregnancy factor (EPF) 173
early pregnancy loss (EPL) see gestational
    trophoblastic disease; miscarriage
ectopic pregnancy 160, 174
education
  by nurses 283–6
  by patient information leaflets 161, 293
ejaculation
  hypospermia 27–8, 43–4, 45, 48, 49–50
  normal 24–5
embryos
  assisted hatching 324
  biopsy 210, 212–14, 303–4
  chromosome abnormalities 210, 217–21, 222,
    325–6, 337
  cryopreservation 140, 156, 191, 194, 246, 304
  implantation rates in older women 193, 243, 321
  sex determination 217–18, 219, 338
  transfer: developmental stage 139, 247,
    324–5; multiple pregnancies 139–40,
    245–6; after oocyte donation 189–90,
    192–3; procedures 135–9, 141, 203,
    247–8; timing 139, 192–3, 203; ZIFT 259–61
emotional aspects of ART
  counselling 270, 271–5
  ending treatment 244
  five-stage response 279–81
endometriosis 102–3, 235–40
  endometriomas 102, 134, 241
  in older women 321
endometrium see uterus
epididymis 24, 29, 45, 51–2
EPL (early pregnancy loss) see gestational
    trophoblastic disease; miscarriage
erectile dysfunction 38
ethics 248–9
  gamete donation 87–8, 268, 332–6
  GIFT 262
  PGD 336–8
  surrogacy 202, 205–7
  treatment for: HIV positive patients 338–9; older
    women 244
ethnicity 3
European Society of Human Reproduction
    (ESHRE) PGD Consortium 212, 336

fallopian tubes
  clinical examination 5, 11–12, 106
  hydrosalpinx 134–5, 234–5

fibroids
    location and ART outcome 227–9
    management 12, 226, 229–31
    older women 321
financial issues
    counselling 282
    donor payment 332–4
    running an IVF unit 290, 291, 314, 316
5-alpha reductase 25, 32
flow cabinets 297–9
fluid balance in ovarian hyperstimulation
    syndrome 147, 148, 156–7, 159
fluorescent *in situ* hybridization (FISH) 210,
    217–21, 326
follicle stimulating hormone (FSH)
    anovulation 6–7
    assays for 121
    controlled ovarian stimulation: alone 108–9;
        with GnRH agonists 116, 118; with GnRH
        antagonists 119; poor responders 244
    FSH GnRH agonist stimulation test 10
    in men 25–6, 30, 35, 41, 82
    ovarian reserve 9, 10, 242–3, 322
    ovulation induction 104
    sources 114, 119–23
follicles
    and ovarian hyperstimulation syndrome 150,
        157
    oocyte retrieval 130, 132–4
freezing *see* cryopreservation

gamete donation *see* donor insemination; oocytes,
    donation; oocytes, sharing
gamete intrafallopian transfer (GIFT)
    comparison with IVF 260–1
    and endometriosis 239
    multiple pregnancies 261–2
    oocyte donation 194, 262–3
    techniques 256–9, 260
GnRH agonist stimulation test (GAST) 10, 322
genetic diseases
    cystic fibrosis 82
    diagnosis *see* preimplantation genetic diagnosis
gestational trophoblastic disease (GTD) 169, 170,
    172, 177–8
GIFT *see* gamete intrafallopian transfer
gonadotrophin-releasing hormone (GnRH)
    in men 26, 30
    treatment of anovulation 104
gonadotrophin-releasing hormone agonists
    (GnRHa)
    controlled ovarian stimulation 113, 114–19,
        239–40, 257, 323
    endometriosis 239–40
    fibroid management 229, 231
    ovarian hyperstimulation syndrome prevention
        151–5
    oocyte recipients 191–2
    ovarian reserve 10, 244, 322
gonadotrophin-releasing hormone (GnRH)
    antagonists
    controlled ovarian stimulation 114, 119, 257

ovarian hyperstimulation syndrome prevention
    154–5
gonadotrophins *see* follicle stimulating hormone;
    human chorionic gonadotrophin; luteinizing
    hormone
goserelin 115
GTD (gestational trophoblastic disease) 169, 170,
    172, 177–8
gynaecomastia 32, 38, 83

hamster oocyte penetration assay 71
hatching, assisted 324
HFEA *see* Human Fertilisation and Embryology
    Authority
HIV positive patients 338–9
HMG (human menopausal gonadotrophin) 114,
    119, 122
HSG (hysterosalpingography) 11, 228–9
human chorionic gonadotrophin (HCG)
    controlled ovarian stimulation: IUI 108; IVF 113,
        114, 130–1
    diagnosis of EPL 172–3
    male infertility 47
    ovarian hyperstimulation syndrome prevention
        150–1, 153
    ovulation induction 104
Human Fertilisation and Embryology Act (UK)
    (1990)
    child welfare 249
    counselling 267
    gamete donation 332, 335–6
    number of embryos transferred 140
Human Fertilisation and Embryology Authority
    (HFEA) (UK)
    Central Register 268
    Code of Practice: counselling 281, 334; gamete
        donation 86–7, 187–8, 333, 334
    as a regulator 211, 278, 293
human leucocyte antigen testing 337–8
human menopausal gonadotrophin (HMG) 114,
    119, 122
human rights 334, 338
hydatidiform moles 169, 170, 172, 177–8
hydrosalpinx 11–12, 134–5, 234–5
hydroxyaethyl starch 157
hypogonadotrophic hypogonadism
    in men 30, 39, 41, 46–7
    in women 103–4, 114, 150
hypospermia 27–8, 43–4, 45, 48, 49–50
hypothalamus
    in men 26, 30
    in women 6–7
hysterosalpingo contrast sonography (HyCoSy) 11
hysterosalpingography (HSG) 11, 228–9
hysteroscopy 12, 230, 233, 260

ICI (intracervical insemination) 94
ICSI *see* intracytoplasmic sperm injection
immunoglobulins *see* antisperm antibodies
implantation of embryos
    in older women 193, 243, 321
    after oocyte donation 192–3

implications counselling 267–9, 270, 334
incubators 295–6, 300–3, 308
infertility
    aetiology: female 2–13, 105–6, 226, 232, 234;
        male 27–37, 80–3
    clinical workup 1–13, 37–46
    definition 26, 100–1
    epidemiology 1, 19, 289
    treatment *see individual techniques*
information technology (IT)
    applications 64–5, 310, 311–15
    hardware 310, 317
    Internet 284
    software 311, 315–17, 318
    training 318
informed consent 268, 283–4, 292, 333, 336
inhibin-A 173
inhibin-B
    in men 26, 42
    in women 10
insemination *see* donor insemination; intrauterine
        insemination
insulin 123
Internet 284
intracytoplasmic sperm injection (ICSI)
    equipment 303
    miscarriage rates 171
    with PGD 210
    sperm quality 56, 77–82, 219
intrauterine insemination
    compared with intracervical 94
    and COS 100–3, 106, 108–9, 322
    and endometriosis 239
IVF chambers 299–300
IVF (in vitro fertilization)
    Bourn Hall procedure 202–3
    controlled ovarian stimulation: endometriosis
        239–40; older women 323; PCO 8, 118–19,
        123; poor ovarian reserve 242–4; treatment
        regimes 112–24, 239–40, 257, 323
    embryo transfer: developmental stage 139, 247,
        324–5; multiple pregnancies 139–40, 245–6;
        after oocyte donation 189–90, 192–3;
        procedures 135–9, 141, 203, 247–8
    factors affecting success 101, 117–18, 247
    maternal age 140, 243–4, 322–3
    oocyte retrieval 129–30; analgesia 131, 135;
        complications 135; immature oocytes 135;
        procedure 131–5; timing 130–1
    surrogacy *see* surrogacy
    ZIFT 141, 259–61, 262–3
    see also oocytes, donation; ovarian
        hyperstimulation syndrome
IVF units *see* assisted conception centres

Johnsen scoring system 23–4

Kallmann's syndrome 5, 30
Kartagener's syndrome 33, 38
kidney 38, 148
King's Fund Centre Counselling Committee Report
    (1991) 266, 267

Klinefelter's syndrome 31–2

laboratory management
    capital equipment 295–6, 297–305
    consumables 305–7
    good laboratory practice 294–5, 297, 305,
        307–9
    IT 314–18
    physical infrastructure 293–7
laparoscopy
    endometriosis 236–8
    fibroids 230–1
    OHSS 155–6, 160–1
    oocyte retrieval 129, 130
    tubal damage 12, 106
laparotomy 230–1
legal issues
    audit 293
    child welfare 249
    counselling 266–7
    gamete donors: anonymity 88, 268, 334–6;
        payment 332
    number of embryos transferred 140
    PGD 211
    software copyright 316
    surrogacy 200, 201, 205
    see also informed consent
letrazole 108
leucocytes, in semen 41, 47, 62–3, 73
leuprorelin 115, 116
Leydig cells 21, 26
LHRH agonists *see* gonadotrophin-releasing
        hormone agonists
LHRH antagonists *see* gonadotrophin-releasing
        hormone antagonists
light 296–7
liver 148
luteinizing hormone (LH)
    anovulation 6–8
    controlled ovarian stimulation 114, 122
    in men 25–6, 30, 41, 83
    recurrent miscarriage 173
    synchronization of menstrual cycles 190–1
    timing of ovulation 4, 95

magnetic resonance imaging (MRI) 228, 230
MAR test 43
maternal age 319
    ART success rates 321–2; assisted hatching 324;
        blastocyst transfer 324–5; COS/IUI 322;
        DI 95, 323–4; GIFT 261–2; IVF 140, 243–4,
        322–3
    causes of infertility in older women: embryonic
        aneuploidy 218, 221, 320, 325–6, 337;
        implantation rates 193, 243, 321; miscarriage
        170, 171; oocyte quality 320; ovarian reserve
        243–4, 319–20; other 321
    counselling 244
    fecundity 2, 106, 319
    pregnancy complications 326
maturation arrest (oligozoospermia) 34, 37, 41,
    47–8

medical history
  men 37–9
  women 2–3, 170
menstrual cycle 2, 321
  synchronization for IVF 190–2, 203
metformin 104, 123
MFPR (multifetal pregnancy reduction) 180–2
micro-epididymal sperm aspiration (MESA) 52, 54, 57
microscopes 300, 303–4
miscarriage
  after ART 171
  diagnosis 172–9
  incidence 168, 169–70
  inevitable 168
  missed 168, 176–7, 178
  recurrent 169, 170, 232–3
  risk factors 170–1, 232–3, 235
  threatened 168
mitochondria 320
mixed antiglobulin reaction (MAR) test 43
mosaicism 218–19, 221
multiple pregnancies
  complications 245–6
  fetal reduction (MFPR) 180–2
  GIFT 261–2
  IVF 139–40, 245–6
  oocyte donation 196
  ultrasound 179–80
mumps 38
myomas see fibroids
myomectomy 12, 230–1

nafarelin 115, 116
National Fertility Association (ISSUE) 244
natural surrogacy 199, 205
nick translation assays 76–7
nurses
  scope of the job 277–8; clinical 286; educational 283–6; emotional support 279–83; treatment programme co-ordination 278–9, 281, 284
  training 277, 286

obesity 123, 248
oestradiol (E2)
  anovulation 6
  monitoring controlled ovarian stimulation 114, 322
  ovarian hyperstimulation syndrome risk factor 149–50, 151
  oocyte donation 188–90, 192, 195–6
  ovarian reserve 9–10
  pregnancy 194
ovarian hyperstimulation syndrome see ovarian hyperstimulation syndrome
oligospermia 34, 219
oligozoospermia (maturation arrest) 34, 37, 41, 47–8
oocytes
  donation: anonymity 334–6; counselling 268,

334; donor characteristics 187–8; egg sharing 333–4; implantation window 192–3; indications for 186–7; maintenance of pregnancy 194–6; to older women 244, 324; outcome 196; priming of recipient 188–92, 245; transfer techniques 194
  GIFT 258–9
  of older women 243, 320
oocytes sharing
  Denmark 333
  France 224, 332
  penetration by sperm 71
  peritoneal oocyte sperm transfer 141
  retrieval: analgesia 131, 135; complications 135; immature oocytes 135; OHSS prevention 156–7; procedure 129–30, 131–5; timing 113, 130–1
  Spain 332
  Sweden 334
oral contraceptives 113, 191, 240–1
ovarian cysts 116, 240–1
ovarian drilling 105, 155–6
ovarian failure 7, 187, 324
ovarian hyperstimulation see controlled ovarian stimulation
ovarian hyperstimulation syndrome
  classification 146–7
  complications 148–9
  pathogenesis 147–8
  patient information leaflet 161
  PCOS 123, 149, 151, 155–6
  prevention 150–8, 161
  risk factors 146, 149–50
  treatment 158–61
ovarian reserve 242–4, 257
  maternal age 243–4, 319–20
  tests for 9–11, 322
ovarian stimulation see controlled ovarian stimulation
ovulation
  assessment of 4–9
  induction 103–5, 239
  see also controlled ovarian stimulation

pampiniform plexus 21
  see also varicocele
paracentesis 159–60
patient information
  leaflets 161, 293
  nurses 283–6
  support groups 269
  see also counselling
PCO/PCOS see polycystic ovary (syndrome)
PCR (polymerase chain reaction) 210, 215–17, 218
pelvic inflammatory disease 2
percutaneous epididymal sperm aspiration (PESA) 49, 53–4, 57
peritoneal oocyte sperm transfer 141
pituitary
  desensitization 113, 116–19; oocyte donation 191–2; poor ovarian reserve 323

function in men 26
tumours 8–9, 30
polar body biopsy 212–13, 220
pollution 294, 295
paint 294
polycystic ovary (syndrome) (PCO/PCOS) 7–8
controlled ovarian stimulation 118–19, 123
ovarian hyperstimulation syndrome 123, 149,
151, 155–6
ovulation induction 104–5, 239
polymerase chain reaction (PCR) 210, 215–17, 218
post-coital test 43, 66–9, 105
Pouch of Douglas 131, 141
pregnancy
complications: ectopic 160, 174; fibroids 226;
future infertility 2, 170; GTD 169, 170, 172,
177–8; miscarriage see miscarriage; older
women 326; oocyte donation 196; see also
multiple pregnancies
steroid production 194–5
preimplantation genetic diagnosis (PGD)
advances in DNA analysis 221–2
defects in: chromosomes 210, 217–21, 222,
325–6; single genes 210, 214–17
embryo biopsy 210, 212–14
equipment 302, 303–4
ethical issues 336–8
genetic counselling 82, 211, 220, 337
indications for 209, 218
patient management 211–12
sex selection 217–18, 219, 338
progesterone
ovarian hyperstimulation syndrome 157, 159
ovulation 4
in pregnancy 172–3, 194; oocyte recipients
189–90, 195–6
prolactin
in men 26, 30, 83
in women 8–9
pronuclei stage tubal transfer 194
puberty, male 25–6, 38
pyospermia 41, 47, 62–3, 73

quality control 293, 305, 307–8

reactive oxygen species (ROS) 63, 72–4
recreational drugs 39
relaxin 173
religion, attitudes to surrogacy 207
renal disease 38, 148
reproductive system, male, anatomy 19–25
respiratory disease 29, 38, 149
Rokitansky–Kuster–Hauser syndrome 5, 205
Royal College of Nursing Fertility Nurses Group 277
Royal College of Obstetricians and Gynaecologists
guidelines 105, 140, 292
The Management of Infertility in Tertiary Care
(2000) 281

safety issues 91–2, 297
salpingectomy 12, 234–5
security 297, 308–9, 315

semen
assessment criteria 27, 63–4
collection of 41
constituents 24–5; see also sperm
leucocytes in 41, 47, 62–3, 73; physical
characteristics 59–60, 61; see also ejaculation
seminiferous tubules 21–2
Sertoli cells 21–2, 26
Sertoli cell only syndrome 32–3
sexing of embryos 217–18, 219, 338
sexually transmitted diseases 11, 41, 88
smoking 3, 30, 76, 248, 283
software 311, 315–17
sperm
antisperm antibodies 42–3, 69–71, 101
asthenospermia 33–4, 47–8
azoospermia see azoospermia
cryopreservation 88–93
donation see donor insemination
GIFT 258
ICSI see intracytoplasmic sperm injection
oligospermia 34, 219
oligozoospermia 34, 37, 41, 47–8
quality: biochemistry 71–7; cervical mucus
interaction 43, 66–9, 70; count 27, 61, 101;
morphology 60, 63–4; motility 61, 64–5,
67–9, 72, 74–5; penetration tests 43, 71;
semen profile 61–2; on thawing 92; viability
65–6
retrieval in the infertile male 53–6
spermatogenesis: failure 30–2, 38, 41, 44, 79–80;
maturation arrest 34, 37, 41, 47–8; normal
22–4, 26; temperature control 21, 35, 39
teratazoospermia 34
Sperm Chromatin Stability Assay 77
sperm survival test 307
spermatids 22, 79–80
staff issues
counselling 269, 275
IVF unit staff requirements 291–2
training 277, 286, 318
see also nurses
steroids
anabolic 39
oocyte donation: maintenance of pregnancy
194–6; priming 188–90, 192
treatment of male infertility 48
see also oestradiol; progesterone; testosterone
subfertility see infertility
superovulation see controlled ovarian stimulation
surrogacy
algorithm 206
counselling 201–2, 205
definitions 199–200
ethical issues 202, 205–7
genetic couple management 200–1, 201–3
indications for 200
legal issues 200, 201, 204, 205
natural 199, 205
success rates 203–4
surrogate host management 201–2, 203

tamoxifen 104
teratazoospermia 34
testis
    biopsy 23–4, 41
    failure 30–2, 38, 41, 44, 54–6, 79–80
    structure and function 20–4
    surgery: as cause of infertility 38; reconstructive
        50–3
    testicular exploration and sperm extraction
        (TESE) 44, 55–6, 79–80
    undescended 37
testosterone 25–6, 32, 41, 83
thawing of sperm 93
therapeutic counselling 269
thrombosis 148, 160
thyroid function 8
training 277, 286, 318
translocations, chromosomal 220–1
transrectal ultrasonography (TRUS) 43–4
transvaso-vasostomy 52–3
triplets 245–6
triptorelin 115, 116
TUNEL assays 77
twins
    chorionicity 179–80
    complications 245–6
    vanishing twins 179, 181
    see also multiple pregnancies

UK
    child welfare 249
    counselling 266–7, 281, 334
    gamete donation: anonymity 87, 334, 335–6;
        payment 187–8, 332, 333; recruitment of
        sperm donors 86–7, 88
    HFEA regulation 211, 268, 293
    number of embryos transferred 140
    surrogacy 200, 201, 205
ultrasound
    embryo transfer 138
    fibroids 228, 230
    hydatidiform moles 177–8
    miscarriage 173–7
    multiple pregnancies 179–80

ovarian hyperstimulation syndrome 150
oocyte donation 189
oocyte retrieval 113, 129–30
USA
    multiple pregnancies in IVF 139, 140
    sperm donation 87, 87–8
    surrogacy 200, 205
uterine artery
    embolization 229–30
    timing of oocyte retrieval 130
uterus
    anomalies 12–13, 232–4
    causes of infertility 3–4, 6, 12–13, 321
    endometrial receptivity 188–90, 245
    fibroids 227–31
    intrauterine haematomas 175
    see also endometriosis

varicocele 34, 35–7, 44, 48–9, 72
vas deferens
    absence of (CBVAD) 28, 43, 49, 82
    obstructions 29–30, 45
    vasostomy 50–3
vascular endothelial growth factor (VEGF) 123,
    147–8, 157–8
vaso-epididymostomy (VE) 51–2
vaso-vasostomy 50–1
vasography 44–6

Warnock Report (1984) 266, 267
weight 3, 104, 123, 248
World Health Organization quality criteria
    cervical mucus 66
    semen 27

X-linked diseases 215, 217–18, 219
XYY syndrome 32

Y chromosome 80–2
Young's syndrome 29

zona pellucida 212, 213, 324
zygote intrafallopian transfer (ZIFT) 141, 259–61,
    262–3